Civil War Pharmacy
*A History of Drugs, Drug Supply
and Provision, and Therapeutics
for the Union and Confederacy*

Civil War Pharmacy
A History of Drugs, Drug Supply and Provision, and Therapeutics for the Union and Confederacy

Michael A. Flannery

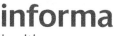

New York London

Informa Healthcare USA, Inc.
52 Vanderbilt Avenue
New York, NY 10017

© 2009 by Informa Healthcare USA, Inc. (original copyright 2004 by The Haworth Press, Inc.)
Informa Healthcare is an Informa business

No claim to original U.S. Government works

Printed and bound in the United Kingdom
Transferred to Digital Print 2011

International Standard Book Number-10: 0-7890-1502-1 (Softcover)
International Standard Book Number-13: 978-0-7890-1502-0 (Softcover)

Visit the Informa Web site at
www.informa.com

and the Informa Healthcare Web site at
www.informahealthcare.com

For Arnold G. Diethelm, MD

ABOUT THE AUTHOR

Michael A. Flannery is Associate Director for Historical Collections, University of Alabama at Birmingham. Besides his duties with the Lister Hill Library of the Health Sciences, he also teaches the history of medicine at UAB. Mr. Flannery received his MLS from the University of Kentucky and his MA in history from California State University at Dominguez Hills. He is editor of the book review section of the journal *Pharmacy in History* and author of *John Uri Lloyd: The Great American Eclectic*. Most recently, he completed *America's Botanico-Medical Movements: Vox Populi,* which he co-authored with Alex Berman, and *Pharmaceutical Education in the Queen City: 150 Years of Service, 1850-2000,* which he co-authored with Dennis B. Worthen; both titles are published by The Haworth Press, Inc.

CONTENTS

Foreword

Civil War historians study the daily lives of men in the ranks; re-enactors identify with army privates and picket skirmishers; and enthusiastic readers attempt to understand the experience of soldiers and civilians in all aspects. With this book Michael A. Flannery adds a new dimension to the study of the Civil War by describing and evaluating for the first time the complete history of pharmacy in both the Union and the Confederacy. Modern readers are dismayed when confronted for the first time with the extent of battle wounds and deaths, but in reality a soldier was two times more likely to die of disease than wounds, and the average man reported sick twice per year. Reading Civil War diaries over the years in my research, I have been impressed that so many times a young man enlisted, healthy and filled with hope, and two or three years later came down with dysentery or some other disease, fought for his life with the aid of the most professional care available, and died within a few weeks. Flannery's path-breaking book provides new perspective on the experiences of these men as well as those who recovered, and the men and women who treated them and those behind the scenes who provided pharmaceuticals. Flannery clears up long-held mysteries, dispels myths, and answers questions that have lingered since 1865.

It is a moment of destiny when a uniquely qualified historian discovers valuable collections of primary sources on a previously unexplored, significant subject. This book is the product of such an experience. Michael Flannery has the background of scholarly experience required for this study. He is a leading authority on the history of pharmacy and the medical history of the United States and an established expert on the eclectic movement of physicians who emphasized botanical medicine as an alternative to the heroic practices of regular doctors. His biography of eclectic John Uri Lloyd is the standard, and he co-authored with Alex Berman the standard one-volume comprehensive history of the botanic medical movements in the United States. He co-authored with Dennis B. Worthen a book on the history of pharmaceutical education in Cincinnati. He taught United

States history at Northern Kentucky University, the history of pharmacy at the University of Cincinnati's College of Pharmacy, and now teaches medical history as Associate Professor at the University of Alabama at Birmingham. He was Director of the Lloyd Library and Museum from 1994 to 1999, and is now Associate Director for Historical Collections, Lister Hill Library of Health Sciences, University of Alabama at Birmingham.

Flannery's background of teaching, publication, and daily work with primary sources gives him the perspective to ask meaningful questions, develop significant themes, and make new interpretations. Until now, historians have been unable to explain why Union authorities removed Surgeon General William A. Hammond in August 1864. He was young, a model of efficiency, and he seemed in the thrust of forward-thinking therapeutics when he removed two prominent drugs from the Union army supply list: calomel, a harsh laxative that caused mercury poisoning, and antimony, a harsh chemical to cause vomiting. The traditional interpretation holds that physicians were ready to drop calomel and antimony and therefore did not oppose Hammond's action. Why then was Hammond court-martialed and dismissed on trumped-up charges? From a medical point of view, it made no sense. But research shows that Hammond was ahead of his time in removing calomel and antimony. These medicines represented regular medicine and physicians continued prescribing them nationwide until around 1900. Flannery's experience in studying the eclectics enabled him to recognize that Hammond's removal of calomel and antimony caught him in the cross fire between the sectarians and the regular doctors. By taking action on the side of the sectarians and attacking the therapeutics of the regulars, Hammond became a traitor to the surgeons who were in control of Union army medicine, and those physicians approved of his removal.

Historians of the Union blockade have concluded that it was effective. Here for the first time, Flannery describes and evaluates the impact of the blockade on Confederate pharmacy; he tells when and how the blockade shut off the supply of international drugs into the South. He relates how talented Confederate Surgeon General Samuel Preston Moore, Confederate pharmacists, and the Southern people reacted by developing substitute medicines from indigenous plants. Flannery provides the first full evaluation of the Confederate indigenous supply table. He evaluates the impact of the Civil War on the development of pharmacy as an industry and profession in the postwar generation that entered the world market.

As a Civil War reader, I have long deplored the myth that Civil War surgeons and hospital stewards were ill-trained bunglers who were flying blind and using remedies that did more harm than good. Flannery demonstrates how far this was from the truth. In reality, Civil War physicians and pharmacists had a well-ordered system based on tradition and developed over generations, and they were intelligent, dedicated individuals who demonstrated their concern for their patients by eagerly seeking and adopting innovations that sometimes proved successful. They proved the value of quinine in preventing malaria, and Flannery particularly admires the Confederates who used substitutes such as mayapple for laxative and raspberry and blackberry for diarrhea, and courageously adapted to the shortages from the blockade, which by 1864 closed their supply of valuable quinine. After describing illnesses and treatments in detail and analyzing the theories involved, Flannery concludes that health care providers on both sides were heroes who performed their duty conscientiously. This work adds a new dimension to the history of the faithful work of Civil War health care professionals.

James A. Ramage
Regents Professor of History
Northern Kentucky University

Acknowledgments

As with a project of this kind, many people played a part in helping to bring it to fruition. First, I would like to thank Dr. Gregory J. Higby and the American Institute of the History of Pharmacy (AIHP), Madison, Wisconsin, for the award of its 2001 Fischelis Grant in support of the present study. Without this essential financial assistance, work on this book could not have begun.

In helping to uncover materials hidden away in long-forgotten files, the author owes a debt of gratitude to librarians, curators, and scholars in several locations, in particular the following: Stephen Greenberg of the National Library of Medicine, History of Medicine Division, Bethesda, Maryland; Rebecca Livingston of the National Archives, Old Military and Civil Records, Washington, DC; Gail McMillan and her staff at Virginia Tech, Blacksburg, Virginia; Joseph M. Ciccone, curator of the Merck Archives, Whitehouse Station, New Jersey; Michael A. Ermilio, archivist for the Joseph W. England Library, University of the Sciences in Philadelphia (formerly the Philadelphia College of Pharmacy); and last but by no means least, Dennis Worthen, scholar-in-residence at the Lloyd Library and Museum, Cincinnati, Ohio, who also served double duty as the ever-encouraging/ever-supportive editor of the Pharmaceutical Heritage series for The Haworth Press. In addition, I would be remiss if I failed to mention my own Historical Collections staff at the Lister Hill Library of the Health Sciences, University of Alabama at Birmingham—Jennifer Beck, Katie Oomens, Tim Pennycuff, and Stefanie Rookis—who each contributed in direct and indirect ways to the completion of this project.

I also wish to extend my appreciation to the many institutions that granted permission to reproduce illustrations for this work. Credit lines appear with each illustration. Special thanks also goes to the AIHP for permission to use a portion of the author's "Trouble in Paradise: A Brief Review of Therapeutic Contention in America, 1790-1864," (*Pharmacy in History* 41 [1999]: 153-163), and to Oxford University Press for permission to use part of the author's "Another

House Divided: Union Medical Service and Sectarians During the Civil War," (*Journal of the History of Medicine and Allied Sciences* 54 [1999]: 478-510), in a section of Chapter 7.

Thanks is also extended to those who read this book in manuscript: David Cowen, Professor Emeritus at Rutgers University; John S. Haller Jr., Professor of history at Southern Illinois University; and James A. Ramage, Regents Professor of History, Northern Kentucky University. I sincerely appreciate their thoughtfulness in reading it, though any errors of commission or omission remain my own. In particular, Dr. Ramage's kind agreement to write the foreword to this book was an honor especially appreciated; I became enthralled by the historical world he opened up to my young and receptive mind some thirty years ago as a student—every author should know the special privilege of calling one's mentor a colleague *and* friend.

Finally, a thousand blessings upon my wife Dona, who accompanied me on several trips to the Alabama Department of Archives and History in Montgomery; one whirlwind excursion looping through the southeastern United States, up to Ohio, and back home to Maylene, Alabama; and two visits to Washington, DC. She has helped in so many ways I hardly know where to begin, but unquestionably her assistance at the National Archives was indispensable. Working together as a team, we were able to plow through documents in a fraction of the time, and I dare say she now knows the U.S. Navy subject files as well as any scholar in the country. This is not the first time she has been my right hand in a research project, so I shall simply say—thanks *again,* Dona.

To all those named and unnamed who helped in the research and/or preparation of this book, I feel duty-bound to admit that I could not have done it without you, a cliché validated by its patent truth.

PART I:
SETTING THE STAGE—
CIVILIAN ASPECTS OF PHARMACY
DURING THE CIVIL WAR

Chapter 1

Civil War Pharmacy and Medicine: Comparisons and Contexts

Civil War pharmacy can be understood in two primary contexts: first, what historians have said about it, and second, the historical milieu in which it took place. With regard to the former something should be said because the issue of pharmaceutical care has received some attention from historians and a modest literature has developed. More important, however, is the fact that nineteenth-century pharmacy and medicine—inseparably linked by ages of theory and practice—existed in a very different world from today. Pharmacy did *not,* as did Athena, spring forth from the head of Zeus. By 1861 pharmacy had hoary traditions born of nature's animal, mineral, and plant kingdoms that grew to compose its time-honored materia medica.

THE HISTORIOGRAPHY OF CIVIL WAR PHARMACY

Histories of Civil War medicine abound. The two classic studies, George Worthington Adams' *Doctors in Blue* and H. H. Cunningham's *Doctors in Gray* set the stage for numerous treatments still emanating from presses at this writing.[1] Yet oddly enough, pharmacy has received comparatively little attention. Civil War historian Allan Nevins noted its conspicuous absence in the literature some thirty years ago.[2] The reasons for this persistent inattention are complex. For one thing, pharmacy is often subsumed within medical histories generally, and Civil War medical histories are no exception. If treated at all, pharmacy is typically relegated to a chapter or perhaps a mere section within a chapter. Both Adams and Cunningham skip lightly over the topic throughout their books. In one of the most recent medical histories of the war, Alfred J. Bollett devotes a somewhat dismissive chapter to what he calls "questionable drugs and 'heroic' therapies."[3] Another reason for the dearth of Civil War pharmacy literature has been simply that there are a comparatively small number of historians working in this field. The subject is so large and the number of pharmacy historians so few, it should be no wonder that major topics such as the Civil War have not been thoroughly covered thus far.

This is not to suggest that no work has been done on Civil War pharmacy. Norman Franke's 1956 doctoral dissertation on pharmacy in the Confederacy was a major contribution to the understanding of drug supply and provision in the South during the war.[4] In 1962 another important addition was made with George Winston Smith's detailed history of the U.S. government laboratories in Philadelphia and Astoria, New York, that were established to provide drugs for the Union Army.[5] For decades these two works formed the substance of historical work on pharmacy during the Civil War. Finally, in 1998, Bruce A. Evans authored *A Primer of Civil War Medicine* devoted to drug therapies of the period. Not strictly a history, Evans chose to present "the essentials of medical therapeutics as they would have been summarized by a reasonably well trained mainstream physician during the years of the War Between the States."[6] Then came Guy Hasegawa's essay surveying the broad scope of pharmaceutical care in the North and South.[7] Hasegawa provided a much-needed overview of the entire subject that was not only objective but also thoroughly researched and fully referenced. Indeed, his work provided many guideposts for the present study.

All of these sources, however, have their limitations. Franke's dissertation covers only Confederate pharmacy; Smith focused only on the Union laboratories; Evans' book provides an interesting perspective and much useful data, but it offers little historical analysis and does not place pharmaceutical care in its larger social, political, and economic contexts; and Hasegawa's article, despite being an extremely helpful start at a comprehensive study, serves principally as a blueprint for further work rather than as the final and definitive word on the subject.

Thus we come to the present work. Not simply a story of drugs and druggists, this book is designed to be a complete treatment of pharmacy care for Union and Confederate forces for four of the most brutal years of conflict ever witnessed by this nation; as such, it will seek to treat the subject in its many civilian and military contexts. It is a story with a cast of many characters: medical purveyors ordering and directing supplies; physicians prescribing medicines; pharmacists (trained and untrained) serving as hospital stewards; businessmen making and selling drugs; adventurers and privateers seeking profit; administrators trying to keep the machinery of health care efficient and functioning; women volunteering their ministrations for the sick and injured; and perhaps most important of all, the thousands of patients for whom all of this effort was directed.

It is a complex story and one that needs telling for a number of reasons, not the least of which is the revolutionary impact of the war itself. Historians have called the war America's "second revolution."[8] Military posturing, saber rattling, battles, skirmishes, intrigues, and strategies are certainly thrilling, but as Charles and Mary Beard long since pointed out, "the core of the vortex lay elsewhere. It was the flowing substance of things limned by statistical reports on finance, commerce, capital, industry, railway, and agriculture, by provisions of constitutional law, and by the pages of the statute books . . ."[9] by which the war, once ignited by the searing flame of slavery, would be truly defined and ultimately determined.

This revolution transformed American life in virtually every way. America came into the war a collection of rural states primarily supported by subsistence farming, which was a speculative trade in staple crops. Towns, villages, and hamlets were inhabited by a comparatively small cadre of professional elites and cottage industry artisans. Compared with European society, America was small and widely diffused. The America that survived the war found itself a nation well on its way to becoming one of the mightiest industrial powers on earth, but it was a distinctly regional development.

A glance at the census data boded ill for the South from the beginning. Although a few Cassandras such as Mexican War hero and Texas Senator Sam Houston (1793-1863) called for cooler heads, most Southern leaders gave no pause to the obvious disparity in numbers and machinery needed to carry out their war for independence. In the South, the largest city in 1860 was New Orleans, with a population of 168,675; the North's largest, New York City, was over six times that size.[10] In manufacturing, Virginia, North and South Carolina, Georgia, Tennessee, Alabama, Mississippi, and Louisiana could muster only 18,945 manufacturing establishments among them in 1860; New York State alone had well over 22,000.[11] Those same eight states had

$89.5 million invested in manufacturing; in contrast, New York had nearly twice that at $173 million.[12] After the war, New York's capital investment would reach nearly $367 million and the state's manufacturing concerns would exceed 36,000, more than the entire South.[13] The imbalance had been growing for some time. Commercial interest and business acumen were clearly not Southern strengths. In a typical year during the 1850s, for example, 421 patents were issued to Massachusetts applicants, whereas in North and South Carolina combined only twenty-six were awarded.[14] The whole of the Confederacy had nothing to match the government armory at Springfield, Massachusetts, a plant employing 3,000 and turning out 1,000 rifles per day, with private concerns producing twice that many for Union troops.[15] Compared to the North, the South's war machine—and the war chest necessary to maintain it—was limited and opportunities to replenish it few. Time was *not* on the Confederacy's side.

Likewise, the Civil War permanently changed American pharmacy, and the roots of that transformation lie in the four years of conflict that created unprecedented demand for mass-produced drugs. Statistics partly tell the tale. In 1860 there were eighty-four chemical manufacturers (including pharmaceutical firms) in the United States, the vast majority of which, as with other industrial concerns, were in the North; by 1870 the number had grown to nearly 300.[16] The product value of drugs rose from $3.4 million in 1860 to $16.2 million in 1870.[17] Williams Haynes accurately summarized the effect of the war's enormously expansive impact on pharmaceutical manufacturing:

> All the familiar war-born influences—shortages, skyrocketing prices, substitutions, hasty improvisation to increase output—stimulated feverish activity. Opium poppies were grown in the Carolinas, Vermont, and California. . . . Hundreds of such typical reactions to the dislocations caused by hostilities met the inflated demands for medicinals. Few of these wartime opportunists persisted, but the able managements of established companies greatly strengthened their positions.

One of the effects of the war was to scatter the industry. Philadelphia remained for years the largest single producer of fine chemicals, but it was no longer undisputed national headquarters. The development of the Mallinckrodt fine chemicals business in St. Louis and the rise of Cincinnati, Indianapolis, and especially Detroit as pharmaceutical centers were out growths of this decentralization which logically flowed westward. Another change encouraged by the four years' struggle was the evolution of alcohol—next to water the most useful solvent—into a prime industrial commodity, a development that culminated in the tax-free denatured alcohol legislation of 1906.[18]

These economic facts are more than just broad trends and statistics; they reflect the aspirations and commercial ambitions of men possessed of an entrepreneurial spirit. So the story of pharmacy in the American Civil War is also a human story. Men such as Edward R. Squibb (1819-1900), Frederick Stearns (1832-1907), Alpheus Sharp (1824-1915), Charles E. Dohme (1843-1911), George D. Rosengarten (1801-1890), Thomas H. Powers (1812-1878), William Weightman (1813-1904), and John Wyeth (1834-1907) built their pharmaceutical manufacturing careers and fortunes (or at least greatly expanded them) on opportunities created by the wartime economy. Others, such as Confederate veteran "Doc" Pemberton, would later give us the formula for what his Yankee veteran counterpart, Frank Robinson, would name Coca-Cola.[19] Another would lend his name even more conspicuously to America's popular postwar beverage industry when James Vernor (1843-1927) began producing the ginger ale that still bears his name.[20] Many more young men—less notable perhaps but nonetheless important in their day—joined in the war effort, and possessed of only a nodding acquaintance with medicine and drugs and their compounding, these men found themselves thrown by circumstance into what first appeared as a sorcerer's den of mysterious potions but what would become a workshop of remedies and they the privileged keepers of its secrets.

Pharmacy in the Civil War is, in short, a story of products, production, and people. As such, it informs the economic and human history of America. More directly it was a significant aspect of health care provision during a period in which the nation was sorely in need of it. Like the legendary twins Cosmas and Damian who symbolize the symbiosis of medicine and pharmacy, this story forms an inseparable part of the American Civil War's medico-pharmaceutical past. It is a story long overdue.

AMERICAN PHARMACY AND MEDICINE AT MIDCENTURY

When hostilities escalated from words to weapons in the spring of 1861, health care fields were profoundly different from the highly professionalized, scientific disciplines familiar to Americans today. Although physicians had finally organized themselves into a coherent body with the founding of the American Medical Association in 1847, pharmacists, struggling to cut themselves from medicine's apron strings, had only recently established the American Pharmaceutical Association in 1852. Many other fields had not even emerged yet. Nursing was nonexistent as a discernable field, for example, though the war would do much to help shape it into what would become a viable profession.

If health care was only beginning to coalesce into something resembling a profession, its aspirations as a science were even more embryonic. Systematic laboratory research tied directly to clinical practice, for example, was still on the horizon, as was rigorous graduate-level training for would-be physicians and pharmacists. In therapeutics a hoary materia medica held on tenaciously, its adherents awaiting the breakthroughs in chemical synthesis and pharmacology that would finally release them from the bondage of time-honored traditions. For physician and pharmacist alike, practice in the 1860s was predicated not on innovation born of research but on the comfortable assurance of precedence.

Yet health care was poised for change. Historians often refer to medicine in this period as "in transition" or "coming of age."[21] These are apt phrases. As John Haller has noted,

> nineteenth-century medicine evolved from a murky antiquity, with traces of its faulty parentage embarrassingly evident. Generations of medical practice clung tenaciously as physicians sought extensions to the boundaries of ancient knowledge. New theories and old habits jostled uncomfortably in the same medical handbags.[22]

Indeed, most practitioners in the 1860s still considered their calling a healing *art* rather than a medical *science*.[23] Theories and speculation on the etiology and treatment of disease were in ample supply, and without any objective test for safety and efficacy save the observations of the physician, virtually any notion was as good as any other. In this context many rose up to challenge medical orthodoxy. Unlicensed and unregulated, so-called allopathic or regular medicine held no hegemony in health care; instead, it faced organized opposition from homeopathic, eclectic, and physio-medical physicians ready and able to attack the therapeutic convictions of their mainstream counterparts. American medicine at midcentury was nothing if not fractious—every group sporting its own peculiar doctrine, every group vying for respectability.[24]

Although pharmacy was not affected by all of these factors in the same ways, this was the milieu in which both pharmacists and physicians—for better or for worse—had to operate. Since the fundamental role of "pharmaceutists" (as the more formally trained often referred to themselves at the time) was to ensure the quality of the ingredients and accuracy of the compounded prescriptions, they served primarily as guarantors and implementers of the materia medica developed from the physician's corpus of knowledge about disease, diagnosis, and therapeutics. In short, what physicians thought about these subjects appreciably affected virtually everything pharmacists did.

It is not enough to merely say that surgeons and assistant surgeons (the designation for all physicians who would serve in the Union and Confederate militaries) knew nothing of germ theory and, hence, little about doctoring. This presentist approach does little to illuminate the nature of medical practice and assumes that physicians faced wartime illness and injury as tabulae rasae. The materia medica and the therapeutics from which it was drawn were the material expressions of theories and concepts old and new. But *which* materia medica would become the standard supply table and *what* therapeutics would be administered to the men in camp and field? Regular physicians were not the only ones with a body of established drugs and drug therapies. The sectarian groups—homeopath, eclectic, and physio-medical—also had their own regimens, stemming from their own theories of disease and its treatment. Still, the materia medica and therapeutics were largely of *regular* medicine. In fact, despite a sizeable organized opposition to allopathic practice, the Medical Department of the Union Army spent considerable time and effort "protecting" the corps against what it viewed as audacious pretenders to the healing art. Irregulars of every stripe were barred from sitting for the surgeon's and assistant surgeon's exams, and a nonregular practitioner discovered among the ranks might be summarily dismissed.[25] Even in the South, where prohibitions against sectarian practitioners was less pronounced, the vast majority of medical personnel was committed to allopathic medicine. For this reason, in order to get into the mind of the nineteenth-century pharmacist, some effort needs to be made in exploring the tenets of regular medical thinking of the day.

Here George B. Wood (1797-1879) (Figure 1.1) serves as an excellent guide, made all the more so by his dual services to pharmacy and medicine. Wood studied medicine at the University of Pennsylvania, receiving his degree in 1818. In 1822 he joined the Philadelphia College of Pharmacy (PCP), founded just one year before as the first school of its kind in the United States. Wood became a key figure in the early revisions of the *Pharmacopoeia of the United States of America* (more commonly referred to as the *United States Pharmacopoeia* or simply *USP*). In 1833 he joined Franklin Bache (1792-1864), a fellow faculty member at the college, in editing the *Dispensatory of the United States of America* (more commonly referred to as the *United States Dispensatory* or simply *USD*).[26] In 1835 Wood resigned his post at PCP to become chair of materia medica and pharmacy in the Medical Department of the University of Pennsylvania. Serving for many years as president of the American Philosophical Society and College of Physicians of Philadelphia, Wood became one of the leading physicians of his age. The name George B. Wood would have been instantly recognized by any worthy American physician or pharmacist of the mid-nineteenth century.[27] His work alone with the *USD* would have guaranteed his fame; this vade mecum of therapeutics passed through fourteen massive editions and some 120,000 copies by the time of his death. But Wood's notoriety was extended into the heart of every medical classroom through his *Treatise on the Practice of Medicine,* a multiedition textbook that became standard fare for the nineteenth-century medical student.

Thus, Wood's *Treatise* becomes an especially useful window into medical practice during the Civil War. Virtually every physician worthy of the name would have had some knowledge of its contents, and

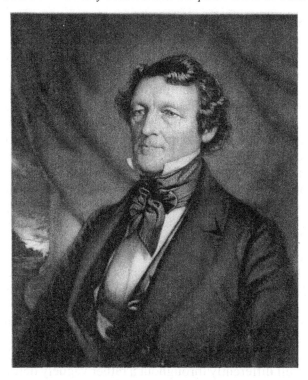

FIGURE 1.1. George B. Wood, physician and early leader of American pharmacy, co-authored with Franklin Bache the first eleven editions of the *Dispensatory of the United States of America* from 1833 through 1858. After Bache's death in 1864, Wood carried on the work through the fourteenth edition issued in 1877. This, plus Wood's two-volume and many-editioned *Treatise on the Practice of Medicine,* made him perhaps the most noted authority on disease, diagnosis, and therapeutics during the Civil War period; his works were consulted by physicians and pharmacists alike. Illustration courtesy of the Reynolds Historical Library, Lister Hill Library of the Health Sciences, University of Alabama at Birmingham.

by 1861 many a newcomer to the field would have had fresh if not fond recollections of the fifth edition firsthand. Using this hefty two-volume text as our guide, then, we might propose to enter into the Civil War physician's mind through the book's contents.

A surgeon (North or South) typically confronted scores—sometimes even hundreds—of sick men every day. Was the man flushed, sweating, hot, or shivering? Clear signs of fever would bring forth the requisite dose of quinine. Was the soldier suffering from diarrhea? Perhaps a regimen of opium or Dover's powder was in order. Were the bowels blocked? A prescription of jalap or a preparation of mercury might answer. If the symptoms were inconclusive, surely calomel could not fail. Was inflammation or irritation the problem? A poultice of cantharides would do nicely. Whatever the malady or the surgeon's success rate, one thing was sure: he did *not* administer to his patients blindly and without established precedence as his guide, and for most Wood's *Treatise* served as the therapeutic compass.

An exhaustive discussion of Wood's book would create a volume in itself, but its salient points can be fairly easily delineated. Wood begins by dividing pathologic conditions into two basic types: those stemming from an "exciting or depressing agency" and those exhibiting "peculiar products."[28] The former he identifies as coming from five sources: irritation, inflammation, depression, congestion, and fevers. The latter comprises tuberculosis, melanosis, cysts, cancer, tumors, and parasites. For the purposes of this study, the first category of pathologies is of greatest interest. Of these, inflammation, according to Wood, was "beyond all comparison the most important of diseased conditions."[29] Inflammation—typically characterized by redness, heat, pain, and swelling—was seen as a condition that would manifest itself differently throughout a rather vaguely defined course of an illness. This could often lead to notions startlingly different from modern protocols of disease management. The appearance of pus, for example, rather than an alarming sign of infection, became for the nineteenth-century physician an unmistakably *good* sign. Wood pointed out the virtues of "*healthy* or *laudable pus,* because it often acts an essential part of the repair of injury, and the restoration of a healthy condition of parts."[30] Although Wood gave paramount importance to inflammation in his pathology, he admitted that others placed congestion as the chief factor in disease.[31]

Wood's views on the etiology of disease were even more opaque and diffused, and he stated that a complete enumeration of "all the possible causes of disease would be an almost endless task."[32] He did outline five though: (1) exterior influences and "moral relations"; (2) "bodily derangements" and those governed by "the will"; (3) "noxious matters within the body"; (4) systemic, functional, or structural problems; and (5) accidental injuries, which include not only trauma but also chemical causes such as "all stimulants [coffee, tea, alcohol, etc.] not essential to health."[33] Into the first category, Wood placed "atmospheric impurity" as "an abundant source of disease"; such impurity could be caused by the effluvia arising from human waste and filth and the decomposition of vegetable matter, to which he attributed so-called "miasmatic" illness, malaria, and "marsh-miasma." As the name would suggest, the culprit was *mal aria* (literally, bad air) created by assorted if somewhat mysterious vapors or gases exuded from the decomposing matter.[34] Wood himself did not identify the precise nature of these bad airs, concluding that in their epidemic forms they operate by some "secret power."[35]

Wood tried hard to understand the manifestations of disease even if he did not have clear notions of its cause. He knew a contagion when he saw one—a disease capable of passing from one individual to another through contact of secretion or exhalation—and admitted the distinction between this and *infection* was so unclear that he proposed the latter term be abandoned altogether.[36] He explained, however, that two theories prevailed as to the nature of contagion. One view held that they consisted of "ferments, which, entering the blood-vessels, occasion chemical changes, that result in a further production of similar contagious matter. . . . This explains the reproduction of the morbific agent."[37] The other theory asserted that the contagion was caused by "organic agents, either animal or vegetable" that enter the bloodstream and multiply as germs, which, in turn, excites the system "into desperate efforts, and throws off the intruders and their whole brood, or perishes in the attempt."[38] Whatever the particular conjecture might be, almost every so-called contagionist agreed that these diseases were distinguished by their uniformity of symptoms and their ability to attack an individual only once; epidemics on the other hand could manifest themselves in a variety of ways and might be contracted multiple times. Others, noting the many instances in which alleged contagions did not behave in these predictable ways, argued against the concept altogether. Throughout the early 1800s contagionists and anticontagionists wrangled over the matter to no clear conclusion.

Enter English physician William Farr (1807-1883). In 1842 Farr merged the contending notions by insisting that epidemic, endemic, and contagious diseases were all similar in their etiologies. In Farr's view they were all spawned by the introduction of some animal poison into the bloodstream of a susceptible host. Farr believed that once this poison was introduced, a "pathological transformation" occurred not unlike a fermentation process. To describe this chemical transformation, Farr chose the word *zymotic* from the Greek *zymos,* meaning ferment. By viewing pathology in this way, Farr could explain disease as being spread by contact or by particular environmental factors, such as heat or moisture, that would make hosts susceptible on the one hand and encourage zymotic activity on the other. Farr was captivated by the numerical methodologies of Pierre Louis (1787-1872), who had taken Condorcet's and Laplace's earlier work on probabilities and put medicine's received wisdom in bloodletting to the test through statistical mortality/recovery-rate analysis of the practice in cases of pneumonia.[39] Similarly, Farr was convinced he could prove his zymotic theory through in-depth and detailed statistical analyses of disease epidemics. Ultimately, perhaps even a set of laws or principles could be established outlining with predictable certainty how epidemics would begin, develop, mature, and eventually wane.[40]

Farr's views had a powerful influence over the medical community on both sides of the Atlantic. Wood provided a lengthy note on zymotic diseases but cautioned against treating "these speculations" as received truths.[41] Still, the concept had attained wide enough acceptance by the start of the Civil War to be included as the first class of diseases discussed in the compendious *Medical and Surgical History of the War of the Rebellion.*[42] This volume identified zymotic diseases as comprising some of the most prevalent during the entire course of the war: diarrhea, dysentery, and a wide variety of permutations of those disorders, such as ulcerative diarrhea, simple inflammatory dysentery, and diphtheritic dysentery.

Wood vis-à-vis Farr offered etiological explanations that highlighted some of the curious precursors to the later definitive germ theory of disease that would emerge in the 1870s and 1880s, explanations that in some limited but fascinating senses might not have been wholly off the mark.[43] The fermentation theory explained in somewhat stilted fashion how bacteria and viruses might multiply; the organic theory gave a rather awkward account of what a modern clinician might view as an immune response. Wood's discussion shows how close and yet how far his generation was from the more complete understanding of bacterial and viral infection. Either idea might in fact explain the basis for contagions, however, it was noted that these hypothetical *causes* of disease could just as easily be the *results.*

It would take Louis Pasteur (1822-1895) and Robert Koch (1843-1910) to establish the paradigms upon which so much of modern medicine would be based. It is ironic that in 1865, the very year America's Civil War ended, Pasteur was asked to investigate the cause of pébrine, a silkworm disease that had been devastating the French silk industry for the past decade. With years of work on fermentation behind him—and an indefatigable passion to disprove the age-old spontaneous generation theory—Pasteur correctly concluded that the worms were infested with a microscopic organism that was both contagious and hereditary. Simply hatch silkworms from eggs free of this microscopic parasite and the problem was solved. From this early research Pasteur then turned his attentions to the higher animal studies that would lead directly to his germ theory of disease.[44] Similarly, Koch's proof that a specific microorganism was responsible for a specific disease through the postulates that bear his name was a mere eleven years away when the Civil War ended.[45]

All of this came too late to help the men in camp or field who served on either side of this great American conflict. By today's standards what Civil War–era medicine *did* have to offer was not much, and the public knew it even then. Medicine's own internecine fighting between regular and sectarian ranks kept its worst features in the public eye; its comparatively weak professional standing made it seem a less honorable pursuit than many others; its wide-ranging speculations created a recondite nosology leading to public distrust and ambiguity as well as confusion among even its most learned practitioners; and its antiquated remedies such as bleeding and dosing with harsh mineral agents caused the public to be skeptical and even fearful of the healing art. Historian Richard Shryock characterized the age nicely by asking an appropriate if not wholly rhetorical question: Compared with the great innovations in commerce, transportation, and industry, what certain benefits could medicine offer to the people of the 1860s?

> No reassuring answer could be made for many years. The very progress physicians were making between 1830 and 1850 made it more difficult for them to offer the public much encouragement. The first generation of critical clinicians had so much traditional trash to clear up, and such difficult foundations to

lay, that it was never able to build a therapeutics that could impress the laity. This was inevitable. Someone had to distinguish between typhoid and typhus before anyone could look for the cause of either. But until causes and even cures were found, the public was conscious of little progress. Someone, again, had to show the futility of bleeding, before attention could be centered upon a search for more effective remedies. But until the latter were discovered, it appeared only as if that little which the patient had, had been taken away. Therapeutic nihilism was really a sign of progress . . . but it discouraged the generation that witnessed its appearance. Hence the paradox, that the most hopeful period in the history of medicine was the one in which the public looked to medicine with the least hope.[46]

If this was the typical mind-set of the patient, so too was it the pall that hung over every physician of the Civil War, and indeed over his compounding and dispensing colleague, the pharmacist. Medicine and pharmacy may be summarized as being practiced in a context of uncertainty, but modern students who assume that because health care providers knew nothing of germ theory or medical microbiology that care was delivered in an intellectual vacuum are in for a shock. Both unfamiliar *and* familiar terms show up in the diaries, casebooks, and diagnosis and prescription records of practitioners. Nomenclature then was *not* the nomenclature now—virus and bacteria *do* appear in the primary sources. A virus, however, was not understood as a microbe smaller than a bacterium capable of replicating and causing serious illness and inappropriate immune responses but simply as a poison and *perhaps* vaguely and nonspecifically as an agent for disease transmission; bacteria were known but were just one broad group of microscopic *animalcule.* Causes of disease, as we have seen, were highly conjectural—assorted effluvia, poorly defined contagions and infections, and mysterious ferments (zymotic or otherwise)—all, some, or frankly none of these might have been the cause of a disease or epidemic. A few could not contain their frustration as when, in an 1860 address before the Massachusetts Medical Society, Oliver Wendell Holmes (1809-1894) complained, "I firmly believe that if the whole materia medica, *as now used,* could be sunk to the bottom of the sea, it would be all the better for mankind,—and the worse for the fishes."[47] But on the whole, physicians and pharmacists—and in desperation, even their patients—were less cynical.

They *had* to do something, and most provided and received care with a conviction built more on tradition and faith than on science. That faith and tradition forms a fascinating and significant story in Civil War health care.

PHARMACY AND MEDICINE IN THE CIVIL WAR: AN OVERVIEW

Such was the state of medicine when hostilities broke out in Charleston Harbor in the early morning hours of April 12, 1861. The Medical Department of the U.S. Army was unprepared to meet the contingencies of war, an expression of administrative incompetence that risks understatement. When the war broke out there was a total force of slightly over 13,000 in the regular army, with a medical staff of 115 including the surgeon general.[48] Of those, twenty-four resigned to join their Southern brethren and three quit (or, alternatively interpreted, were dismissed from) the service altogether, refusing to serve on either side.[49] There was no hospital system to speak of; no ambulance corps; and no war-ready infrastructure for medical supply and distribution. In fact, there was very little in the way of medical service at all. The surgeon general at the time of the siege of Fort Sumter was Thomas Lawson (1789-1861), an old and ailing career man who died one month later. His replacement, Clement A. Finley (1797-1879), whose forty years of service was his chief claim to the post, personified an ossified military system based more on seniority than merit.[50]

A mounting struggle of such monumental proportions would call for a medical department ready and willing to improvise and innovate quickly to meet the needs of a large standing army. In the spring of 1861 it was not up to the task. John H. Brinton (1832-1907), who would later distinguish himself as a surgeon for the Union Army, gave a revealing description of Dr. Simons, the medical director at Cairo, Illinois, where Brinton first reported for duty in September 1861. Dr. Simons typified the "old fogies" who peopled the early U.S. Army Medical Department. He had served in the military since 1839, viewed himself as "a typical soldier," disliked the practice of medicine, and, according to Brinton, seemed "more an army man than an army surgeon."[51]

The men of this department were a reflection of the general economic and administrative lethargy that had settled over the military in the years following the Mexican War. For the whole of the medical corps even as late as July 1861, the entire budget consisted of $241,000, of which over 80 percent had already been spent on medical stores.[52] Far from urging the Medical Department on to extraordinary effort to fill the demands of the national emergency, the army, on May 22, 1861, supplemented the ranks with a mere sixty-two appointments and an additional 110 were added as "brigade surgeons" who would not belong to the regiments.[53] President Lincoln's 75,000 volunteers provided their own surgeons based on state appointments of dubious merit. Although some states such as Ohio, New York, and Vermont took their medical appointments seriously, others did not. Some even defended the practice of filling surgeon and assistant surgeon positions with men holding little—in some cases *no*—medical training.[54] While Surgeon General Finley dawdled, the Women's Central Association of Relief and other concerned citizen groups petitioned to create an organization to supply matériel relief to the gathering troops. Believing it to be "a monument of weak enthusiasts, and of well-meaning but silly women," Finley and his officer cohorts reluctantly agreed provided that "the operations of the Commission should be confined to the volunteers."[55] On June 9, 1861, Secretary of War Simon Cameron gave the order establishing the United States Sanitary Commission.

Part of the problem stemmed from a general attitude outside the medical corps that downplayed the significance of "the Southern problem." When the President issued his initial call for 75,000 volunteers he seemed to view the matter as little more than an extended policing activity. Signing them on for only three months' service, the commander in chief simply claimed the "combinations [of the South] too powerful to be suppressed by the ordinary course of judicial proceedings or by the powers vested in the marshals by law."[56] Lincoln further minimized the crisis by convening Congress not immediately but in eighty days. The young Confederacy scorned Lincoln's response. "The Administration labor under the delusion that they will soon strike terror into the South," taunted *The Charleston Mercury,* "and that the war thus begun will be a small and a little one. They have been deceived."[57] How right the *Mercury* was!

It would soon become evident that Ft. Sumter was the beginning of a long, protracted war. The early failures of the U.S. Army Medical Department in 1861 spawned reform early the next year. In January 1862, Edwin M. Stanton replaced the ineffectual Cameron as secretary of war. By April, Congress replaced the seniority system with promotion based on proven ability and competence, leaving the way open for the young, ambitious William A. Hammond (1828-1900) (Figure 1.2) to be appointed Surgeon General on April 25, 1862.[58] Hammond's role in revitalizing the Medical Department was immense, despite his military career coming to an unfair and unfortunate end in a politically motivated court-martial that will be discussed later.[59] By the time the equally youthful medical director of the Army of Potomac, Jonathan Letterman (1824-1872), implemented his reor-

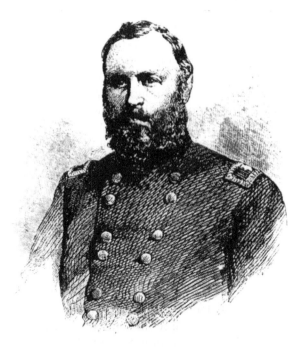

FIGURE 1.2. Surgeon General William A. Hammond's ambitious reforms of a tradition-bound U.S. Army Medical Department earned the talented administrator a court-martial. Exonerated of all charges years later, Hammond nevertheless rose to prominence in medical circles and was the founder of the American Neurological Association. From *Harper's Weekly,* 1863. Illustration courtesy of the National Library of Medicine, History of Medicine Division.

ganized field hospital and medical supply systems by the fall of 1862, the Union medical corps had developed into an efficient, war-ready unit.[60] By war's end the Union army had appointed 547 surgeons and assistant surgeon volunteers, 2,109 volunteer regimental surgeons, 3,882 volunteer regimental assistant surgeons, 5,532 acting assistant surgeons, and seventy-five acting staff surgeons.[61]

Pharmacy care was delivered through a system of physicians appointed as medical purveyors whose principal charge was to manage the distribution of drugs and other medical supplies. Beneath them were hospital stewards who served as noncommissioned officers holding a rank equivalent to ordnance sergeant and charged with compounding and dispensing of drugs; the role of these stewards will be more closely examined in Chapter 4. As will be seen, despite the fact that these men were not given officer rank, they held positions of considerable responsibility and they commanded the respect of officers and enlisted alike. Even medical students viewed assignments as hospital stewards as choice appointments; there, they could gain much needed experience in their field.[62] Regimental surgeons of volunteer units followed the time-honored tradition of selecting their stewards from their own ranks, with one allowed for each battalion.[63] At the height of the war there were more than 700 hospital stewards serving in general hospitals alone, and many more were stationed in the field.[64] In the navy a comparable position was that of surgeon's steward holding the rank of petty officer. There was a higher "professional" position called a medical storekeeper, who technically held the rank of first lieutenant. Created to act as "skilled apothecaries or druggists," their number never exceeded five, and they were largely regarded as civil appointments that failed to earn the respect of the regular medical staff.[65] As such, the storekeeper never attained a position of importance during the war.

In the South, the provisional congress at Montgomery, Alabama, established a Medical Department on February 26, 1861, consisting of a surgeon general, four surgeons, and six assistant surgeons. As wartime necessity dictated, this number would greatly increase. After a couple of unsuccessful appointments, the surgeon general's position fell upon the sturdy shoulders of South Carolinian Samuel Preston Moore (1813-1889) (Figure 1.3) on July 30, 1861. An able administrator but a man fastidious about rules and protocols, Moore would head the Confederate Medical Department for the duration of

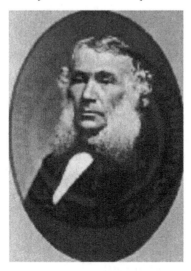

FIGURE 1.3. Surgeon General Samuel Preston Moore was responsible for all Confederate pharmaceutical operations. During his brief but illustrious tenure Moore operated a system of laboratories, developed a supply table of indigenous remedies, and attempted to acquire drugs from foreign suppliers amidst an ever-tightening blockade. Photo courtesy of the National Library of Medicine, History of Medicine Division.

the war.[66] Faced with the huge task of creating an efficient department from scratch, Moore built a unit regarded in retrospect as "among the most efficient in the Confederacy."[67] The Medical Department mirrored the structure of its Union counterparts. It too included hospital stewards and storekeepers, positions created by act of the Provisional Confederate Congress on May 16, 1861.[68] It is very difficult to determine the exact number of stewards who served in the Confederate military (a considerable portion of the Confederate Medical Department records were destroyed in the burning of Richmond at war's end), but the total number of medical officers in the Confederate Army has been estimated at 834 surgeons and 1,668 assistant surgeons; there were an estimated seventy-three medical officers in the Confederate Navy.[69] Unlike the Union Medical Department initially bogged down with old hangers-on, the Confederate medical corps had no traditions placing its officers in an administrative straitjacket. Their challenges would be different, and these will form a significant part of this book.

THE ROLE OF DISEASE

Whether serving the North or South, those charged with the duty of supplying, compounding, and dispensing drugs were kept busy throughout the conflict largely because of the nature of maintaining the health of any large-standing military organization in the nineteenth century. Health and healing during this war—indeed in every war until World War I[70]—was defined more by combating disease than by repairing injuries. Despite the popular images of wholesale amputations, bullet extractions, fracture repairs, and wound closures of every grizzly description, the real debilitater was illness. Among Confederate troops as many as two-thirds of their 600,000 men were under treatment for illness by war's end.[71] Union troops fared better, but the stark reality was that even for the victorious the average soldier was about twice as likely to die of a disease contracted in camp than of a wound acquired in battle.[72]

The chief culprits in order of prevalence were diarrhea and dysentery (euphemistically referred to by its victims as "the Tennessee trots" or "Virginia quickstep"), accounting for more than 1.3 million cases and some 35,000 deaths; malaria, typhoid, and assorted camp fevers came next; then respiratory ailments (catarrh, bronchitis, and so-called lung inflammation [pneumonia]); and, finally, assorted digestive disorders.[73] The Federal numbers of wounded versus disease tell the story: there were approximately 425,000 traumatic cases (consisting primarily of wounds and injuries); the number of nontraumatic cases (basically disease diagnoses and treatments) was slightly more than 6 million.[74]

Regimental losses detail the sad toll from disease during the war. Consider Colonel Edwin C. Mason's 1,100-man regiment of the 7th Maine Infantry: it was so depleted by disease that at the Battle of Antietam (September 1862) it was able to send only 182 men into the field.[75] Total deaths from disease in that regiment were nearly double those killed in combat.[76] Similarly, George P. Foster's Vermont Brigade, 4th Vermont Infantry, suffered 280 deaths from disease compared with 162 from wounds incurred in the field.[77] Henry Lawton's regiment belonging to Grose's Brigade, 30th Indiana Infantry, lost 275 of its 1,126 men to sickness and 137 in battle.[78] Regimental statistics on disease mortality rates among the Confederates are not available, but a tally of deaths compiled from the incomplete muster rolls of the Confederate Archives by U.S. Provost Marshal General James B. Fry at the end of the war revealed 59,297 deaths from illness, considerably more than twice those listed as "died of wounds." [79]

Among African-American troops disease was even worse. Camp fevers topped their sick list, with 892 cases per 1,000; there were 839 cases per 1,000 of diarrhea/dysentery. Respiratory ailments were 354 per 1,000, and digestive complaints were reported at 295 per 1,000.[80] In each category incidents of illness appreciably exceeded that for white troops, suggesting that medical care in camp and field was sub-standard compared with that provided for whites. It has been pointed out that black soldiers had virtually all been exposed to, and therefore had acquired some resistance to, malaria; in fact, death from that dis-ease, including typhoid fever, was 18.72 percent compared with a 23.34 percent mortality among whites.[81] But blacks were obviously not fever-free. African-American soldiers' exceedingly high fever rates may be attributed to the more nebulous "intermittent," "peri-odic," or "continued" fevers and to the equally vague "crowd poison-ings."[82] The conclusion of one historian that blacks served "under conditions of considerably greater distress than their white compatri-ots" seems supported by indisputable evidence.[83]

Given the high disease rates throughout the war, the medical con-text for the Civil War, then, was *not* one principally of saws and su-tures but of mortar and pestle. It was truly a question less of surgical skill and more of pharmacy care. Hospital stewards would implement the prescriptions of physicians from materials supplied by purveyors, all of whom were groping to understand the nature and cause of the invisible enemies—*pneumococcus, streptococcus, staphylococcus, E. coli, Entameba histolytica, Vibrio cholerae,* and many others—decimating their comrades worse than the rifle and canon fire of their adversaries. Subsequent chapters will examine this process in some detail. Whether or not these medical purveyors were effective—and it will be seen that it should *not* automatically be assumed that they were not—is probably of less significance than that they tried, and in so doing permanently transformed the nature of pharmacy in Amer-ica. In terms of overall medical care during the Civil War, this is a big and important story.

Chapter 2

The State of Pharmacy
in America, 1861

Although a general overview of the state of health care and the relationship of pharmacy to medicine has been given in Chapter 1, a
more complete picture of pharmacy itself needs to be rendered in order to understand its role and relative position during the Civil War. In
education, manufacturing, and community practice, pharmacy in the
1860s bore little resemblance to what it would become in the next
century. Although each topic could easily fill a volume of its own, a
brief overview of each of these important aspects of pharmacy in civilian life should aid in establishing the context of pharmacy care in
the military.

EDUCATION

In 1861 there were only six colleges of pharmacy in the entire
United States. These early schools, the first of which was established
at the Philadelphia College of Pharmacy (PCP) in 1821, emanated
from local apothecaries who banded together in mutual self-interest
to form associations. In order to raise the standard of practice and
help create a reliable labor pool, these associations promoted the establishment of formal schools in pharmacy. In addition to PCP, the
model institution, were the following: Massachusetts College of
Pharmacy, established in 1823; the College of Pharmacy of the City
and County of New York, 1829; Maryland College of Pharmacy,
1840; Cincinnati College of Pharmacy, 1850, the first west of the Al-
legheny Mountains; and Chicago College of Pharmacy, 1859.[1] Typical curricula included course work in chemistry, medical botany, and
the materia medica for which George Fownes' *Elementary Chemis-*

try, Asa Gray's *Gray's Lessons in Botany and Vegetable Physiology,* Edward Parrish's *Introduction to Practical Pharmacy,* and Wood and Bache's *United States Dispensatory (USD)* were standard texts. All instruction was didactic, with opportunities for clinical or laboratory experience few to none.

The eruption of open hostilities caused no small alarm among college faculty. "In times like the present, when the regular routine of society is threatened with convulsion, and the arrangements of today may be soon altered by the pressure of circumstances," cautioned William J. Procter Jr., editor of PCP's *American Journal of Pharmacy,*

> it behooves the rising generation to avoid, as far as possible, the evil results by securing a business education, fitting them to meet the exigencies which may surround them on their entry into manhood. . . . The able mechanic, the thorough bookkeeper, the earnest physician, and the qualified pharmaceutist, are much more likely to find employment than the pretender or half educated.[2]

William C. Bakes, a trustee for PCP, noted early that he was "repeatedly called on" for men to serve as hospital stewards in the army and navy.[3] There is little doubt that the huge diversion of young men into the military had an appreciable effect on all these pioneer colleges of pharmacy. The college at Cincinnati managed to keep its doors open during the war, but just barely. During the war, a young Charles T. P. Fennel (1854-1942) recalled attending the Cincinnati school with his father in classes that had been reduced to small roundtable lectures. Meeting in the evenings above Gordon's drugstore at Eighth Street and Western Row, Fennel was introduced to the field with "classmates many years my senior."[4]

Formal training in pharmacy was clearly not considered essential for the ordinary druggist, nor did established practitioners always appreciate it as useful. Procter chided his New York colleagues for not giving proper support to the city's college of pharmacy, saying, "We cannot doubt the success of the New York School of Pharmacy, if the pharmaceutists of that city can be properly awakened to the importance of the instruction to be obtained at its lecture hall."[5] With the exception of PCP, other schools remained embryonic at best. The Massachusetts College of Pharmacy offered only sporadic courses, and did not embark on a regular curriculum until after the war.[6] Without licensing or state board exams, pharmacy was generally considered a trade; on-the-job training from a more experienced practitioner was seen as wholly sufficient. Thus, a standard two- to three-year apprenticeship was the mainstay for the vast majority of nineteenth-century pharmacists. Indeed out of the 11,000 pharmacists practicing in 1860, less than 5 percent had graduated from any formal course work.[7] Even by century's end only 12 percent of those in practice had anything beyond basic apprenticeship training.[8]

Unlike schooling today that typically *precedes* practice, formal course work in pharmacy in the 1860s was generally concomitant *with* practice. Classes at all the early pharmacy schools were held in the evening, with instruction normally delivered by physicians.[9] Historian Gregory J. Higby has accurately described formal education in this period as a "finishing school" whereby apprentices took a few courses to "round out" or polish their skills as compounders and businessmen.[10] Typical was Chicago's pharmacy school, whose students were described as "earnest young fellows, employed in drugstores during the day" with courses presented "in the briefest manner" given three evenings per week for twenty weeks.[11] The ability to detect adulterations in crude drug products, shoddy merchandise, and substandard drugs were the most common expectations of most pharmacy students in these classes. Even the preeminent PCP reflected this finishing-school model. From the college's beginning in 1821 until 1869, the school could count only slightly more than 700 graduates out of 3,000 total registrants.[12] Clearly, apprentices (perhaps at the promptings of their mentors) were attending courses to fill out their more practical hands-on training with little regard for completing the degree requirements. In short, of those calling themselves variously pharmacists, pharmaceutists, druggists, or apothecaries, those with no course work were common, those with some course work rare, and those graduated from a full curriculum rarer still.

It would be unfair, however, to characterize pharmacy education as lagging behind the rest of the country's educational standards. In contrast to Europe, where strong central control and well-established universities created rigorous pharmacy curricula, America was in the throes of educational growing pains. All American education in the first half of the nineteenth century was primarily didactic, based on rote memorization, and founded on a faith in English traditions that emphasized classical learning in Latin and Greek. Scientific training in pharmacy and medicine could not be sustained by private and proprietary effort alone; state and federal support would be essential. The Morrill Act establishing the land-grant colleges upon which the state university system would be based was not passed until 1862. This act reflected a significant shift in public attitudes toward education. Rather than higher education serving an elite of class and privilege, large-scale educational reform was rooted in the belief that university training should be available to all interested and capable students, that the applied sciences should be given special attention, and that publicly supported colleges and universities would be uniquely suited to supporting the needs of an increasingly complex society.[13] The land-grant college system would have an appreciable effect on the development of pharmaceutical education, for it was Albert B. Prescott at the state-supported University of Michigan who would first institute a modern academic pharmacy curriculum that broke the old finishing-school mold. But in 1861 all this lay in the future.

MANUFACTURING

Similar to education, pharmaceutical manufacturing in antebellum America was underdeveloped compared with its European counterparts. Although Glauber of Amsterdam and London's Worshipful Society of Apothecaries had had large-scale drug manufacturing operations since the seventeenth century, and many French pharmacists joined in similar enterprises in the eighteenth and early nineteenth centuries, the industrialization of American pharmacy still loomed on the horizon.[14] Evan Ellis tells of his father's modest laboratory in Philadelphia:

> We fitted it [the laboratory] up with a steam boiler in the cellar, jacketed copper pans, stills, a press, and in fact all the equipment of a pharmaceutical laboratory as known at the time. Numbers of open furnaces for divers operations were around, and there were drying rooms on the second floor.[15]

Although the war would do much to turn America toward mass-produced, mass-marketed pharmaceuticals, the 1860s still saw most medicines either compounded by the physician or pharmacist. Pre-packaged patent medicines—though gaining in popularity—would not become the ubiquitous product of consumers' choice until after 1865. Ellis provides an interesting description of domestic medicine during the prewar years:

> At this period there were comparatively few patent medicines— not one perhaps where there are 100 to-day [1903]; and it was also the habit with families to purchase drugs in their crude, or original state, and prepare from them the various compounds known as domestic remedies. As to patent medicines, the public, especially the rustic community, had most of their ailments satisfied with a lot of old English things, whose proprietary right had run out or somehow they had become public property, and they apparently covered the ground. And if any one of you think the modern quack audacious in advertising his wares, I would have you read the original English wrappers that came with all these, and which some druggists adhered to. . . . Here they are: Godfrey's Cordial, Bateman's Drops, Dalby's Carminative, Harlem Oil (a vile concoction); and so large was the sale of such things that it constituted the greater portion of the business of many of the wholesale druggists of the 30s and 40s, and their apprentices (as one who came to us after he served two years said) knew nothing else than putting up these, supplemented with filling vials of laudanum, castor oil, etc.[16]

Because his family members were Quakers, Ellis admitted that his father—despite the fact that throughout the Civil War "every old thing was salable in the way of drugs"—could not out of principle take advantage of the lucrative government contracts that would become available with the conflict.[17] Others could, and did. As we shall see, it was on the crest of the tidal wave of war trade that much of the American pharmaceutical industry was born.

Although there was nothing like the industry giants of the postwar years, it is not correct to conclude that no antebellum manufacturing occurred in America. In the larger cities such as Cincinnati—the so-called Queen of the West—a fairly sizeable wholesale drug trade had developed with pioneer firms established by T. C. Thorp, William S. Merrell, George M. Dixon, William J. M. Gordon, and F. D. Hill.[18] Although still comparatively small-scale with regional distribution outlets, companies in Cincinnati, Louisville, St. Louis, and Chicago actively competed with Eastern and even European rivals for the physician's business. The French firm of Garnier, Lamoureux, and Company advertised their sugarcoated pills as a popular and convenient way to make the disgusting remedial agents more palatable.[19] Competition in the East was even more intense. In the 1850s, New York City had twenty-four wholesale drug establishments; Philadelphia had twenty-one; Boston, nine; and Providence, three.[20]

One of the larger and more interesting manufacturers during this period was Tilden and Company of New Lebanon, New York. Founded in 1824 by an intelligent and industrious Connecticut Yankee, Elam Tilden (1781-1842), this business was greatly expanded by his son Henry A. Tilden.[21] Pharmacy pioneer William Procter Jr. (1817-1874), invited by Tilden to view his New Lebanon facility in 1851 (Figure 2.1), gave this interesting and detailed account of one of the largest antebellum drug manufacturers—certainly the preeminent botanical house—then in operation:

> Their factory is an extensive, oblong, three storied building, in the basement of which is a powerful steam engine which performs the double duty of propelling the powdering apparatus, and of driving a double acting air pump connected with their vacuum evaporators.
>
> The recent plants collected for extracts are brought to the mill from the gardens, reduced to a course pulpy state by a pair of chasers [a type of grinding mill], and subjected to a powerful screw press to extract the juice. This is clarified by coagulation, strained, and the pure juice introduced into the large vacuum apparatus, holding several hundred gallons, where it is concentrated rapidly to a syrupy consistence, at a temperature varying 110°–130°, almost entirely free from the deteriorating influence of the atmosphere. In the construction of this apparatus, they have had a view to great extent of tubular steam-heating surface, so as to be able to accomplish the very large amount of evaporation their business demands. The finishing apparatus is analogous to the vacuum pan of sugar refiners. We witnessed the operation in progress with the thermometer standing at 112° F. They make annually about 8,000 pounds of extracts from green plants and roots, consisting chiefly of Conium 2,000 lbs, Dandelion 2,000 lbs., Lettuce 1,200 lbs., Stramonium 500 lbs., Butternut 800 lbs., Belladonna 500 lbs., Hyoscyamus 500 lbs., and so on. These extracts in the aggregate according to Mr. Tilden's

estimate, are derived from about 300,000 lbs. of green material, and require the evaporation of more than 20,000 gallons of juice.

Besides these, a considerable amount of extracts are made from dry materials, both foreign and indigenous as Gentian, Rhubarb, Chamomile, May-apple, Horehound, Cohosh, etc. They are also about engaging largely in the manufacture of extract of Liquorice from foreign root.

In the powdering department they run burr stones [probably a Buhr-stone mill] and chasers, and use bolting and dusting apparatus. They powder large quantities of material on contract, besides that for their special business, amounting annually to from 50 to 60,000 pounds.

In the herb department, the quantity of material handled is very large. The plants are brought from the gardens into a large room in the factory building, where a number of girls are employed in picking them over to remove other plants accidentally present, and separating the decaying parts and the stems when desirable. They are then placed on hurdles [a portable framework often loosely latticed], and exposed in the drying room till properly desiccated. Two presses are kept in operation, by which 2,000 pounds of material are sometimes pressed in a week, and about 75,000 pounds per annum, including near three hundred varieties of plants.[22]

Tilden did not market his products directly to the public. His entire inventory was sold strictly to physicians or pharmacists. Tilden published books designed for practitioners in "putting up of officinal formulae" from company stocks. By the start of the war Tilden listed an impressive array of dosage forms containing over 140 pages of botanical extracts, fluidextracts, tinctures, syrups, wines, mixtures, and pills with explicit instructions for their use and preparation.[23]

Procter had a very favorable impression of the Tilden Company, calling it, "*directly* beneficial to the medical interests of the country."[24] The firm employed thirty men and five women.[25] Even Tilden, however, would be dwarfed by modern standards. Squibb, a company that would soon derive great impetus from wartime drug demands, would employ over 6,000 workers nearly a century later and produce 400 products yielding sales of $60 million.[26] Similarly, Merck and Company, successor to the Philadelphia-based Powers and Weight-

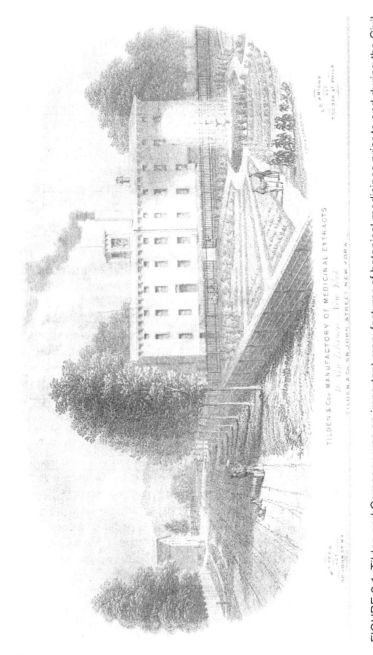

TILDEN & Cº. MANUFACTORY OF MEDICINAL EXTRACTS

TILDEN & Cº 98 JOHN STREET NEW YORK

FIGURE 2.1. Tilden and Company was an important manufacturer of botanical medicines prior to and during the Civil War, and as such was a leading standard-bearer of quality tinctures and extracts. It was one of the very few important pharmaceutical firms not located in Philadelphia. Illustration from the 1861 Tilden catalog, courtesy of the Reynolds Historical Library, Lister Hill Library of the Health Sciences, University of Alabama at Birmingham.

man firm that manufactured the bulk of the quinine sulfate for the Union Army, would 100 years later have more buildings than Tilden had employees and produce some $68 million in sales for its 6,000 stockholders.[27]

Nonetheless, Procter's description of the Tilden factory illustrates a number of important points about nineteenth-century pharmacy. First is that despite the use of large steam engines to automate the process, much of the work was still labor-intensive. Second, the materials worked were botanical. Although some companies—including Powers and Weightman, Rosengarten and Sons, and the Edward R. Squibb laboratories—made chemical products, the fact that a firm such as Tilden could sustain and even expand its business to such a scale from a wholly herbal inventory speaks to the importance of the vegetable materia medica in the mid-nineteenth century. For the most part, the Tilden Company grew its own crude drug product rather than purchasing it on the open market or importing the materials. Finally, although some solids were prepared, most available dosage forms were alcohol-based fluids. From this, mid-nineteenth century pharmacy in America may be characterized as a laborious undertaking chiefly comprised of indigenous plant remedies delivered in liquid dosage forms. This becomes even clearer when community pharmacy is examined.

COMMUNITY PRACTICE

For all the drug wholesalers and fledgling manufacturing concerns, the bulk of pharmacy care took place in either the physician's office or, in more cosmopolitan settings, the apothecary shop. Even by the beginning of the twentieth century, the majority of physicians still dispensed their own medicines.[28] They prescribed and compounded a wide variety of vegetable, mineral, and animal substances, but a review of the 1860 *United States Pharmacopoeia (USP)* indicates that 587 (or 67 percent) of the total number of 871 medicinal substances listed therein were botanical.[29] Some of the more popular were: cinchona, sometimes referred to as Peruvian bark, and its refined counterpart, sulfate of quinine, both used as antiperiodics[30]; opium from *Papaver somniferum*, the powerful narcotic and anodyne (i.e., pain reliever) of choice for many physicians of the day, as well as its refined alkaloid constituent, morphine, discovered by Friedrich Wilhelm Sertürner in 1804[31]; mayapple from *Podophyllum peltatum,* a cathartic so often used as a substitute for mercurous chloride that it earned the dubious sobriquet "vegetable calomel"[32]; *Taraxacum officinale,* or dandelion, used as a tonic and diuretic thought "to have a specific action upon the liver, exciting it when languid to secretion"[33]; geranium, from *Geranium maculatum,* considered "one of our best indigenous astringents"[34]; and jalap, from *Ipomea jalapa,* "highly popular in the United States in bilious fever."[35] But there were some time-honored mineral agents commonly dispensed as well: calomel (mercurous chloride), iron sulfate, sulfate of copper, sugar of lead, and an assortment of salts such as bicarbonate of soda, cream of tartar (bitrate of potassium), carbonate of potassium, citrate of potassium, and the ever popular tartar emetic (antimony potassium tartrate), to name but a few.

This materia medica was delivered in a number of solid or liquid dosage forms. The most common solid preparation came as pills. Pills were spherical masses usually bound together with honey, molasses, or gum arabic as excipients. Not to be confused with more modern disk-shaped tablets that are molded or pressed in dies, pills circa 1861 were regarded by the leading pharmacy textbook of the day as "the most popular and convenient of all forms of medicine."[36] It should be pointed out that since the term tablet was not used until Burroughs Wellcome applied it to their brand of compressed pills in 1878,[37] the Civil War pharmacist or hospital steward would have regarded a reference to tablets as slabs bearing inscriptions, such as those in the Bible. Pills were another matter. They were normally made by reducing the active medicinal agent to a powder, adding a binding agent, rolling the mass into a pilular consistency, carefully apportioning it into units on a measured pill tile, and rolling them out into spheres. Pills typically weighted from 0.10 to 0.30 g and contained four to five grains of vegetable powder or five to six grains of heavy metal.[38]

Powders were an intermediate step in the pill-making process. Sometimes medicines remained in powdered form, and there were specific advantages to this. As a powder, all the proximate principles of the active ingredient could be administered without a menstruum (i.e., a solvent or suspension medium). Usually wrapped in papers in a measured dose, they could be easily mixed in water or some other liquid at the time of oral administration. However, powders held particular disadvantages. They were extremely sensitive to moisture and humidity, often tasted bad, and were light-sensitive.[39] Nevertheless, a few powders had attained honored status. Dover's powder was particularly popular throughout the Civil War, and consisted of one part each of ipecac and opium mixed in eight parts of potassium sulfate. This "useful and admirable compound" was frequently prescribed in cases of rheumatism.[40] Alfred Stillé (1813-1900), professor of medicine at the University of Pennsylvania and author of the first American textbook on general pathology, recommended Dover's powder in full doses for what he called "other inflammations" such as pleurisy, pneumonia, bronchitis, enteritis, and dysentery.[41] Another traditional favorite was Seidlitz powders. This laxative, according to Parrish's instructions, was made up in two parts: (1) a mixture of bicarbonate of soda, tartrate of soda, and potassium and (2) tartaric acid.[42]

Some medicines were simply too distasteful to dispense as powders. In such cases, a number of ingenious methods had been devised—some of ancient origin—to administer the offending article. Dried herbs might be powdered but then combined with syrup or honey and made into an electuary or confection.[43] Other means for making otherwise obnoxious medicinal plants more palatable might be to candy or preserve the whole root. These dragées date from an eighth-century Arabian process.[44]

There were other solid and semisolid preparations—plasters, suppositories, ointments, resins, poultices, and so on—and these too were used singly and in combination. Perhaps most obnoxious from a modern perspective was the use of the cantharis beetle (specifically, *C. vesicatoria*) or Spanish fly. Premised on the notion that applying a second or counterirritant could relieve primary ones,[45] these bright green beetles native to central and southern Europe would be crushed and applied to the afflicted surface. In such a state these beetles produce a toxic substance known as cantharidin that becomes a powerful blistering agent upon administration.[46] Stillé reported a surprisingly wide range of external—and internal—applications for cantharides.[47] Most commonly, however, it was made into an ointment, producing "after the lapse of one or more hours," explained Stillé, "some degree of redness, a feeling of numbness in the part, and afterwards a stinging and burning pain, which is not, however, apt to be severe unless it is aggravated by the contact of external objects with the inflamed skin."[48]

When not being dosed with pills, powders, poultices, or plasters, the patient was more often than not treated with a variety of liquid preparations. Today's highly concentrated chemotherapeutic agents are more readily delivered in tablets or capsules, often in time-released form, but in the 1860s the so-called Galenical solutions were extremely popular dosage forms. Tinctures were the oldest, dating from the thirteenth century. These hydro-alcoholic solutions were most commonly used as a medium for botanical substances.[49] By the time of the Civil War, fluidextracts, which first appeared in the 1850 *USP,* had come into their own. Ideally they were made so that one part of the drug equaled one part of the fluidextract, although there were admitted departures from this basic principle.[50] The idea was to simplify the administration of drugs by making the dose equal to the active drug. Fluidextracts were regarded as especially American preparations, since they were developed and perfected by such pharmacy notables as William Procter and Edward R. Squibb.[51] Elixirs, the sweetened alcoholic preparations designed to improve or mask the unpleasant flavor of the many bitter-tasting botanicals, would largely be a postwar phenomenon that would ultimately lead to the establishment of the *National Formulary* in 1888.[52] There were a few elixirs in the 1860s, but by and large, tinctures and fluidextracts comprised the liquid dosage forms most commonly in use during the war years.

Just as drugs today have broad classifications—such as analgesics, antibiotics, antidepressants, antiseptics, diuretics, etc.—so too did the drugs of the 1860s. Stillé's magisterial work on therapeutics lists twelve broad categories: lenitives designed to "allay irritation"[53]; astringents causing contraction or constriction[54]; tonics that generally strengthen and enervate the body[55]; general stimulants that, unlike tonics, "*temporarily* . . . increase the vital activity of the whole system"[56]; cerebrospinal stimulants, which are medicines directly affecting the nervous system[57]; an odd and rarely referenced category called tetanica or spinants, which allegedly operated "exclusively upon the spinal marrow"[58]; general sedatives that reduced the activity or the power of one or more parts of the body and affected both circulatory and nervous systems[59]; arterial sedatives that acted directly on the heart or circulatory system[60]; nervous sedatives acting directly on the nervous system[61]; evacuants, the largest single category listed, which comprised any agent causing discharge (this included diuretics, expectorants, emetics, cathartics, etc.)[62]; and, finally, alteratives, an admittedly vague term that referred to any medicine tending in proper dosage to "correct all morbid qualities in the body."[63]

There was also a class of therapeutics designated as depletive. Consisting primarily of bleeding (or cupping) and various dietary manipulations, these did not directly employ medicinal substances and discussion of their application is not appropriate under consideration of pharmaceutical remedies. However, the practice of leeching was common during and well after the war as "the least painful and in many instances the most effectual means for the local abstraction of blood. They [leeches] are often applicable to parts which, either from their situation or their great tenderness when inflamed, do not admit of the use of cups."[64] The use of the leech *(Hirudo medicinalis)* for such purposes was over 2,000 years old and had become the apothecary's special responsibility; by the nineteenth century pharmaceutical advice on the care and dispensing of these invertebrate "physician's helpers" was commonplace.[65]

These categories take on added importance when it is realized that they served essentially as a pharmaceutical nosology whereby items specifically within the materia medica could be organized. Examples of lenitives included mucilaginous substances—such as gum arabic, flaxseed, and slippery elm bark—and other fatty, gelatinous, or saccharine substances. Examples of popular astringents included minerals such as alum, lead, and zinc as well as herbs like catechu, logwood, and the barks of white and black oak. Some of the irritants were chlorine water, chlorinated soda, chlorinated lime, assorted acids, and the aforementioned cantharides. Common tonics were the barks of cinchona, willow, dogwood, and wild cherry. Among tonic remedies were the appropriately named "bitters" that comprised columbo root, gentian, and yellow root (*Xanthorhiza simplicissima,* not to be confused with *Hydrastis canadensis,* which had similar properties and was a favorite of eclectic practitioners).

Stimulants presented special problems that need some explanation. Stimulants often included items surprising to the modern student: alcohol, opium, and other narcotics. Believing alcohol and narcotics to be stimulating rather than depressing, Stillé separated the obviously dulling properties of these agents from what he called their "medicinal action." Making some peculiar hairsplitting distinctions in order to accommodate his theory, Stillé asserted that the sedative properties of these substances represented a "secondary operation" to their primary stimulant effects. The intoxicating and depressant action, he insisted,

> has no relation to the medicinal action of narcotics, which is primarily stimulant in every case. It is not even proportioned to this action, for opium, which is the most powerful narcotic, is decidedly less stimulant than belladonna or stramonium, whose hypnotic virtues, on the other hand, are comparatively feeble.[66]

The mere fact that Stillé had to expend so much ink in defense of his position indicates some differences of opinion. Indeed, the noted authority on the therapeutic action of drugs, Frederick William Headland, considered alcohol only "nearly" stimulant and opium to be "intermediate between stimulants and sedatives" that first "stimulates slightly" but then "acts as a sedative to a greater extent."[67] In both cases of alcohol and opium it is interesting to note that Headland considered narcotics separate and distinct from stimulants, placing them under *narcotica inebriantia* and *narcotica somnifera,* respectively. For purposes of Civil War pharmacy, whatever the merits or demerits of these respective positions, most surgeons clearly considered alcohol a stimulant and opium and many other narcotics as stimulant anodynes.[68]

The remaining categories were a bit clearer. Digitalis, American hellebore, and lobelia were all regarded as sedative. The largest single class, evacuants, included: emetics such as ipecac and antimony; cathartics such as colocynth and mayapple; expectorants including cimicifuga and balsam of Peru; diaphoretics (causing perspiration) such as Dover's powder and sassafras root; diuretics including copaiba and juniper; and anthelmintics (i.e., vermifuges) such as santonica *(Artemisia pauciflora),* and the aptly named wormseed *(Chenopodium anthelminticum).* Finally, come those medicinal agents producing demonstrable—sometimes dramatic—physiological alterations in the human body, examples of which include arsenic, iodine, and the ever-popular mercury in its various forms.

This was pharmacy as virtually every American practitioner of the 1860s would have known it. Whether right or wrong, efficacious or downright dangerous (as it sometimes was), one point seems incontrovertible: pharmacy practice was not simplistic or haphazard. When a medicine was prescribed and compounded it was not without some basis in therapeutic theory, and making up the desired remedy took no little skill. This point has often been lost on historians, who frequently paint nonsurgical medical practice during the Civil War with a broad and bland brush. Such a facile reading of wartime therapeutics has led to the wholesale dismissal of nearly *all* the materia medica as worthless, unnecessary, or even dangerous.[69] The administration of numerous natural products proceeded on "so little knowledge regarding their use," claimed one Civil War authority recently, "that their application was often little more than wishful thinking."[70] This issue will be taken up at length in Chapter 10 in an appraisal of the Confederate materia medica. For now it should be said that the usefulness of the remedies in question were extremely variable; no sweeping generalization does the subject justice. Nor is it appropriate to mistake blind wishful thinking for rational therapeutic faith. Blind wishful thinking was the purview of the quack and charlatan, whereas rational therapeutic faith rested upon generations of theory exemplified in a nosology tied to a well-ordered-if-not-always-effective materia medica developed over generations of practice. True, this was called the age of therapeutic nihilism, and as we have seen Oliver Wendell Holmes wanted to see all the drugs thrown into the sea; but not many of Holmes's colleagues agreed, and the Massachusetts Medical Society very nearly censured him for his harsh criticism.[71] Until something better came along, the vast majority of physicians and pharmacists alike clung to the formal theories and protocols they had learned from their mentors, much of which was exemplified in their materia medica and dosage forms.

The classification and structure of the materia medica and its various dosage forms speaks to the formal framework of pharmaceutical practice. What is missing, however, is something of the color of a pharmacist's day-to-day life. Whatever else may be said of nineteenth-century pharmacy, it was arduous work. Typical was A. E. Magoffin of Bainbridge, Ohio, who recalled the laborious daily grind of his youth as an apprentice:

> One of my first duties in the drug life was the making of tinctures, syrups, etc. I can shut my eyes now and look back to the later [eighteen] fifties and see a row of half-gallon and one-gallon specie jars sitting on a shelf in our back room, and am re-

minded of the seven and fourteen day maceration periods—then straining through a cloth (no filter paper then that I call to mind). How I'd squeeze and squeeze those cloths to get out all the liquid. We knew nothing of tincture presses.

A wonderful difference has made itself evident in these fifty years [Magoffin is writing in 1907]. We saved not only six to thirteen days in manufacture, but also a large amount of loss by evaporation, as well as a lot of hard and tedious work.

Then I can recall the luscious compound cathartic pill—that good old-fashioned cure-all for everything but amputated legs. My stunt was usually 2,000 every month, sometimes oftener. My! Oh, my! How I hated that job; and while I am writing I may say I am tasting the colocynth—whew! How nasty. No sugar-coating in ours, then, thank you; just plain pill, taste included. Along in 1871 or 1872 I bought a small sugar-coater, guaranteed to coat 200 pills at a time, but it was no good.

Then I remember that old—not sachet—powder called "hicry picry" by our patrons [Hiera Picra (powders of aloes and ca-nella), a popular unofficial preparation with an extremely bitter flavor]. How's that for taste in the mouth, you old fellows? Do you recall it? I do almost as good as "fetty" [asafetida, also called "devil's dung" for its especially foul odor and taste]. I ground my own spices up till about 1874. In fact, I did so in the eighties, and guaranteed them pure.[72]

For those physicians who did their own compounding—and as we have seen this was the vast majority—all these sundry manipulations and tasks would have been very familiar.

Our overview of pharmacy in 1861 might conclude here but for one important aspect that particularly affects an understanding of its provision during the Civil War: *Southern* distinctiveness. To disregard the regional aspects that had come to surround health care rendered in a Southern context would be to miss a large part of the uniqueness of the period. By 1861 regionalism in all things—economics, politics, social mores, and even the health sciences—had come to play a significant role in defining professional and public life. No less so in pharmacy.

SOUTHERN MEDICINE AND PHARMACY

One particularly insightful Civil War historian has made a telling statement that runs as a sad, if not chilling, leitmotif throughout the bloody conflict. "As a force in human affairs," writes Michael C. C. Adams, "what is believed to be true may be more instrumental than the truth itself. Whether a view is right or wrong may be less relevant than the fact that a man acts upon it."[73] One of those views was the concept of Southern medical distinctiveness, which by the advent of open hostilities had seized the attention of the Southern medical intelligentsia. The notion that climatic and geographic factors played a major role in health and disease is ancient, but as a sense of growing Southern nationalism emerged, many medical men suggested a unique brand of practice premised on a distinctly Southern medico-geographic and racial argument.[74]

Leading physicians such as Josiah Clark Nott (1804-1873) of Alabama and Mississippi's Samuel A. Cartwright (1793-1863) argued that blacks were entirely different from whites in that they had important anatomical differences, and were afflicted with their own peculiar disease entities. Although it is true that some diseases follow racial lines—such as sickle cell anemia, which affects blacks rather than whites, or yellow fever for which blacks have comparative immunity—Nott and Cartwright took racial distinctions in medicine to absurd lengths. These polygenists claimed that the unity of creation as described in Genesis was allegorical and that, in fact, each race represented a unique species. Such notions gave the aura of "scientific" justification for the South's *Herrenvolk* democracy and lent credence to notions that blacks not only *could not* but indeed *should not* have a voice or even legal position in civic affairs.[75] Medical fire-eaters such as A. P. Merrill of Tennessee and A. F. Axson of Louisiana quickly added their names to the polygenist theory. Others thought the idea speculative at best and unbiblical—if not heretical—at worst. But almost every Southern physician agreed that geographic and climatic conditions peculiar to their region required that students planning to practice medicine along with them receive training in the South. Although the alleged medical differences between whites and blacks were built more on inherent beliefs in Caucasian superiority than on science, the argument that the South had it own unique diseases had some truth, considering the prevalence and endemic character of maladies such as malaria, yellow fever, pellagra, and hook-worm. All of this combined to form a "States' Rights Medicine," which was fairly well defined if not always scientifically coherent.[76] The impact of the combined onslaughts of vocal and vehement fire-eaters was immediate, causing an exodus of Southern sympathizers out of the New York, Boston, and Philadelphia medical schools into those below the Mason-Dixon line in the years 1859 to 1861.[77] North Carolinian William Cozart echoed this sentiment when he declared, "[A]s the northern diseases differ materially in their characters from the southern, the advantages therefore, southern students have by at-tending southern Colleges are no doubt considerable."[78]

Given all the particularism and special pleadings for a distinctly *Southern* medicine, it would be unreasonable to assume that phar-macy was singularly unaffected. In fact, as historian David L. Cowen has pointed out, Southern pharmacy *was* different from the North in at least three major respects: first, its commercial aspects; second, its regulatory environment; and third, its relationship to the South's brand of *Herrenvolk* medicine and the political fallout that issued therefrom.[79]

Commercial pharmacy dates from colonial times, and may prop-erly be said to have originated in the South. The warm climate of the Southeast suggested that certain commercial advantages might be obtained from growing economically useful plants in that region. In 1732 The Worshipful Society of Apothecaries of London sent physi-cian Sir Hans Sloane and East India Company representative Charles DuBois to the Royal colony of Georgia. The next year a "Trustees Garden" was established at Savannah that produced several varieties of medicinal plants: jalap, sarsaparilla, sassafras, and snakeroot among them.[80] Although by 1751 the venture had apparently been aban-doned, it is important to note that this was the first systematic effort of any pharmaceutical group in the American colonies to grow medici-nal crops for commercial purposes.[81]

This did not end medicinal plant activity in the South. By 1770 John Ellis produced a catalog of some fifty plants from the Orient and Tropics that he regarded as well suited for cultivation in the South.[82] The early botanical expeditions through the Southeast undertaken by scientific adventurists such as William Bartram, Mark Catesby, Johann David Schöpf, and others established the South as an important source of indigenous medicinal plants early on. Although the South would never become a significant manufacturer of mass-produced drugs, it certainly *did* became a center for crude drug products. That the South became an early and important resource for medicinal plants is demonstrated in British importation data. One of the more important indigenous American medicinal plants exported to mother England was sassafras (chiefly, *Sassafras officinale* but perhaps also white and red sassafras, *Sassafras alibidum* and *S. molle,* respectively). By 1770 England was importing 76½ tons of the plant, with a value of £2,142 (approximately £186,073 in modern currency).[83] The other American plants commonly exported to England were Southern medicinals such as ginseng *(Panax quinqefolium)* and snakeroot (most likely *Aristolochia sepentaria*).[84]

Before synthetics began to dominate the market, pharmacists still tied to the vegetable materia medica considered the South as an important resource well into the twentieth century. "In locating her laboratories in different parts of the world," acknowledged Henry C. Fuller,

> nature selected, as one of them, a vast wilderness in the mountainous region which one day was to be the southern United States. Here, in what is now southern Virginia and North Carolina, there gradually developed through the ages a wonderful flora. . . . Out of this Blue Ridge section of the Southern Appalachian System now comes 75 per cent of North America's contribution to the drug supplies of the world.[85]

The second aspect of Southern pharmacy relates to its legal and regulatory environment. Earlier it was noted that pharmacy was largely unlicensed, virtually unregulated, and considered more a trade than a profession. Although this is true as a generalization, there was some regulation prior to the Civil War, primarily in the South. Given the comparatively frontier conditions then prevalent throughout the Southeastern states, this is something of a surprise. Nevertheless, that the region was an early center of regulatory activity has been well documented by the research of David Cowen. Prior to 1861 only four states required the examination and licensing of pharmacists, all of them in the South: Louisiana, Georgia, South Carolina, and Alabama.[86] Although South Carolina repealed the penalty clause of its pharmaceutical licensing law in 1838, and evidence of enforcement in the other states seems weak, the fact that the legislatures of these states gave attention to the matter at all is worthy of note. Interestingly, Georgia required not only the licensing of botanic physicians but of botanic apothecaries as well.[87] The South was also the vanguard in legislation, passing laws concerning adulterated drugs and the sale of poisons. Louisiana enacted its drug market regulations in 1803, and Missouri, Georgia, and Alabama all followed with similar statutes in the 1830s.[88] The reasons for this early activity are unclear, but Cowen suggests that perhaps it can be traced to "some Carolinian yet unknown; who perhaps trained in France, who had friends and connections in New Orleans."[89]

The French influence among the Southern elite was particularly strong in Louisiana, and the wave of Huguenots from western and northern France who emigrated to the American colonies in the 1680s settled mostly in Charleston, South Carolina.[90] This infusion of French heritage and culture would have a direct impact on pharmacy practice in the Southern states, especially in terms of the progressive legislation that the South adopted. The reasons for this are fairly clear. French pharmacy in the nineteenth century, particularly in Paris, was well regulated, and France had long since seen the separation of the *pharmacien* from the *médecin* as distinct professionals.[91] That this would have accrued to the benefit of Southern pharmacy, as Cowen suggests, is quite likely. Eighty percent of the Civil Code of Louisiana, for example, was taken directly from the Code Napoléon.[92] In Charleston no greater example of French influence is to be seen than in medical botanist/physician Francis Peyre Porcher (1824-1895) (Figure 2.2), who would make significant contributions to the Confederate Medical Department (see Chapter 9). Although Porcher took his medical training in his native South Carolina, he was the fifth generation of proud and prosperous French Huguenot stock. Porcher was fluent in French and spent more than a year studying in Parisian hospitals, where the French clinical school was leading the way in medical progress.[93] Many of Porcher's South Carolinian colleagues undoubtedly also carried the French impress into practice, accruing to the benefit of pharmacy and medicine alike. Although it cannot be said that this influence pervaded the South, its presence was palpable enough to mark it as distinct from that of the North.

The third and final feature of pharmacy in the South was less enlightened but unmistakably present: namely, its relationship to slavery. An economic system built on the forced labor of nearly 4 million

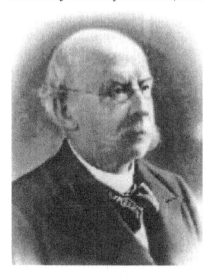

FIGURE 2.2. Francis Peyre Porcher was from one of the prominent families of Charleston, South Carolina. His *Resources of the Southern Fields and Forests* was the basis for the Confederacy's indigenous supply table, and is today considered a classic of American medical botany. Photo courtesy of the Waring Historical Library, Medical University of South Carolina.

human chattel owned by less than 400,000 slaveholders presented obvious problems.[94] One of the most telling was the paranoia it engendered among the white population. Concern over a repeat of the Denmark Vesey conspiracy that occurred in 1822 or the Nat Turner insurrection in 1831 made the South, in historian Kenneth Stampp's words, "a land troubled by a nagging dread."[95] In response to the Vesey incident the citizens of Charleston gave voice to their fears in an open petition to their legislature: "We should always act as if we had an enemy in the very bosom of the state prepared to rise upon and surprise the whites, whenever an opportunity afforded."[96] These slave uprisings, as terrifying as they might have been, could be responded to and dealt with swiftly and collectively. More disquieting were individual or subtler forms of subversion—a slave might select his white victim and violently murder him or her or, perhaps more frightening, a black house servant or servants might secretly poison the white residents. This fear of poisoning was not confined to the Deep South but, in fact, was evident wherever slavery was to be found. Even the border state of Kentucky affords examples of convictions based on little more than circumstantial evidence fueled by fear: a young slave girl was accused of lacing the meal of her master's Louisville family with arsenic; a house servant named Harriet was executed for allegedly poisoning her master's coffee; when a family became ill after breakfast suspicions were immediately directed to the slave cook; and the sudden death of an infant under a youthful slave's care resulted in her subjection to speedy "justice."[97]

Whether real or imagined, this fear was ever present, and efforts to mitigate it translated into specific pharmacy legislation dating from colonial times. Since the only difference between many a medicine and poison was the dose, the apothecary shop or doctor's office could be a veritable arsenal for a disgruntled slave. Virginia took great pains to keep its enslaved population away from the resources for revenge. As early as 1748 a provision was added to its slave act prohibiting blacks from preparing or administering medicines, except by order of their masters, on penalty of death.[98] Similar laws were passed in Georgia and South Carolina.[99] In 1753 Alexander Garden, writing from South Carolina, nervously confided to Charles Aston of Edinburgh,

> The Negroe slaves here seem to be but too well acquainted with the Vegetable poisons (whether they gain that knowledge in this province, or before they leave Africa I know not, tho I imagine the Latter) which they make use of to take away the Lives of y[r] Masters, who they think uses them ill, or indeed the life of oy[r] person, for whom they Conceive any hatred or by whom they imagine themselves injured.[100]

By the nineteenth century these disquieting admissions had turned into an open frenzy of paranoia. In Georgia an 1835 statute prohibited any "person of color," whether slave or free, from being employed in an "apothecary shop or druggist's store" where there were poisons on hand.[101] Barring blacks from professional fields—teaching, law, and the formal clergy—was premised on what seemed evident to most white Southerners: Africans, slave or free, were inferior and therefore less capable than whites. In pharmacy and medicine, however, whites tacitly conceded the skill and proficiency of their African chattel in medical botany by legally preventing them from engaging in that pursuit. By 1860 pharmacy in the South was a legally mandated white activity, giving proof to the fact that, despite the most strident fire-eaters' claims for the superiority of their Southern culture, the one thing their "peculiar institution" *did* unmistakably foster was abject fear.

SUMMARY

These were the curious contours and socioeconomic contexts of pharmacy in 1861. Pharmacy went to war as unprepared as the rest of the country. The preceding pages have established the essential conditions of the field as they existed, and they warrant the following conclusions:

- Pharmacy was considered essentially a trade and, except for a few pockets in the South, was unregulated.
- The separation of pharmacy from medicine had barely begun in 1861.
- The industrial capacity to mass-manufacture drugs was still in its infancy.
- The practical aspects of pharmacy—compounding, dosage forms, and sundry manipulations of an extensive materia medica—were complex and not as simplistic and haphazard as often assumed by modern analysts.
- The correlation of pharmacy practice to medical theory was equally complex.
- There were discernable regional differences in American pharmaceutical practice.

All of these factors will play important parts in this unfolding story. Some will explain the relative status and working conditions of individuals attempting to provide some modicum of pharmaceutical care under extremely trying conditions; others will define the larger context of drug supply and provision in the North and South; and still others will demonstrate the pivotal role that the war had in setting the stage for pharmacy in the years to come.

Chapter 3

Angels of Mercy:
Women and Civil War Pharmacy

Women's contributions to the war effort formed an appreciable link between civilian and military pharmacy care. That care, however, took place within two very different contexts. In the North, the vast majority of women who actively participated in the war effort did so under the aegis of the U.S. Sanitary Commission. In the South, attempts at establishing a coordinated relief effort took place on a regional basis but nothing comparable to that of the nationwide Sanitary Commission. This fundamental difference highlights a distinction that would characterize the provision of health care between Union and Confederate forces throughout the war. That the concerted efforts of women in augmenting the provisioning and care of soldiers made an important difference in maintaining the health of the armed forces will become clear in Chapter 4.

THE WOMEN'S ROLE:
"A CALL TO PLAIN POSITIVE DUTY"

Francis Henry Underwood (1825-1894) described his generation as "wearing all unconsciously the masks which custom had prescribed."[1] In the 1860s, those "masks" were clearly marked and rigidly fixed by race, class, and gender. The war would do much to transform the racial masks that custom had prescribed, and masks of class would change as the middle class and nouveau riche emerged out of the surge of business and industry in the postwar years. The war would also affect the conventions of gender. Women would make unprecedented contributions to the war effort, and yet the resistance of tradition-bound officials would not make their path easy. Patriarchal society, bound up in generations of primogeniture, mores, and custom, would not yield readily to the notion of women taking an active role outside the home.

Jane West (1758-1852), author of the many-editioned *Letters to a Young Lady* (among her other epistles of nineteenth-century manners and taste), described the "mask" of domesticity women were expected to wear throughout the era. Speaking for the women of her age, the ubiquitous "Mrs. West" declared that marriage was

> the most extended circle in which (generally speaking) Providence designed us to move. Nor is that circle so circumscribed as to give cause to the most active mind to complain of want of employment; the duties that it requires are of such hourly, such momentary recurrence, that the impropriety of our engaging in public concerns becomes evident, from the consequent unavoidable neglect of our immediate affairs. A man, in most situations in life, may so arrange his private business, as to be able to attend the important calls of patriotism or public spirit; but the presence of a women in her own family is always so salutary, that she is not justified in withdrawing her attention from home, except in some call of plain positive duty.[2]

The armed forces of both the North and South held to this notion and allowed women to assist the troops through the provision of extra supplies or nursing but *not* directly attached to the units they would serve—something that would not occur until the next century. During the Civil War, women's role would consist of civilian service.[3] Yet by 1861 many women did, in fact, see their active involvement in the war effort as a plain positive duty. At least 3,200 would serve as salaried nurses, and many more gave aid and relief to soldiers on a voluntary basis.[4]

Women specifically served in three capacities, each of which entailed some modicum of pharmaceutical care. The first was as *vivandiéres,* sometimes referred to as *cantiniéres. Vivandiéres* was a term derived from the Napoleonic campaigns when the French army decided to regularize the female camp followers by allowing them to sell food and drink to the troops.[5] In the American Civil War the word had lost its pecuniary aspect and instead became a vague and roman-

ticized Francophile borrowing meaning virtually any kind of feminine military support. Many *vivandiéres* were wives or daughters of
officers in Union or Confederate volunteer regiments. Although not
officially recognized by the armies of either side, the issuance of
vivandiére uniforms for volunteer regiments implies that the regular
army brass tolerated their presence. They provided much-needed
nursing care, and their ever-present flasks of spirituous "stimulants"
show that their ministrations took on at least the rudimentary form of
medicinal relief.[6] About the *vivandiéres* little more need be said.
Their existence warrants some mention, but their numbers were few
and their appearance was more of a novelty than a regular means for
enlisting feminine aid in the machinery of war.

The second and more significant capacity in which women performed service in the war was through organized effort. In the South
this was primarily through community societies and associations that
were formed at the church, city, or county level. In the North, women
contributed their energies and skills to similar organizations but most
importantly through the U.S. Sanitary Commission (see Figure 3.1).
Unlike the other relief agencies, the Sanitary Commission had a truly
national character.

The third way for women to assist in the war was through individual contributions: the setting up of relief stations near encampments;
gathering together a few interested neighbors to establish a hospital in
a donated building or even a home; wild-crafting remedies in the woods;
or growing or foraging medicinal plants in the surrounding country-
side. This was common throughout the South and by far the most
prevalent assistance rendered by the mothers, sisters, and daughters
of the Confederacy.

Both organized and individual contributions would be the two
main avenues open to women who wanted to assist in the war effort.
As will be seen, these two very different contexts of service were
founded on social expectations largely determined by geopolitical
distinctions peculiar to the North and South. Of the two, surely the
most remarkable was the Sanitary Commission. Historian Allan Nevins
has called this "the most powerful organization for lessening the horrors and reducing the losses of war which mankind had thus far produced."[7] Actually, as will be explained, *womankind* was chiefly responsible for this progressive agency.

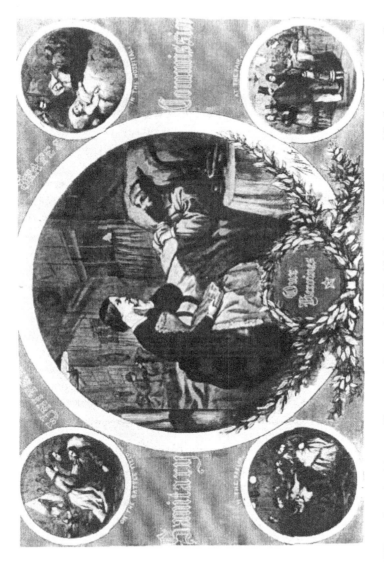

FIGURE 3.1. Despite this maudlin portrayal so typical of the Victorian period, the contributions of women through the U.S. Sanitary Commission were deeply appreciated, as showcased in this illustration from *Harper's Weekly.* Image courtesy of the National Library of Medicine, History of Medicine Division.

THE UNITED STATES SANITARY COMMISSION

Alexis de Tocqueville (1805-1859), the renowned commentator on nineteenth-century American life, noted "the extreme skill" with which the young Republic would seek "a common object" and the success this object had "in inducing [Americans] voluntarily to pursue it."[8] He further observed that Americans

> feel a natural compassion for the sufferings of one another, when they are brought together by easy and frequent intercourse, and no sensitive feelings keep them asunder, it may readily be supposed that they will lend assistance to one another whenever it is needed. When an American asks for the co-operation of his fellow citizens, it is seldom refused; and I have often seen it afforded spontaneously, and with great good will.[9]

This spirit of philanthropy and charity was epitomized in the U.S. Sanitary Commission. Immediately after President Lincoln's call for 75,000 volunteer troops, three days after the attack on Fort Sumter on April 12, 1861, women throughout the North rallied to provide assistance. That same day the women of Bridgeport, Connecticut, met to plan relief efforts, and ladies in Lowell, Massachusetts, and Cleveland, Ohio, soon followed.[10] The organization that would form the nucleus of the commission, however, was the Woman's Central Relief Association of New York, led by Louisa Lee Schuyler (1837-1926), who had already made her reputation for charity through her work with the Children's Aid Society.[11]

The association had as its primary organizer Unitarian minister Henry Bellows (1814-1882). After Bellows had a chance meeting with Dr. Elisha Harris (1824-1884), superintendent of Staten Island's quarantine hospital, the two men met with fifty prominent ladies at the New York Infirmary for Women to discuss ways of aiding the mobilized and mobilizing troops.[12] The result of that meeting was a call for all women of New York City to meet at Cooper Institute on Monday, April 29, to discuss ways in which "the nature and variety of the wants of the Army" might be gathered and how "the overflowing zeal and sympathy of the women of the nation" might find "a careful channel" in which to offer their benevolent services as nurses.[13] This call yielded a plan of organization signed by more than ninety women.[14]

A joint committee comprising Bellows, Harris, and a few select New York physicians was formed to take on the delicate task of approaching the government about the project. The suggestion for an organization composed primarily of women to assist and advise the government, especially the military, struck officials as presumptuous if not downright impertinent. But Surgeon General Thomas Lawson and Secretary of War Simon Cameron, tiring of Bellows' persistence, decided to adopt a paternalistic "there, there" attitude toward these "charming neophytes," an approach that eventually put the proposal on Lincoln's desk. The President appeared to hold a similar opinion, and after letting the recommendation sit on his desk a few days he finally gave his unenthusiastic signature on June 9, 1861, stating that this curiosity might serve as "a fifth wheel to the coach."[15] The new surgeon general, Dr. Clement A. Finley, who assumed the post with the death of Thomas Lawson on May 15, was never fond of the organization but was talked into grudging acceptance by the pleading Bellows. William Quentin Maxwell, the commission's modern-day historian, has summed up the government's attitude thus: "Neither good nor bad could come from this group. Destiny would give it a short life; at the end of its span this commission of inquiry and advice would stand in monumental mockery of well-intentioned philanthropists and silly women."[16] How wrong they were!

With Bellows as president, George Templeton Strong (1820-1875) as treasurer, and Frederick Law Olmstead (1822-1903) as secretary general, the commission would receive able administration. The commission probably would never have received an official ear if it had not been proposed and promoted by such prominent and persuasive men. They were in some ways titular heads of a charitable relief agency whose size had never before been seen on the North American continent. The *real* laborers were thousands of women all across the country whose single-minded devotion to their cause grew into an organization capable of dispersing more than $4.5 million worth of supplies, relief, and publications through the course of the conflict.[17]

The women who dealt with the Sanitary Commission on a daily basis best tell the story.[18] "The object of the Sanitary Commission," recalled Mary Livermore (1820-1905) (Figure 3.2),

> was to do what the government could not. The government undertook, of course, to provide all that was necessary for the soldier. . . . But, from the very nature of things, this was not

possible, and it failed in its purpose . . . from occasional and accidental causes.[19]

Having toured many camps in November 1861 on behalf of the commission to ascertain their needs, Livermore knew firsthand what the government could not provide.[20] Its lack of preparedness for provisioning and caring for a large standing army was painfully evident throughout the early war years.[21] The commission was under orders not to "interfere" with the regular troops. Its charge was to provide whatever may be requested and to assist in provisioning those heeding the president's call for immediate enlistments. As Katharine Prescott Wormeley (1830-1908) points out, "it [the commission] was to inquire into the *matériel* of the volunteer army, to inspect recruits, and examine the working of the system by which they were enlisted; it was to keep itself informed as to the sanitary condition of the regiments" and "on the information thus acquired it was to base such suggestions to the Medical Bureau and the War Department as should bring to bear upon the health, comfort, and morale of the army the

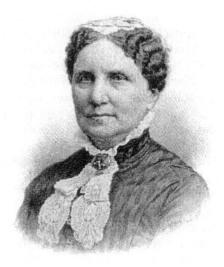

FIGURE 3.2. Mary Livermore became a central figure in the U.S. Sanitary Commission through her leadership of the Northwestern branch at Chicago. Image from her memoir, *My Story of the War* (1888), courtesy of the Reynolds Historical Library, Lister Hill Library of the Health Sciences, University of Alabama at Birmingham.

fullest teachings of sanitary science."[22] Thus, the dual duties of the commission were to supply deficiencies where needed and advise the government on improvements to camp conditions and other matters affecting the health and welfare of volunteer troops.

The commission was divided into eastern and western departments, and worked through a network of supply depots (see Figure 3.3). Livermore, who along with Jane Hoge (1811-1890) took charge of the Chicago branch of the Sanitary Commission, provides an informative glimpse into its operations:

> Whence came these hospital supplies, or the money for their purchase? They were gathered by the loyal women of the North, who organized over ten thousand "aid societies" during the war, and who never flagged in their constancy to the cause of the sick and wounded soldier. As rapidly as possible, "branches" of the United States Sanitary Commission were established in Boston, New York, Philadelphia, Cincinnati, Chicago and other cities— ten in all. Here sub-depots of sanitary stores were maintained, and into these the soldiers' aid societies poured their never-ceasing contributions. The supplies sent to these ten sub-depots were assorted, repacked, stamped with the mark of the Commission, only one kind of supplies being packed in a box, and then a list of the contents was marked on the outside. The boxes were then stored, subject to requisitions of the great central distributing depots, established in Washington and Louisville. Through these two cities, all supplies of every kind passed to the troops at the front, who were contending with the enemy.[23]

Under this distribution system it was generally acknowledged nearly all supplies got to their intended recipients with only minor cases of misdirection or pilfering.[24]

The supplies of food, clothing, housing, and numerous other amenities provided by the commission have been well documented in Charles Stillé's official report of 1866 and ninety years later in Maxwell's contemporary history of the organization. The commission's role in pharmaceutical care, however, has not received adequate attention. In fact, Maxwell dismisses its pharmaceutical activities. Explaining that the early shortages of drugs experienced by many regiments early in the war arose from internal requisition problems that were the military's responsibility and not due to any real de-

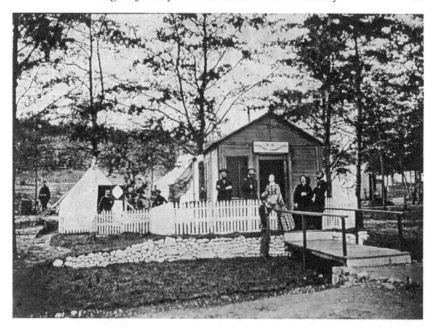

FIGURE 3.3. The central role of women in the U.S. Sanitary Commission is depicted in this photo of a U.S.S.C. depot near Brandy Station, Virginia. Image courtesy of the National Library of Medicine, History of Medicine Division.

ficiency of supply, he concludes that the commission shied away from offering to rectify that which should have been handled through the U.S. Army Medical Department. The commission

> frowned on making a temporary expedient a fixed policy. . . .
> Neither systematic nor desultory provision of needed medicines
> by the commission would solve the difficulty. Responsibilities
> would have been greater than it could meet; they would call for
> the employment of a staff of apothecaries at each depot and a
> doubling of expenditures. . . . The problem was one for the sur-
> geons to solve.[25]

This conclusion is easy to draw from a general perusal of the literature both by and about the commission. Most of the Sanitary Commission reports give scant information on drug supplies and pharmacy care, and Stillé's stodgy account says nothing in this regard.

The impression is that the commission offered only food, clothing, shelter, and general nursing care with little or no drug provision or pharmaceutical care throughout the course of the war. A more careful perusal uncovers a different story.

Postwar accounts from the women who had actually *done* the work suggests that commission nurses in the hospitals delivered drugs and pharmacy care to the sick and wounded. Katharine Wormeley, undoubtedly in the absence of a surgeon or assistant surgeon, took it upon herself to administer morphine when she felt it necessary.[26] Before eyebrows are raised at this assumption of authority, it should be noted that Wormeley was working on hospital boats on the York and Pamunkey rivers in Virginia, where men fresh from the battlefield were transported for immediate care until they could be delivered to the general hospitals. Nearly all were in need of attention, and the sheer numbers—as many as 4,000 in one week[27]—allowed no time to await the instructions of equally overworked physicians. But even in cases where surgeons and assistant surgeons were on hand and readily available, it was not unheard of for commission women serving in the hospitals to administer the medicines ordered.[28]

Of course there were physicians so opposed to women in the medical field that they refused to let them so much as apply a topical remedy. Elvira Powers, for example, was prevented from administering a mere mustard plaster by a hospital surgeon who reminded her that "the men nurses do that."[29] Powers thought the refusal came not from the request but from the manner in which she had made it. Perhaps, but her experience shows that women nurses had to deal with attending surgeons and assistant surgeons with extreme caution. Surgeon General Finley thought that the presence of women contributed to military disorder, and many physicians considered them "a useless annoyance."[30] Surgeon John H. Brinton (1832-1907), admitting no lack of enthusiasm on the part of women to assist in the war effort, called it "a craze."[31] "[T]his female nurse business was a great trial to all the men," he concluded, "and to me at Mound City [Illinois] soon became intolerable;" his solution was to replace the female nurses with nuns from Notre Dame in Indiana.[32] Brinton's comments and actions show that it was not just a matter of gender bias. Inexperienced women armed only with conviction and a sense of moral superiority could become nuisances. Others, however, became quick studies and valuable adjuncts to the health care system. The best of these nurses were unquestionably superior to many of the male caregivers. Some had to persist in their ministrations, even against "wiser" counsels from "experienced" males, as when one anonymous woman continued the administration of "nourishment and stimulants," saving a patient who had been given up for dead.[33] Patriarchal resistance and condescension aside, it may be stated with some confidence that women did provide useful pharmaceutical care with some regularity.

The precise nature of that care becomes clearer from an interesting hospital instruction manual issued by the Women's Central Association early in the war and undoubtedly used by many nurses (male and female) during the conflict. The Women's Central Association commissioned a committee of physicians in New York City to prepare a guide

> intended to supply the Nurses of the Army Hospitals explicit and intelligible directions for the *preparation* [emphasis added] of proper articles of drink and diet for the sick, and also for the preparation and application of such external remedies as may be directed by the medical attendant.[34]

This little, twenty-page booklet included instructions on the preparation of poultices made from bread and milk, brewer's yeast, powdered cinchona bark, ground slippery elm, slippery elm and flaxseed combinations, digitalis, conium, stramonium, opium, and "where the discharges are offensive, powdered charcoal or Labarraque's disinfecting fluid are useful additions to the poultice."[35] It also gave directions for the preparation of fomentations (externally applied hot cloths) steeped in solutions of hops or chamomile flowers as well as the application of leeches.[36] Some of the most complex preparations included the enemas. These comprised polypharmacy purgatives made from senna leaves, chamomile, olive oil, castor oil, powdered aloes, turpentine, and other ingredients.[37] The skill and attention of the attending nurse in the preparation and administration of these enemas was critical, since they could also include potentially dangerous substances such as opium, tincture of laudanum, and belledonna.[38]

This manual served as a linchpin between the dual functions of the commission: that of providing direct care, which these instructions were clearly designed to do, and that of advising, something this diminutive guide also does. This latter aspect also serves to underscore the important function the commission assumed in pharmaceutical therapeutics. Since camp sanitation was such an ever-present commission concern, it quite expectedly gave extensive recommendations on disinfectants, many of which were a part of the *USD*. Rather than confront physicians with presumptive advice on matters with which they should have been well familiar, the commission (recognizing that many physicians were not well familiar) appended a list of disinfectants such as sulfate of lime, quicklime, chloride, bromine, and others for "the convenience of persons who may have occasion to refresh their memory with the more practical facts relating to special disinfectants, and the best method of their application."[39] The commission had to handle the Medical Department with such kid gloves that it cautiously issued its pamphlet on the subject as "hints."

Although many Sanitary Commission reports gave advice on camp conditions and hygiene, they also recommended medicinal agents to combat many of the most severe maladies experienced in camp and field.[40] Perhaps the most important of these was Report No. 31 on *Quinine As a Prophylactic Against Malarious Diseases*.[41] By the end of 1861 the commission reported to the secretary of war that it had "issued to regimental surgeons, at their request, two hundred and twenty gallons of the solution sulphate of quinine in spirits ('quinine bitters') for the use of their men, under their own supervision."[42] Much more will be said in Chapter 7 on the use of quinine during the war, however, this example illustrates that the commission not only advised on pharmaceutical matters but also supplied drugs directly to the troops.

Commission agents charged with inspecting hospitals and camp conditions—some of which were women (Mary Livermore, Jane Hoge, Eliza Harris, and Annie Turner Wittenmyer, to name a few)—often dealt with pharmaceutical issues on the basis of camp inspections. Sometimes it was not a question of supply but of the persons responsible for prescribing and dispensing them. Although improvements in the medical staff would be instituted under the leadership of Surgeon General William A. Hammond, the administration of Finley was lackluster at best. No thought to the quality of physicians appointed to the volunteer units was given, and only a few states sought to oversee the process with any degree of effectiveness. One commission inspector, for example, found a surgeon appointed to a volunteer unit who had not been examined by a medical board. The appointee described himself as "a barber" and "an occasional cupper and leecher," and the inspector found his prescriptions "rudely written" and consisting "chiefly of tartar emetic, ipecacuanha, and epsom salts, hardly favorable to the cure of the prevailing diarrhea and dysentery."[43] Lack of medical preparedness early in the war forced the commission to sometimes cobble together a functioning hospital. At one hospital in Wheeling, soon to be *West* Virginia, the commission arranged for a "Doctor" Logan, also a "respectable druggist," to serve as post surgeon. In order to obtain competent staff, the commission paid little attention to the U.S. Army's reservations about employing women at the bedside. For example, the commission contracted with the local Sisters of Mercy "to receive and attend to the sick at $3.50 each per week."[44] Logan employed a physician to treat the patients and supplied medicines from his own drugstore stock.[45]

If staffing was problematic, so was supply. Mary Livermore complained that early in the war there was "no prompt supply of proper medicines."[46] Fortunately, Sanitary Commission inspectors were specifically charged with the duty to "discover and remedy defects" in drug supplies.[47] As in the Wheeling hospital case, the use of community resources was not uncommon elsewhere. When a hospital at Gallipolis, Ohio, found itself without the necessary medicines, the commission arranged for their purchase from an apothecary in the vicinity. In some cases drugs were proximate but unobtainable, as when one surgeon found his medicines locked up in a chest unreachable in a baggage car; the commission obtained "for him such medicines as immediate needs required."[48] The problem of supply was widespread. The New York agency of the commission, for example, found the medical purveyor's storehouse nearly empty and promptly provided him with twenty-five wagon loads of "stimulants" (i.e., whisky), undefined "medicines," thirty barrels of bandages, 3,000 bottles of wine and cordials, along with other "hospital conveniences."[49]

Further anecdotal accounts demonstrate that the U.S. Sanitary Commission did provide medicines when and where required and, furthermore, gave specific therapeutic advice when and where needed. Supplies need not and, in fact, did not come from a staff of pharmacists in the employ of the commission but rather from community sources that, under the direction of volunteer commission physicians, came from solicitations of the various relief agencies comprised of women from across the country. The alacrity with which these indefatigable women could obtain much-needed medical stores was remarkable. From the outbreak of hostilities, Rebecca Rouse (1799-1887) and her Soldiers' Aid Society of Cleveland, for example, acquired in just eight months time over 5,800 pounds of bandages, pads, and compresses along with 106 bottles of assorted stimulants.[50]

By war's end the commission could look with pride at providing essential medicines to Union forces. Details of the nature and extent of that activity commissionwide are unfortunately not available, since governing board member Dr. H. A. Warriner never completed his supply service report.[51] But by 1871 Dr. John Strong Newberry (1822-1892), secretary of the western department of the Sanitary Commission, could report that his agency alone had distributed over 100,000 bottles of whisky and other stimulants, 5,500 medicine wafers, nearly 40,000 ounces of chloroform, 2,055 pounds of disinfecting powders, 978 bottles of bitters, 775 bottles of patent medicines, 317 ounces of quinine, 137 pounds of blackberry root, 103 pounds of alum, 56 pounds of slippery elm bark, 40 pounds of gum arabic, 19 pounds of camphor, and twelve boxes of assorted medicine.[52] When this is added to the value of supplies acquired elsewhere by the commission through its thousands of aid societies, the total value of pharmaceutical supplies provided by this benevolent institution throughout the four-year conflict may be roughly estimated at $285,000 (in 1860s values).[53] Although this is nearly a tenth of the $2,114,541 in drugs manufactured at the U.S. Army Laboratory in Philadelphia,[54] it must be remembered that the commission's disbursement policy was to provide materials *where most needed,* not general replenishment of stocks. Thus, it can be said that this value—targeted as it was—may be multiplied exponentially by the exigencies it satisfied.

Women throughout the North worked with surgeons and assistant surgeons, medical purveyors, and hospital stewards in contributing to Civil War pharmacy. But their activities were not one-sided. Women of the Confederacy viewed the aid and comfort of their men with the same urgency as their Union counterparts.

WOMEN IN THE SOUTH

The provision of drugs and pharmaceutical care in the South was quite different from the North. For one thing, nothing resembled the U.S. Sanitary Commission through which Southern women could channel their energies for the benefit of the whole Confederacy.

There was a Women's Relief Society of the Confederate States headed by a Nashville organizer, Mrs. Felicia Grundy Porter, but its work never approached the comprehensiveness suggested by its ambitious-sounding title.[55] Yet women *were* involved in aiding their war for independence in other ways. Throughout the South various Ladies Auxiliary Christian Associations and Soldiers' Relief Associations were established. In Fairfield, South Carolina, the Ladies' Relief Association collected numerous medicinal agents: turpentine, slippery elm, patent medicine, chloroform, ginger root, arrowroot, wine, and gum camphor.[56]

The rosters of hospital attendants and nurses are full of notable Southern women. Fannie Beers first provided nursing care in Georgia hospitals and then took to the field when Union troops occupied the area; Susan Leigh Blackford worked in the famous Chimborazo Hospital in Richmond; Almira Fales stored medical supplies, and upon South Carolina's secession distributed over $150,000 worth of goods; Ella King Newsom Trader cared for the sick and wounded at several points in the western theater, and after the Battle of Shiloh her services were sought by several Confederate surgeons; pistol-packing Phoebe Pember was Chimborazo Hospital's administrator, the first woman to hold such a position; and Sally Tompkins headed Robertson Hospital, also in Richmond.[57]

Much of the medical care provided to confederate soldiers took place in makeshift hospitals that the women themselves established and staffed under the aegis of their own local aid societies. This work sometimes involved directing and managing soldiers who had been detailed to assist in the wards (and who likely were nonplussed as to the exact requirements of their positions). Ellen P. Bryce reminisced to a doctor in Tuscaloosa, Alabama, of her work:

> In the spring of 1864 an Ala. Regiment was encamped here. I recollect we had the 41st Ala. Reg.—much sickness among the soldiers, measles got in amongst those country fellows, then camp fever. We ladies then had a Society of which Mrs. Isabel Pratt, Dr. Pratt's Mother (he was Prof. at the University of Ala)—Mrs. Isabel Pratt was President of the Soldiers Aid Society. Mrs. Lizzie Lee . . . was Secretary. I was Treasurer. We got the Trustees of the Ala. Ins. Hosp. to lend us one wing of the building for our Hospital, and we had a kitchen in the center

building where we had our food for the sick soldiers to be
cooked . . .

It is a pity we have no record of our Hospital. We got our supplies from the Headquarters where the officers and Generals and
soldiers stayed. . . . I became a Nurse to a Ward. I was 22 years
old. I had 18 men in my Ward. I lost 5 by death—that that awful
camp fever took them off. I shall never forget my experience—
our nurses to do the necessary work, were soldiers detailed from
Camp, we had two in each Ward, beside the lady nurse & the
Surgeon & Matron.[58]

Perhaps the most famous woman nurse of the South was Kate
Cumming (1828-1909) (Figure 3.4). Although few Southern women
wrote detailed accounts of their relief work during the war, Cumming's
extensive narrative provides an intimate glimpse into the duties they

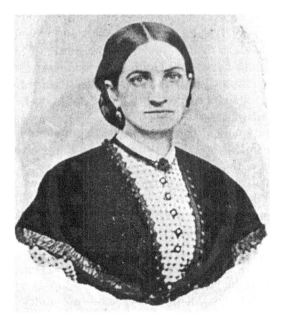

FIGURE 3.4. Kate Cumming was born in Scotland but moved at an early age to
Mobile, Alabama. Although few Southern women wrote accounts of their wartime service, Kate Cumming's *Journal of Hospital Life in the Confederate Army
of Tennessee* (1866) is a notable exception. Cumming served in hospitals in Mississippi, Tennessee, and Georgia. Image courtesy of the National Library of
Medicine, History of Medicine Division.

commonly performed.[59] In it she describes making therapeutic beverages like hot toddies (sweetened spirituous drinks normally flavored with nutmeg) and administering them to the men. While male hospital stewards and volunteer pharmacists typically performed compounding and dispensing functions, Cumming's familiarity with the culinary arts, something taught to every girl of her generation at an early age, served her well in compounding preparations. One interesting example was her experience with administering arrowroot. Arrowroot, a plant native to the West Indies, was a substance listed in the *USD* and was widely considered a nutritious, easily digested flour especially suited for the sick and particularly useful in febrile conditions affecting the stomach and bowels.[60] Its value was unquestioned; getting it down the men was another matter. Cumming wrote:

> We have a quantity of arrow-root, and I was told it was useless to prepare it, as the men would not touch it. I thought that I would try them, and now I use gallons of it daily. I make it quite thin and sometimes beat up a few eggs and stir in while hot; then season with preserves of any kind—those that are a little acid are the best—and let it stand until it becomes cold. This makes a very pleasant and nourishing drink; it is good in quite a number of diseases; will ease a cough; and is especially beneficial in cases of pneumonia. With good wine, instead of the preserves, it is also excellent; I have not had one man to refuse it, but I do not tell them of what it is made.[61]

It is likely that nearly every experienced female nurse working in the Southern hospitals had her favorite remedy.[62] Mrs. A. F. Hopkins, who had charge of caring for the Alabama regiments in Richmond, prepared a "convalescent bitters" from slippery elm, quassia, gentian, columbo root, sugar, and "good" whisky.[63]

These women sometimes did more than compound and dispense medicines; they often ordered large stocks to maintain their hospital stores. This function was deemed so important that Sally Tompkins became the first woman to ever officially serve in an American army when she obtained a captain's commission from President Jefferson Davis so that she might more easily order supplies for Robertson Hospital from the medical purveyor.[64] Mrs. Hopkins also was not shy in requesting drug supplies. She requisitioned large amounts of Jamaica ginger, ginger, fluidextract of uva ursi, laudanum, sweet nitre, blue mass (mercury), rhubarb, cloves, allspice, and green tea for her Alabama patients.[65]

As the war progressed the South increasingly felt the effects of wartime shortages brought on by the Union naval blockade. As the grip tightened and port after port closed, Confederate access to foreign resources markedly diminished and drug supplies naturally suffered. One of the most acute shortages was in the supply of opium, which normally was imported from Far Eastern and Turkish sources. In response, Surgeon General Samuel Preston Moore issued a circular on March 19, 1863, asking "the ladies of the South to interest themselves in the culture of the garden poppy [*Papaver somniferum*, from which opium is obtained]."[66] Medical purveyors were instructed to provide poppy seeds to any lady on demand, orders that were apparently filled as requests began to flow into the purveyors' depots.[67]

Surgeon General Moore tried to meet the expected shortages by encouraging reliance on medicinal plants native to the southeastern states. He formalized this plan with the commissioning of Francis Peyre Porcher's *Resources of the Southern Fields and Forests* (1863), about which more will be said later. Yet even before this, just one year into the war, orders were received in the medical purveyor's office in Richmond enlisting civilians (this would imply women mostly, since most of the men had gone off to war) in the foraging and cultivation of medicinal plants. Each purveyor was instructed to employ

> from one to three trustworthy agents to go through the country in their districts, to collect and encourage the Country people to cultivate, collect, and prepare the indigenous plants needed. A special list of such indigenous plants as may have been collected, will be forwarded monthly to this office in order that when necessary the plants may be sent to the Laboratory that preparations may be made from them.[68]

Of course this assumes a certain familiarity with medical botany among the general populace, an assumption not unfounded. It was in this manner, in fact, that a considerable amount of pharmaceutical care was delivered on a less formal, more time-honored basis. Domestic herbalists, many of them women, provided indigenous remedies. Dr. C. Kendrick, who lived in Mississippi during the war, recalled that these "sure enough doctors" took charge of treating the sick.[69] Following "the botanic practice," they gave emetics such as lobelia and boneset; purgatives such as Culver's root, mayapple, and white walnut bark; and prepared decoctions of willow, poplar, holly, sassafras, plum, locust, wild cherry, black haw, oak, snake root, and other local flora.[70] Similarly, Joseph Jacobs reported that a veritable apothecary was to be had in "every good housewife's pantry" and how "the grandmothers of those days revived the traditions of Colonial times."[71] Moreover, these women knew from oral traditions handed down to them for generations when to gather the plants. They knew, for example,

> that barks were best gathered while the sap was running, and when gathered the outer and rougher portion should be shaved off and the bark cut thinly and placed in a good position in the shade to dry; that roots ought to be gathered after the leaves are dead in the fall, or better, before the sap rises; that seeds and flowers must be gathered only when fully ripe, and put in a nice dry place, and that medicinal plants to be secured in the greatest perfection should be claimed when in bloom and carefully dried in the shade.[72]

So it may be said with some assurance that Southern women contributed to Civil War pharmacy but certainly in less formally structured, though no less important ways, than their Northern counterparts laboring through the commission. Nevertheless, there can also be no doubt that this lack of structure and organized effort had some effect on the ability of the Confederacy to supply medicines on a regular basis. Without a formal Confederatewide association capable of directing activities, there was no way for civilian contributions and services to be systematically directed and rendered when and where needed. This was a principal strength of the Sanitary Commission, and it was something wholly lacking in the South. Shortages created by the blockade exacerbated the situation for the Confederacy. Northern analysts noted this disparity and derided the "Southern ladies" who allowed their zeal to cool and "contented themselves with waving their handkerchiefs to the soldiers, instead of providing for their wants."[73] They concluded that "the gifts and sacrifices of Southern women to their army and hospitals, were not the hundredth, hardly the thousandth part of those of the women of the North to their countrymen."[74] Southerners noted this problem too. Kate Cumming berated her Confederate sisters for not flocking to the hospitals, complaining that "a lady's respectability must be at low ebb when it can be endangered by going into a hospital."[75] But this lack of public work belies the contributions of Southern women who foraged in field and meadow for the most effective remedies they knew from their mothers, grandmothers, and great-grandmothers. Nor does it take into account the assistance women provided at the request of their surgeon general to gather and forward crude drug product on to the medical purveyors. It is unfortunate for the men of the South that this activity did not take place under the supervision of a Sanitary Commission–like body devoted to that purpose, but it does not mean it did not occur at all.

The reasons why there was no comparable Confederate relief organization are rooted in demographics, social conventions, and political ideas peculiar to the South. To begin with, the South was an agrarian economy never much more than one step removed from a frontier setting.[76] This kept families relatively isolated, a condition aggravated by a slave economy that tended to make plantations, both large and small, models of insular self-sufficiency. Such social conditions tended to reinforce the cult of domesticity to which women were born. Girls were commensurately raised to conform to these expectations. When women did routinely gather—at church, at weddings, or the occasional visits of friends and relatives—this normative culture was again solidified in discussions of child rearing, household duties, husbands, and (if allowed the luxury) fashion. The slave system was even held up as a positive benefit to Southern woman. "If then, slavery is morally corrupting," asked the Reverend Robert L. Dabney of Virginia,

> Southern ladies should show the result very plainly. But what says the fact? Its testimony is one which fills the heart of every Southern man with grateful pride; that the Southern lady is proverbially eminent for all that adorns female character, for grace, for purity and refinement, for benevolence, for generous charity, for dignified kindness and forbearance to inferiors, for chivalrous courage, and for devout piety.[77]

Of course, this idealized "Southern lady" never really existed in fact.[78] More accurate was Dabney's careful prefatory remarks reminding his reader that all this elevated character was to be displayed wholly within the domestic sphere.[79] The woman's place was in the home. In such an environment it was difficult, if not impossible, for women to network and organize on a broad scale; gathering in the cause of social activism was unthinkable.[80] The Southern political culture also implicitly argued against a large-scale organized women's relief movement. For all of the fire-eaters' saber rattling in the name of "The Cause," the concept of nationalism was an inchoate ideal rather than a definite goal rooted in specific principles. Lacking distinctions in language, religion, and history, Southern nationalism was built on the "shallow foundations" of geography and economics and became a chief reason for the failure of its bid for independence.[81] In the North the call to arms become one of defense of the Union and aroused a nationalism that had slumbered (waking only occasionally over xenophobic nightmares and jingoistic manifest destiny) since the ratification of the Constitution. In contrast, the South had no similar rallying cry. "At least to the same degree to which specific states remained the focus of American loyalties after independence," writes Liah Greenfeld, "the state, rather than the Confederacy, remained the focus of Southern loyalties."[82] Thus, in the South a broad and comprehensive effort at relief simply did not accord with the allegiances of its citizens. No wonder that the well-intended Mrs. Porter's Dixie-wide Women's Relief Society never really took shape.

The political climate in the North was quite different. Women had already begun to organize in the cause of abolitionism and their own rights. By 1861 a few militant women had already come together thirteen years before at Seneca Falls, New York, to discuss and rectify their second-class status. Interestingly, this landmark convention was conceived when one of its organizers, Lucretia Mott (1793-1880), was denied a seat at an antislavery conference in London on the sole grounds of her gender. Teaming up with Elizabeth Cady Stanton (1815-1902), the meeting drew 240, forty of which were men, most notably the ex-slave and abolitionist Frederick Douglass.[83] As a result of these activities Northern women, even those not actively involved in the woman's movement, were no strangers to the idea of organizing toward some common altruistic end. Though America was still predominantly agrarian, the cities of the Northeast and Midwest were growing rapidly, more women lived in cosmopolitan areas, an environment that lent itself well to concerted, organized effort. In contrast, the unmistakable association of the woman's movement with abolitionism was sufficient to cause most Southern women (the

Grimké sisters being notable exceptions) to recoil at the very notion of venturing beyond hearth and home. Even after the war, the women of the so-called New South were, in historian George Rable's words, "unaffected by a growing feminist activism elsewhere in the country."[84] Given these two very different social milieus, the more individual and domestic contributions of women in the Confederacy are readily explained.

WOMEN AND CIVIL WAR PHARMACY: AN APPRAISAL

Any overall assessment of women's pharmacy care during the war must be prefaced by the observation that their roles in military service were ill-defined and embryonic at best. Not formally a part of the army or navy organizations, women worked in a male-dominated arena. Estimates of the female-to-male nurse ratio in the North are generally accepted to be about one to five.[85] In the South, males also predominated, although the first Confederate Congress noted that when females were in attendance at hospitals the mortality was cut in half.[86] Indeed, women often practiced their bedside pharmacy as part of their nursing duties, formally or informally assumed, and therefore both are essentially inseparable. First and foremost, the men who received their care, North and South, appreciated them. An unidentified missive signed simply "A Soldier" wrote appreciatively to Cornelia Hancock at Camp Bradford, Maryland,

> You will please excuse a Soldier for writing a few lines to you to express our thankfulness for your kindness to our poor wounded comrades after the late battle. You little know the pleasure a Soldier feels in seeing a woman at camp.[87]

Some injured and sick soldiers found themselves in women's homes, such as Absalom Robley Dyson (1832-1864), who served with the 5th Missouri Volunteers, CSA. Writing home to his wife Louisa, Dyson wrote thankfully,

> I am at a private house in this place and could not be better treated were I at home. . . . May God bless the ladies of Raymond [Mississippi] and surrounding country. I could write a

volume about the kind treatment which the wounded soldiers receive from the hands of ladies but suffice it to say that . . . many a poor fellow that is now living would have been dead, had it not been for the kindness of those fair creatures.[88]

Another young soldier wrote of the women in the hospital, "This seems like having mother about."[89]

It is interesting to note that women not infrequently provided care to whomever needed it, disregarding whether the soldier's affiliation was with the North or South.[90] But prejudice and partisanship was certainly not unknown, and the practice of placing the Union and Confederate wounded side by side tested the patience of many a woman. One nurse working in a Union hospital in North Carolina was so incensed at the prospect of treating the enemy's wounds that she had all of the Confederate wounded removed from her ward.[91] Unfortunately for the Robert Dabneys of the South who believed their women to be of a higher order and above reproach, certain ladies proved themselves to be victims of less noble traits. One hospitalized Union casualty, refusing to identify himself, wrote pleadingly to John Mulhallan Hale, quartermaster in Nashville:

> Will you allow a soldier to say a word in behalf of the sick and wounded in the over crowded hospitals of Nashville where there is a great deficiency in the sanitary stores and where there is no kind female hand to administer in the hospital to the sick and suffering.

The author of the letter complained of never having but "one or two visits from the ladies of Nashville" and those exhibited a "want of sympathy" and were "in sad contrast with the noble conduct of Union ladies in other places who have so freely brought their aid to the wounded and suffering from the Confederate ranks who have fallen into the hospitals of our own army."[92]

These incidents should not tarnish the reputation of the many women who provided all kinds of relief and assistance during the most devastating conflict in American history. Although the majority of pharmaceutical work was accomplished through medical purveyors and hospital stewards, the women's contributions should not be forgotten. It was through the U.S. Sanitary Commission that thousands of women contributed personnel and materiel that directly assisted in the effort to provide medicines and pharmaceutical care to 2,100,000 Union soldiers and sailors. Moreover, the women impressed the war effort with a truly *national* stamp, overcoming petty sectional rivalries and state jealousies. It may be said with some confidence that their pharmacy contributions were as important as the other forms of relief they provided. Never before had women been so involved in pharmaceutical affairs through the acquisition, distribution, and administration of therapeutic agents in an institutional setting.

Despite this excursion into a traditionally man's world, it was not recognized or appreciated by those most closely involved. The fact that the military could relegate their invaluable work to mere services rendered "in connection with extra diets, the linen-room and laundry" becomes a reductio ad absurdum needing no further comment.[93] Even the Sanitary Commission itself dismissed the role their women had played, stating that the female nurses "owed their usefulness" to the fact that they were "docile enough and wise enough to respect the superior knowledge and authority of the Surgeons."[94] Yet perhaps *because* pharmacy was traditionally regarded as a masculine field (although pharmacy degrees earned by women have exceeded men since 1985),[95] women's contribution in this regard went largely unnoticed. Even William Maxwell's *Lincoln's Fifth Wheel* portrays the commission as an effective, benevolent agency made so by the guidance of Henry Bellows, Elisha Harris, Frederick Law Olmstead, and other men on the governing board. While their work is not to be discounted or diminished, where are the women who formed the lifeblood of the commission? It is revealing that of the forty-two figures listed in the book's biographical notes, only two women (Schuyler and Wormeley) are mentioned.

As discussed earlier, women who provided pharmacy care for Confederate troops did so largely without the benefit of an organizational network. Theirs was one of ad hoc assistance, when and where needed. What is most fascinating is that where women *did* provide assistance with the acquisition, preparation, and dispensing of drugs they seemed, in part because of more pressing demands, to have a freer hand in their work. The commissioning of Sally Tompkins into the Confederate Army knew no corollary in Northern ranks. As the foregoing discussion has shown, women laboring in Union ranks had to constantly tiptoe around sensitive surgeons quick to take offense;

physicians were all too often making certain their domain was not intruded upon by some presumptuous female. Curiously, Southern examples are certainly there but harder to find. The reason probably stems from the very fact that these women provided their care in such nonthreatening ways, without the menacing power of institutional largesse; this may have allowed certain freedoms without impugning the viability of the prevailing social order.

The bias against women serving in medical roles was a double-edged sword that cut to the ultimate disadvantage of those needing care the most—the soldiers in camp and field. The Sanitary Commission permitted women to channel their resources and build an infrastructure of care of unprecedented proportions. Yet that very same commission was viewed warily by a patriarchal society. The women of the South were given greater relative freedom in their pharmacy care, but at the price of fewer resources and less overall direction. The men who had a stake in the nurse's ability to render care—the sick and wounded—knew best. "That little gal that used to come to us every day," declared one hospitalized soldier, "I tell you what, she's an angel if there ever is any."[96] The authorities had decided that these angels of mercy might minister to the sick and wounded, but they had best do so without carrying even the hint of equality as a concealed motive. The brief entry of women into Confederate health care proved to have few long-term effects on their status in the postwar South. As George Rable has pointed out, "Former nurses found few opportunities to apply their administrative [and therapeutic] skills outside the home and instead returned to domestic life. Although a few later became the subjects of syrupy obituaries, most died in obscurity."[97]

During the four-year shortage of available male resources, some civilian pharmacists took to hiring women as clerks; but following the war the vast majority of women receded back into their domestic roles.[98] This included the female nurse who had taken her impromptu pharmacy practicum in hospital, camp, commission depot, transport vessel, and supply car. The resumption of their prewar roles is indicated by the 1870 census, which listed only 34 women out of 17,369 traders and dealers in drugs.[99] Just as Cincinnatus returned to his plow after admirably serving his country, women of the North and South returned to their homes to once again don "the masks which custom had prescribed."

PART II:
PHARMACY IN THE UNION

Chapter 4

The Principals: Medical Purveyors and Hospital Stewards

Having examined civilian pharmacy during the Civil War, our attentions are now directed to the military aspects of providing medicines to soldiers and sailors of the largest military machine North America had ever seen. We begin with the U.S. Army. The administration of military drug supply and distribution was the responsibility of medical purveyors. Hospital stewards provided pharmacy care in hospital, camp, and field. In order to understand pharmacy in the Civil War an appreciation of the roles played by these two positions is crucial.

OFFICIAL DUTIES AND RESPONSIBILITIES OF MEDICAL PURVEYORS

There were, in fact, two positions responsible for maintaining drug supplies and distributing stores to Union troops: medical purveyors and medical storekeepers. About the former, more will be said momentarily. Medical storekeepers were skilled pharmacists who served as commissioned officers established by a law approved on May 20, 1862.[1] General Order No. 55 set forth the requirements, duties, and responsibilities of these storekeepers.[2] Successful candidates for appointment had to be between twenty-five and forty years of age, "of good moral character," and pass an examination "in the ordinary branches of a good English education, in pharmacy and materia medica, and to give proof that they possess the requisite business qualifications for the position."[3]

The experience of Robert T. Creamer gives an interesting glimpse into the operations of the Medical Department with regard to the appointment of medical storekeepers. A pharmacist in New York City, Creamer had to solicit recommendations from physicians and colleagues attesting to his fitness for duty as medical storekeeper.[4] Almost three months later he had heard nothing and inquired as to the status of his application.[5] Finally, no doubt crossing in the mails, word came of his commission two days later on August 25, 1862.[6] But Creamer's problems were not over. According to Provision 12 of Circular No. 7 outlining the storekeeper's responsibilities, each appointee was required to post a bond "in such sums as the Secretary of War may require, with security to be approved by him."[7] But with notification of his commission came no explanation as to the specifics of his duties (though he already knew generally that it was a pharmacist's post) and no explanation as to the precise nature and amount of the bond required of him.[8] Finally, in September, apparently instructions were received and his bond was sent in. By October 8 he reported to the surgeon general that he was at his post as acting medical purveyor and storekeeper.[9] The fact that it took from May to October (in a state of war) to get a man nominated, commissioned, bonded, and in the field is indicative of the bureaucratic malaise and inefficiency that plagued the military during the early years of the war. Surgeon General William A. Hammond would do much to change this, but in May, when Creamer was first nominated, Hammond had only recently been appointed and it would take some time to chisel away at the Medical Department's ossified administrative structure and reticence to change.

These kinds of delays would undoubtedly affect the practical operations of the Medical Department in providing reliable, accurate, and timely drug supplies. Medical storekeepers had considerable responsibilities. Once at their post they were charged with the responsibility of storing, guarding, issuing, and accounting for drugs and medical supplies at a salary of $124.16 per month.[10] But their numbers and powers were limited. The General Order only authorized medical storekeepers "not to exceed six in number"; despite the hyperbolic claim that they held positions "of considerable magnitude and responsibility," they held no definite rank (often given the sobriquet "captain"), were not line officers, and were considered civil appointees, thus denying them and their families of any claims to a pension.[11] They had a uniform that was largely ignored and the fact that four out of the six storekeepers were given assignments to serve as acting medical purveyors demonstrates that the position never really took hold within the structure of the U.S. Army Medical Department.[12]

Indeed it was with the purveyors that the duties of drug supply and distribution resided. Medical purveyors were drawn from the surgeon's ranks of the regular army whenever possible,[13] though, as we have seen in the case of Creamer, by 1862 that was becoming increasingly difficult. Purveyors had chief responsibility for the procurement, quality, distribution, and packing of all medicines.[14] The substances for which they were responsible were enumerated in the official standard supply table (see Appendix A). There is a temptation to view the supply table as a restrictive list of medicinal substances from which neither the purveyor nor the medical officer could veer or vary. Initially that was, in fact, the case. Surgeon General Finley insisted that no unlisted, nonstandard medicine could be issued without his personal approval.[15] But his progressive replacement, William A. Hammond, liberalized this policy and from 1863 through the duration of war, surgeons and purveyors had some discretion on what and in what amounts they ordered. Hammond had made the standard supply table exactly that—a list of standards to use as a guide for what should be kept on hand and in what quantities. "Individual preferences," the Medical Department advised, were to be "indulged at the discretion of the Medical Director or the Surgeon General."[16] However, the purveyors were instructed to adhere "strictly" to the official classification, order, and nomenclature of the table.[17] Any and all irregularities in the quality and quantities of drugs arriving into hospital, camp, and field were to be reported by the medical officers to the surgeon general. When troops were on the move, field purveyors accompanied them and requisitioned the medical supplies from the closest issuing depot.[18] Purveyors were not always on hand, however. In such cases the army permitted quartermasters to order drugs and medical supplies, but it discouraged the practice by burdening the process with red tape. Requisitions had to be issued in triplicate on two separate forms specially designed for that purpose, a requirement undoubtedly designed to reduce such requests to genuine need.[19]

Drug supplies came through the principal purveying depots or the subordinate departmental or field depots. Orders from the former were to be placed for three-month supplies only; orders from the smaller depots could be made at the medical director's discretion on an as-needed basis.[20] The problem with this arrangement was that it tended to encourage lockstep quarterly orders to the main depot, which could leave regiments with surfeits and surpluses of drug stocks, depending upon the health of the men. Prior to the war the army distributed all of its medical supplies through one depot at New York City, then linked to regional subdepots. With the outbreak of hostilities, however, a more complete network of main depots and subdepots had to be established. By the close of 1861, Philadelphia, which was the nation's leading pharmaceutical manufacturing center, was added to New York as a principal depot. From these two points medicines were distributed to the total of 30 subdepots established in: Washington, DC; St. Louis, Missouri; Cairo, Illinois; Baltimore; Hilton Head, North Carolina; Fort Monroe, Virginia; New Orleans; Memphis; Nashville; Louisville; and Chicago.[21] The effectiveness of this system will be discussed in Chapter 5; for now it can be stated that it functioned reasonably well, though not without its glitches.

This was the supply and distribution side of pharmacy; the care and dispensing side was the responsibility of the hospital steward. While the duties of the purveyor were straightforward and clearly circumscribed, those of the hospital steward were extensive and varied.

OFFICIAL DUTIES AND RESPONSIBILITIES OF HOSPITAL STEWARDS

The official duties and responsibilities of hospital stewards were set down by Joseph Janvier Woodward (1833-1884) in *The Hospital Steward's Manual*.[22] Because the hospital steward had, under the direction of the surgeon, general supervision over all aspects of the entire hospital,[23] the manual covers not only his duties but those for whom he was responsible: wardmasters, nurses, female nurses, cooks, and laundresses. Virtually everyone, except physicians, reported to the steward, who served as the hospital's chief administrator. On the instructions of the senior medical officer, all issues of order and security, light and ventilation, quality and quantity of food, cleanliness and orderliness of the wards and grounds devolved to the steward. In accordance with the breadth of his responsibilities, he was to receive "obedience from all non-commissioned officers, enlisted men, and citizen nurses in the hospital."[24] As part of the steward's regular duties, he was also supposed to make thorough inspections of the entire hospital under his charge at least twice a day and in the evening he was to "inspect the condition of the lights and fires."[25]

The number of hospital stewards was established as one steward per general hospital; but in hospitals that exceeded 150 patients more were allowed.[26] Troops in the field were permitted one steward, one cook, and one nurse per company (about one hundred men). That was the "official" allowance. In reality, there were probably no more than two to three medical care personnel per regiment (about 1,000 men).[27]

The probable reason why the number of hospital stewards never approached the number allotted was the special nature of this position. As many and as varied as the steward's duties were, his core function was to serve as pharmacist. Besides having to be between the ages of eighteen and thirty-five, "of honest and upright character" and "temperate habits," he was also to "have sufficient practical knowledge of pharmacy to enable him to take exclusive charge of the dispensary."[28] This requirement was emphasized in the manual's discussion on reading of prescriptions. In bemoaning the many ways in which different surgeons may abbreviate "the officinal names for convenience,"[29] Woodward refused to add a list of approved abbreviations since

> no person shall be enlisted a hospital steward unless he is *sufficiently skilled in pharmacy* [italics in the original] for the proper performance of his duties, it is presumed that such a list would be unnecessary here. Most of the abbreviations, moreover, at once explain themselves to anyone familiar with the officinal names of the articles, as the steward should certainly be with those on the army supply table.[30]

Responsible not only for compounding preparations on order of the surgeon or assistant surgeon, the hospital steward was also given explicit instructions on the maintenance of the dispensary. Preparations were to be kept together as to type and dosage form—arranged alphabetically within their groups—with morphine, strychnine, veratria, and the other "powerful alkaloids" secured under lock and key.[31] (Details on the precise nature and extent of the steward's pharmaceutical duties, as well as Woodward's suggestions on the performance of those activities, are provided in Appendix C.)

The steward's other primary function was to manage the medical supplies. This included the maintenance of all hospital equipment and surgical instruments, along with supervising the medicinal stores. Although the manual made it clear that requisitions for all medical supplies (especially drugs, excipients, and liquors) were to be made by the medical officer in charge, the steward was to keep an accurate and up-to-date inventory of medicines on hand and report any short- ages to the surgeon. In actual practice, however, it is most likely that the steward did most of the ordering because the manual states, "it is frequently convenient for the hospital steward to make out the requi- sitions in accordance with the foregoing form, and carry them to the surgeon for his approval and signature."[32]

Although the general question of how effective the purveyors were has been deferred to the analysis of drug supply and provision, the same question in terms of hospital stewards may be best answered here, for it will highlight the disparity between the "official" role he played and that which he actually assumed in practice. The adjutant general made hospital steward appointments in the regular army, but the military did not formally recognize the function of pharmacy dur- ing the Civil War. Caswell Mayo, who conducted interviews with many ex-stewards, indicated that the majority who attained this posi- tion were either wholly or partly lacking in the knowledge and skills of pharmacy.[33] In the many volunteer units, the chief surgeon merely assigned a man or men to the post. This permitted a great deal of dis- cretion and variation in each individual steward's particular fitness for his position. Charles Beneulyn Johnson (Figure 4.1), who joined Company E of the Illinois 130th Infantry Volunteers in August 1862 and served for three years, provides an interesting account of his ap- pointment in his memoirs:

> Our first Hospital Steward was James M. Miller, of Greenville, Ill., where he had served an apprenticeship in his father's drug store, and where he now resides [1917] and has the reputation of being the wealthiest man in his county. As Ward Master of the Regimental Hospital I served a sort of apprenticeship under Hos- pital Steward Miller, and later, when he saw fit to become a com- missioned officer in a colored regiment, I succeeded to his posi- tion. This was not because I was as well qualified for the place as I should have been, but because I was the best fitted for it of anyone who was available. I had had a little Latin, a little chemistry, a lit- tle physics, a little higher mathematics before joining the army, and very shortly after I entered I began familiarizing myself with

drugs and chemicals, and with such other duties as might fall to the lot of a hospital attaché. Indeed, I studied so hard that sometimes things became confused in my mind. . . .

We had a few medical books, among which I recall "Pareria's Materia Medica," "Mendenhall's Vade Mecum," a work on chemistry; "Parish's Pharmacy," and "Gray's Anatomy," then a new work just out.[34]

In similar fashion Jonathan Wood, of the 14th Regiment Ohio Volunteer Infantry, was clearly serving in the capacity of a hospital steward, though listed officially on the rolls as a private.[35] Wood's unit had extensive duty throughout the South, seeing action in Kentucky,

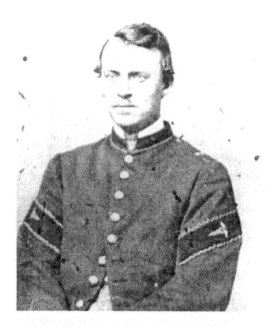

FIGURE 4.1. The hospital steward served as the military pharmacist during the Civil War in Union and Confederate armies. This photograph of Charles Beneulyn Johnson, who served with the 130th Illinois Infantry Volunteers, shows the distinctive chevrons worn by stewards. Johnson's published work *Muskets and Medicine* is one of the most detailed accounts of a hospital steward's duties and life with the U.S. Army. Photo courtesy of the Reynolds Historical Library, Lister Hill Library of the Health Sciences, University of Alabama at Birmingham.

Tennessee, Mississippi, Georgia, and North Carolina. When he was finally detailed as a hospital steward to a general hospital, he was too ill to assume the position he had unofficially served for so long and was discharged at Chattanooga with a surgeon's disability certificate.[36]

Such irregularities naturally led to some stewards who were clearly unfit for the position. Sometimes the volunteer units gave evidence of wholly incompetent stewards. George E. Cooper, medical purveyor of a depot "with supplies enough for 30,000 men," wrote plaintively to his superior:

> I have had turned over to me the debris of Medical Stores of the three months [volunteer] troops. And each a mess. Had Dr. Lawson [probably a reference to Surgeon General Thomas Lawson, who had died some four months earlier] been about & come in when I was unpacking he would have caused a hole in the ground. The medicine chests are in the finest condition of all. The stoppers have come out of many of the bottles and ipecac, quinine, tartar emetic . . . have made a most strange and curious compound. In truth none of them, save one, which has never been opened, are in condition to use again without sending them back to N. York to be re-filled.[37]

Although such slovenly goods were ultimately the responsibility of the unnamed unit surgeon, some grossly incompetent steward was probably the most directly culpable party.

Sometimes incompetence bred dishonesty. Disreputable, drunk, and ignorant contract surgeons, of which there were more than a few early in the war,[38] not infrequently permitted gross abuses of stewards through lack of interest or oversight. Such instances usually caught the vigilance of an attending nurse. A. H. Hoge, associate manager of the northwestern branch of the U.S. Sanitary Commission, noted the problems that "incompetency, unfaithfulness, and frequent change of . . . medical men" created for hospitals.[39] The matron in charge at Union Hospital found the situation so bad that the hospital steward there was openly profiteering in goods and supplies at the expense of the patients, spurring her to notify Secretary of War Stanton, who launched a full investigation leading to the imprisonment of both the steward and chief surgeon.[40] Similarly, assistant surgeon Thomas Winston protested to the hospital steward that his hospitalized men of the 149th Illinois Volunteers were being fed only "crackers, coffee, and sugar" and when presenting his complaint, "[c]ould get nothing but imputance [sic]."[41]

Of course these were exceptions to the rule. Katharine Wormeley noted that both the government boats she worked on, the *Louisiana* and the *State of Maine,* had "excellent hospital stewards."[42] Although a great many hospital stewards had been pharmacists, apprentices, or pharmacy clerks in civilian life, some became quick studies. Edwin Witherby Brown of the 81st Ohio Volunteer Infantry described himself as a "journeyman carpenter" who found himself first wardmaster and later hospital steward for the men of his unit.[43] Brown's two-volume account of his experiences during the war shows diligence and care in his concern for the sick and wounded, characteristics that sent extra responsibilities his way. Brown recalled

> The officer in charge of the camp was so overwhelmed with work that he was compelled to use everybody that he could trust to help, and so I got all sorts of jobs—acted the doctor and got into all sorts of trying positions. . . . How many, many of these poor people I cupped and mustard plastered I can never tell. I did my very best to help them.[44]

At one point he was detailed to assist with the examination of ex-slave enlistees before they were to be mustered into service. Brown took this duty particularly seriously.

> They were brought perfectly nude, three at a time, into a room for examination: So that I had an unusual chance to see and know for myself the exact condition they were in. And I want to testify here that three-fourths of them had by lash or brand been brutally treated.[45]

Spencer Bonsall, hospital steward for his 81st Pennsylvania Volunteers, also demonstrated concern for his comrades.[46] Bonsall's letters to his wife Ellen give an interesting account of his unit's activities during the Peninsular Campaign and the bloody Battle of Fredericksburg. Bonsall's descriptions are also punctuated with comments on his daily activities. With stoic diligence, he writes, "I have been busy all day getting our books, etc. all up, compounding prescriptions, making pills, powders and potions, and attending to various other matters."[47]

Not a few hospital stewards were physicians who were either waiting to take their examinations before the medical board or had taken them unsuccessfully. Once passed, these stewards could become assistant surgeons. Other likely candidates were medical students, who welcomed the opportunity for some practical experience, something their didactic medical school curricula typically failed to provide.

Besides hospital stewards there was one other group designated to provide pharmacy care. These were the variously titled "stewards, chemists, apothecaries, and purveyors" of the Marine Hospital Service, predecessor to the U.S. Public Health Service.[48] Dating from 1798, the Marine Hospital Service was the largest military health care system prior to the Civil War. In twenty-seven hospitals located at major seaports such as Boston, Baltimore, Charleston, and Staten Island as well as major inland waterways in Cincinnati, Chicago, Louisville, and Memphis, each hospital had someone assigned to administering the hospital, managing its supplies, and providing pharmacy services to its patients. These hospitals provided care for soldiers and sailors stationed along inland and coastal waterways.

RANK AND STATUS OF MEDICAL PURVEYORS AND HOSPITAL STEWARDS

The rank of a medical purveyor stemmed not from his position as purveyor but from his position as a physician within the Medical Department of the U.S. Army. Physicians' positions and ranks, established in 1847, were as follows: surgeons were commissioned as majors, signified by a gold leaf on each shoulder strap; first assistant surgeons were commissioned as first lieutenants, designated by four bars on each shoulder strap; and second assistant surgeons were commissioned as second lieutenants, shown by wearing two bars on each shoulder strap. As the war went on, the need for a cadre of regular medical inspectors became apparent, and by 1864 some sixteen had been commissioned as lieutenant colonels.[49] That said, the respective ranks of military physicians had never been formally clarified, so they were typically referred to by their position rather than rank.[50]

The hospital steward was a noncommissioned officer holding a rank equivalent to ordnance sergeant and was the immediate superior of the first sergeant of a company.[51] Hospital stewards were paid $30 per month, a sizeable increase over the private's and corporal's meager salary of $13 a month. Still, such a salary was not that great compared with what the steward might make in civilian life. Edwin Witherby Brown, the hospital steward for the 81st Ohio Volunteers, could have expected to make $38 per month as a carpenter. Skilled shoemakers could make as much as $50 per month, and even unskilled laborers could command more than the steward's salary.[52] Hospital stewards were designated by two green chevrons decorated with yellow piping and caduceus emblems worn on each sleeve. In 1862, about 400 stewards were known to be serving in general hospitals, a number that would rise steadily through the course of the war.[53]

One of the serious problems with the position of hospital steward was that it allowed for no promotion. No higher rung in the steward career ladder existed, unless one transferred out of the medical corps and into a regular line position, and that is just what some did. Caswell Mayo's postwar survey of stewards notes this preference for those "who were of an active and aspiring nature."[54] Not everyone avoided the position or saw it as a springboard to line duty. John N. Henry of the 49th New York Infantry started as a nurse, but upon receiving his appointment as hospital steward, he wrote elatedly back home to his wife, "My position is the best for me of any in the Reg. My whole duty is one of assistance to sickly, feeble & suffering men. In many respects my position is more independent than that of a line officer."[55] Despite Henry's excitement over his new post, the position remained problematic from an organizational standpoint.

The main issue, as mentioned earlier, was that the U.S. Army did not officially recognize pharmacy. Farming out the work of pharmaceutical care to whomever might seem capable, and consigning the functions of acquisition and distribution to surgeons as purveyors, left no one in the medical corps or elsewhere able to meet basic proficiencies in the things that mattered most in pharmacy—knowledge of the materia medica, medicinal chemistry, compounding, and dispensing. Although clearly some individulas performed pharmaceutical functions for the military (some quite adequately, others not), no one was specifically charged to serve as a pharmacist. This was partly a problem with the status of pharmacy itself. As we have seen, pharmacy in 1861 was only recently emerging as a distinct discipline; until well into the twentieth century, physicians would perform many of the routine and ordinary functions of pharmacy.

Yet it *did* gall members of the emerging profession that pharmacy carried so little status within the military. Toward the war's end many were calling for a professionalization of pharmacy within the U.S. military. Hospital stewards serving in the U.S. Army forwarded a petition appealing to Congress for an increase in pay and rank for their position.[56] In it they insisted: that their duties required greater skill and knowledge than those of other noncommissioned officers, such as ordnance sergeants and quartermasters; that despite their relatively low rank and pay, they were expected to pass an examination as to their qualifications (although this was *not* always administered when immediate needs demanded otherwise), something required of no other noncommissioned officer; that the army gave tacit admission "of the injustice" by the fact that requests for their resignation would be favorably considered, and regulations prohibited their reduction in rank; that clerks in the quartermaster and ordnance departments were paid "double, treble, and even quadruple" the pay of hospital stewards; that in the course of their duties stewards were "compelled to enforce obedience over two noncommissioned ranks above them, a fact contrary to the spirit of regulations"; that despite a ruling from the War Department that enlisted men were to receive extra pay when on detached duty, hospital stewards were routinely denied it; and that there was no opportunity for promotion as a steward.[57] The hospital stewards were not without their allies, most notably the Philadelphia College of Pharmacy. The college formed a special committee to investigate and recommend solutions. On March 1, 1864, the Committee on Military Affairs issued the following report:

> The Board of Trustees of the Phila[delphia] College of Pharmacy, understanding that a petition from Hospital Stewards has been referred to your honorable committee, would respectfully represent that the care of and dispensing of medical supplies for regimental and hospital purposes can be properly entrusted only to the charge of persons acquainted with medicines and believing that the efficiency of the medical department of the army would be advanced by increasing the qualifications and rank of those placed in such charge, do earnestly recommend—

1st That applications for Pharmaceutical position[s] in the army be subjected to an examination as to qualifications in knowledge of pharmacy, materia medica and chemistry.

2nd That the persons so appointed have assigned to them a rank sufficient to command respect and be eligible to promotion in the same manner as Surgeons as high as the rank of captain.

A regulation embodying the above, would, we believe, materially increase the standard of efficiency in that corps, and correct great abuse of the materials necessary to promote the sanitary condition of the soldier.

signed, Robert Bridges, chairman of the Board of Trustees[58]

Another ally came in the form of an interesting communication from a mysterious "M." (The speculation that "M" might stand for John Maisch is unconfirmed but is quite plausible given the breadth of his experience with the U.S. Army Laboratory in Philadelphia). M declared

What is needed to supply the wants of the Medical Department of the Army in this respect is a corps of thoroughly educated apothecaries—not drug clerks, whose whole knowledge consists in knowing how to "make a bundle." A thoroughly educated apothecary will know how to keep accounts, and experience will teach him how a hospital should be conducted. Constitute them as a separate corps under an apothecary-general, instead of purveyor-general, with two deputy-apothecary generals.[59]

M went on to detail the structure of an apothecary corps, noting, "The corps would prove less expensive then [sic] the present system of assigning medical officers as purveyors, who are often very much dependent on their clerks in the discharge of their duties, living, naturally enough, ignorant of the drug business."[60]

Despite the cogency of their arguments, Congress (always interested in not rocking the ever-sensitive military administrative boat) chose to do nothing. Interestingly, some forty years later Caswell Mayo used the egregiously low pay and rank of hospital stewards during the Civil War to issue a renewed call for improvement in their status through the establishment of a corps very similar to that of M's. As in the Civil War, Mayo's call went unheeded. Though the surgeon general's assistant, Major J. R. Kean, admitted the U.S. Army might find the services of a half-dozen pharmaceutical chemists useful, he objected to the establishment of an elaborate corps.[61] The title "pharmacist" over the old "hospital steward" designation was not recognized until 1902, and a pharmacy corps would not be created until World War II (by an act of Congress in 1943).[62] In the military, old habits die hard and new perspectives are often slow in coming.

Chapter 5

The Supplies: Drug Distribution and Manufacturing

Medical purveyors, storekeepers, and hospital stewards constituted the human resources of Civil War pharmacy, however, developing an efficient and reliable system of drug provision was as important as adequate personnel in effectively supplying medicines to soldiers spread out over two massive theaters of war. The problem was exacerbated by the necessity of providing care to an ever-increasing number of sailors attempting to maintain an effective blockade along more than 3,500 miles of Confederate coastline. It was an attempt to subdue and occupy 750,000 square miles. The challenges of supplying the military with medicines were considerable, since the army would grow from a tiny force of 16,000 in April 1861 to over 960,000 by April 1865. Equally daunting was the task of providing medicines for the navy, a branch that started with a mere 7,500 men and would reach 51,500 by war's end.[1] Creating a viable infrastructure of supply would require more than just men and material; it would necessitate creating an organization that would facilitate rather than frustrate the delivery of pharmacy care on an unprecedented scale.

DRUG ACQUISITION AND SUPPLY: ORGANIZATIONAL AND OPERATIONAL ASPECTS

In order to understand how drugs were provided in the U.S. Army during the war, it is helpful to know something of how the medical corps was organized to provide for the sick and wounded. It is a shocking fact that early in war, virtually no general hospitals had been established. Surgeon General Lawson had established the first general hospital in Washington, DC, in January 1861, and when war broke the Medical Department cobbled together a hodgepodge of such facilities in the nation's capital.[2] The debacle at the first Battle of Bull Run on July 21, 1861, created a public outcry. Hacks, stable boys, and assorted lowlifes hired out to transport injured men from the field either broke into liquor stores and got drunk, fled in fear, or both. The rest of the medical corps was no better. The entire army's medical care was supported by regimental hospitals that shadowed their units on the march. There was no ambulance corps, and litter-bearers were usually regimental musicians pressed into service to carry the wounded off the battlefield. These musicians knew little about and cared even less for their newly imposed duties. Medical care for Union troops early in the war was a shameful mess.

Jonathan Letterman (1824-1872), who replaced Charles S. Tripler as medical director of the Army of the Potomac in June 1862, changed all of that by reforming the medical corps at the division level. Letterman established a functional ambulance corps that answered to him directly, rather than to regimental line officers; he ordered a hospital supply wagon for each regiment, and a wagon for bulk supplies for every brigade; and he created a field hospital system for each division (see Figure 5.1). Letterman's extensive reforms in the medical supply and distribution systems, along with his reorganization of the medical personnel within them, yielded results, first at the Battle of Fredericksburg and later throughout the war.[3]

Letterman's contributions put in place a reliable three-tiered hospital system that served the Union troops during the war. Field hospitals provided the most immediate care to their units. They were to be located at or near points of engagement and were officially described as "temporary shelters for sick and wounded in the field."[4] Next came post hospitals "intended for the sick and wounded belonging to the garrison of the post, and of such prisoners as may be there confined."[5] Finally, the larger and more permanent general hospitals were "intended for the reception of sick and wounded soldiers belonging to all arms of the service, and serving in all parts of the United States."[6] These division hospitals were under the general administration of the surgeon general and his office and were "entirely independent in their internal arrangements and discipline."[7]

In terms of pharmacy care this translated into a network of regimental hospital stewards (or those designated to function as de facto stewards) either in the field and post hospitals (see Figure 5.2). When

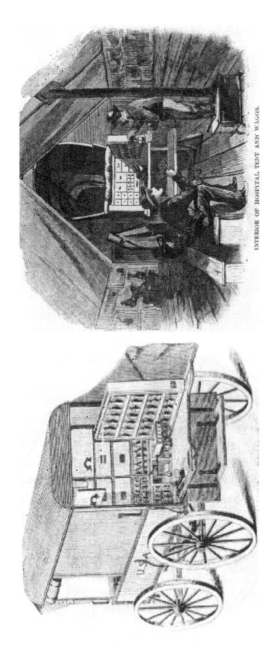

INTERIOR OF HOSPITAL TENT AND WAGON.

FIGURE 5.1. The Autenrieth wagon (left) was introduced late in the war and served as an effective portable apothecary. The "hospital tent and wagon" (right) shows a hospital steward and his assistant at work. Illustrations courtesy of the National Library of Medicine, History of Medicine Division.

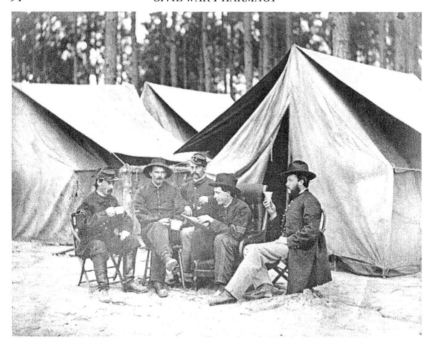

FIGURE 5.2. Hospital stewards of the 2nd Division, 9th Corps camped at Peters-
burg, Virginia. Photo courtesy of the National Library of Medicine, History of
Medicine Division.

large numbers of a particular regiment were wounded or ill and sent
to the general hospital, the steward often was assigned to general hospital duty. In any case, the medical director could detail his stewards
wherever he felt the need greatest. Although this system was a tremendous improvement over what the army had before, it was not perfect, as hospital steward Charles Beneulyn Johnson described his regimental hospital setup with the 130th Illinois Infantry Volunteers:

> In the field the Regimental Hospital Department was allowed
> two small tents for the officers, medicines, etc.; another small tent
> for the kitchen department and supplies, and a larger one for the
> sick. This last, known as the hospital tent, was about fourteen
> feet square and was capable of containing eight cots with as
> many patients.
>   In the field we almost never had sheets and white pillow
> cases, but made use of army blankets that were made of the

coarsest fiber imaginable. In warm weather the walls of the tent were raised, which made it much more pleasant for the occupants.

However, the policy that obtained was to send those who were not likely to recover quickly to the base [general] hospitals, though this was not always to the patient's best interests, for these larger hospitals were oftentimes centers of infection of one kind or another, especially of hospital gangrene [pyemia], which seldom attacked the wounded in the field.[8]

Johnson went on to describe the medicine employed in the field hospitals. During a campaign Johnson's materia medica was restricted to "standard remedies" such as opium, morphine, Dover's powder, quinine, rhubarb, Rochelle salts, Epsom salts, castor oil, sugar of lead, tannin, select tinctures, syrup of squills, whisky, assorted wines, and a few other items.[9] These were unpacked and placed on makeshift shelves of box lids; when marching orders were again received, the medicines were quickly put up in their boxes and packed with "old paper" to prevent breakage.[10] Johnson pointed out that most medicines of that day were in powdered or liquid dosage forms; the powders would be mixed with water, and in the case of quinine, Dover's powder, and tannin the resulting concoction was a bitter brew.[11]

Although the previously mentioned medicines were among the most common on hand, actually getting these drugs when and where needed was another matter. Because medicines were quite costly to supply and replace, army regulations on their care and maintenance were spelled out clearly. Each regimental surgeon was to keep a Register and Prescription Book and a careful record of "all cases excused from duty on account of sickness during the day." Each incident was to be continued until the final disposition of the case could be reported. On each entry any prescription given was to be entered into the book.[12] This not only provided a record of the health of each regiment, it also permitted the surgeon or hospital steward to review the usage of various items in the standard supply table, make an inventory of amounts on hand, and issue a requisition to the medical purveyor, who in turn filled the order from his stock or found another depot or subdepot that could provide the requested item or items.

This was the ideal or "official" protocol for obtaining medicines. Actual wartime situations, however, often dictated that surgeons and stewards go outside these regular channels to obtain desperately needed drugs. *The Army Surgeon's Manual* tacitly admitted to this fact by stating "when a private physician is required to furnish medicines, he will be allowed, besides the stipulated pay, from 25 to 50 per cent on it, to be determined by the Surgeon General."[13] Acquiring drugs from supplies other than the medical purveyor, while not the norm, was not an unheard-of occurrence. Spencer Bonsall sometimes had to get medicines—and writing paper—for his 81st Pennsylvania Volunteers where he could obtain them, even recording his diary on the letterhead stationery of John B. Hall of Fredericksburg, Virginia, "wholesaler and retail dealer of drugs, medicines, chemicals, dyes, paints, oils, window glass, perfumery, etc., etc."[14]

The reasons why a surgeon or steward might have to obtain medicines from a civilian source were many and varied. A few typical examples include breakdowns in supply, poor communications, pilferage, substandard quantity, and quality of the drugs provided. E. McClellan, assistant surgeon at Fort Monroe, Virginia, wrote frantically to the purveyor's office in Baltimore in the summer of 1864 that he needed "as soon as possible" (among other things) 100 ounces of quinine and 600 bottles of brandy, and that surgeon McCormick needed 400 bottles of castor oil, 600 pounds of sulfate of manganese, and 600 bottles of sherry "for immediate use."[15] John C. Carter writing from the purveyor's subdepot in West Virginia complained about "erasures" made by surgeon J. V. L. Blaney to his requisition, and certain "discrepancies between [the] packer's list and supplies received."[16] Similarly, an annoyed J. H. Janway noted the "discrepancies between invoices and packer's lists of medicines" that had been shipped to him.[17] Sometimes it was more than a "discrepancy"— whole orders occasionally turned up missing. The assistant surgeon for the 51st Pennsylvania Volunteers located at Weldon R. R., Virginia, reported that he never received his requisition for supplies, although he did receive invoices. He believed them to be in the hands of the quartermaster at Annapolis.[18]

A major problem was—predictably enough—with "stimulants" or alcohol. F. H. Patton, acting medical purveyor at Harpers Ferry, complained of a "discrepancy of 48 bottles of whiskey" and stated, "the frequent losses of stimulants during transportation demands investigation."[19] There was no doubt what happened to surgeon J. H. Shields' stimulants for the 1st Delaware Cavalry. He found his order "50 bottles short, one barrel having been broken in to."[20] If liquor was not missing, it was sometimes substandard, as when E. Buck wrote in disgust to the Baltimore purveyor's office that the sherry he received was in his opinion "adulterated with whiskey and water"; he called for a "board of survey for the purpose of having it inspected."[21]

Beyond these problems was the ordering system itself. It will be recalled from Chapter 4 that three-month orders to the main purveyors' depots were encouraged, with other orders placed to the subdepots as needed. This looked good on paper but frequently failed in practice. The subdepots often could not provide the needed items from their limited stocks, especially if a major battle had been fought or, more frequently, a major epidemic of dysentery, fever, or influenza had struck the region. This sent subdepot purveyors scrambling to their main suppliers and placed undue strains on a supply system already severely taxed. This led not to a situation of absolute drug shortages but rather to selective surfeits in those substances least needed at the time. Typical was hospital steward John N. Henry's complaint that he had plenty of medicines "not needed but little that is needed."[22]

As exasperating as these problems could be, they were the exceptions to a system that ran reasonably well. To assume that the purveyors could provide every medicine on demand in every instance to an army of nearly a million men without some loss, damage, theft, or quality issues would be unrealistic. None of these problems were endemic to the system, however, and when issues of quality, quantity, and delivery were raised, the army seemed to take notice and address the grievance. The fact that all the incidents mentioned above occurred in the last two years of the war should be sufficient to prove the point that certain inefficiencies could never completely be eradicated from an otherwise reasonably efficient medical supply system.

But who could supply the products in such massive quantities? As in the past, the medicines of the U.S. Army war machine were fueled at first entirely by the private sector. As battle lines were drawn and men were mobilized, the business community took notice. No less interested were those leaders of the relatively small and fledgling pharmaceutical industry.

FREE ENTERPRISE JOINS THE WAR: CIVILIAN SUPPLIERS

The mainstays of the U.S. Army's drug supplies were the manufacturers and wholesalers in the private sector, and in 1861 they were comparatively few. It was (and would remain throughout the nineteenth century), in historian Dennis Worthen's words, an eponymous industry—an industry of personalities, of strong-willed entrepreneurs who directed every aspect of their firm's operations.[23] But in the 1860s they were just emerging. The names that would ring familiar through the latter half of the nineteenth and into the twentieth centuries—Mallinckrodt, Norwich, Parke-Davis, Lilly, Searle, Upjohn—had not been born yet. Indeed many firms were embryonic, such as William R. Warner's modest apothecary on the corner of Philadelphia's Second Street and Girard Avenue that would one day become one of the industry giants as Warner-Lambert.[24]

Production values give some sense of proportion. The total value of the U.S. chemical industry output, of which drugs were included, was only $3.2 million in 1860; fifty years later that figure would rise to nearly $118 million.[25] But who represented this $3.2 million? As we have seen, by the beginning of the war Tilden and Company had an established reputation as a manufacturer of high-quality botanicals; many other pharmacists who had success running their drugstores were trying their hand at small-scale manufacturing and billing themselves as wholesalers. In Philadelphia, the nation's pharmaceutical capital, small manufacturers such as the Charles Ellis Company and Dulles, Earl, and Cope were producing a few select items for the wholesale trade. Burgin and Sons, another family firm in the City of Brotherly Love, specialized in the manufacture of bicarbonate of soda, sal soda, Rochelle salt, and Seidlitz powders.[26]

But other more familiar names were taking their first steps toward greatness.[27] A company that emerged from an eighteenth-century apothecary was Schieffelin of New York City. From 1828 to 1859, Henry M. Schieffelin (b. 1808) brought his business to prominence. In 1833 Charles M. Olcott would pair with John McKesson (1807-1893) to start their New York firm, which changed its name to McKesson and Robbins when Daniel C. Robbins replaced Olcott upon Olcott's death in 1853. In 1849, in a one-story wooden building, Charles Pfizer (1824-1906) started the Brooklyn operation that would bear his name. Alpheus Sharp (1824-1909) and Louis Dohme (b. 1837) formed their joint partnership in 1857. All of these enterprises grew to be major pharmaceutical companies in part because their businesses were appreciably stimulated by wartime demands.

One particularly interesting example came not from Philadelphia or New York but from Detroit. There, Frederick Stearns (1832-1907) arrived from Buffalo and bought out Higby's interest in Higby and Stearns, a company established in 1855. On orders filled as medical purveyor to the state volunteer troops of Michigan, Stearns built a major manufacturing concern. After the war the Frederick Stearns Company became involved in the popular patent medicines craze, an exercise that would earn Stearns expulsion from the American Pharmaceutical Association for producing a "sweet quinine" tonic made not from quinine at all but from its crude drug derivative, cinchona. Yet Stearns was neither a charlatan nor villain, for in 1872 his firm became one of the first to list the active ingredients on its products—thirty-four years before the Food and Drug Act would mandate it.[28]

Although nearly all these businesses were poised for greatness, throughout the war three laboratories outshone them all: Rosengarten and Sons, Powers and Weightman (Figure 5.3), and Squibb. Not surprising, two out of the three come from America's nineteenth-century pharmaceutical center, Philadelphia. The firm of Rosengarten and Sons had almost comic beginnings.[29] When nominal partners Charles Seitler and Carl Zeitler had a dispute in 1822—one speaking only French, the other only German—George D. Rosengarten (1801-1890), fluent in French, German, *and* English, mediated. Just two years later it was the mediator, not the disputants, who held title to the company. During the early years, Rosengarten's business was touch and go until he was joined by N. F. H. Denis, a Frenchman who had studied under the famous chemist Pierre-Jean Robiquet. Denis also knew the intricacies of processing quinine, a demonstrably effective febrifuge about which much more will be said later. The secret to George Rosengarten's success is told by his descendant Adolph G. Rosengarten Jr.:

> Now quinine is a natural substance found in the bark of the cinchona tree [native to South America]. And the genius of the business was to buy up the cinchona—Peruvian bark as they called it—at the cheapest possible price and then extract the qui-

nine, by the most efficient process, make it into sulfate and sell it. Marketing was no problem. Quinine [i.e., fever] was endemic in the South and the supply usually was less than the demand. They made a good deal of money out of the business in the 1850s. He [Denis] went back to France and lived on his capital. My great-grandfather continued.[30]

But Rosengarten would have his chief competitor in another Philadelphia firm, Powers and Weightman, which also grew out of the manufacture of quinine. Powers and Weightman actually had its birth with the firm of Farr and Kunzi, located on the north side of Arch Street.[31] John Farr was a precocious English chemist fascinated with the possibilities of improving the botanical drugs that predominated the materia medica of the nineteenth century. In 1818 he and a Swiss colleague, Abraham Kunzi, established a small drug wholesale establishment engaging in the preparation of various herbal drugs. In 1820, French chemists Pierre-Joseph Pelletier and Joseph-Bienaimé Caventou had isolated and described the plant alkaloid quinine extracted from cinchona bark, and by 1823 the firm of Farr and Kunzi was the first to manufacture quinine sulfate in the United States.[32] In December 1837 Thomas H. Powers (1812-1878) (Figure 5.4) and Farr's nephew William Weightman (1813-1904) (Figure 5.5) joined in partnership under the name John Farr and Company.[33] In 1841 the firm became Farr, Powers, and Weightman; with John Farr's death on March 1, 1847, the name was changed to simply Powers and Weightman, by which it would be known until 1905.

Much more of Rosengarten and Powers and Weightman will be said in the discussion of quinine in Chapter 7. In terms of providing pharmaceuticals to Union troops, it should be stated here that both companies contributed mightily. Nearly one year into of the war Rosengarten and Sons was marketing more than 350 different items (see Table 5.1). Known for the high quality and purity of their merchandise, both Rosengarten and Sons and Powers and Weightman had won numerous awards and special notices throughout the 1840s and 1850s from The Franklin Institute, a prestigious independent scientific association of Philadelphia.[34] Like its competitor Rosengarten, Powers and Weightman was manufacturing a wide range of medicinals and was able to report (with the exception of 1861) unprecedented profits during the war years.[35]

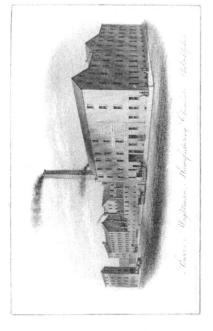

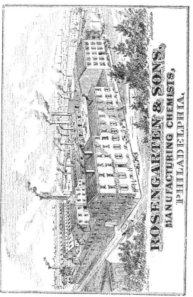

FIGURE 5.3. Rosengarten and Sons and Powers and Weightman as they appeared in the 1860s. These firms were two of the country's largest pharmaceutical manufacturers during the Civil War. Both located in Philadelphia, they established themselves with the production of quinine sulfate, one of the most important medicinal substances of the war used against malaria. George D. Rosengarten (1801-1890) established his firm in 1822. Although Farr and Kunzi—out of which Powers and Weightman grew—were the first Americans to manufacture the precious quinine sulfate in quantity in 1823 (one year before Rosengarten), Thomas Powers and William Weightman did not go into partnership until 1837. When John Farr died ten years later, the firm assumed the name by which it would be known through the remainder of the century. Eventually acquiring the Rosengarten firm, Powers and Weightman would finally be absorbed by Merck in 1927. Illustrations courtesy of Merck Archives, Merck & Co., Inc., Whitehouse Station, New Jersey.

101

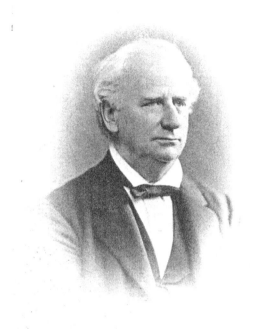

FIGURE 5.4. Thomas H. Powers, one of the founding partners of Powers and Weightman, a major pharmaceutical producer in Philadelphia. Photo courtesy of Merck Archives, Merck & Co., Inc., Whitehouse Station, New Jersey.

As prosperous as these old Philadelphia firms were, their preeminence was about to be challenged by an ambitious physician named Edward Robinson Squibb (1819-1900) (Figure 5.6). There is some irony in the fact that Squibb received his medical degree in 1845, the same year William T. G. Morton publicly demonstrated the use of ether as an anesthetic, because Squibb built his career on ether. Squibb's research set the standard for quality ether, exceeding even those set by the *U. S. Pharmacopoeia*.[36] In 1856 he gave the world a much-improved ether still apparatus capable of batch-producing ether of much purer and uniform strength.[37]

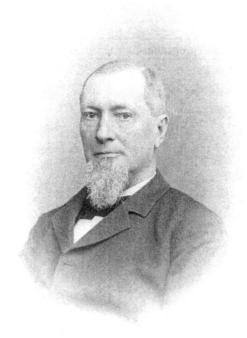

FIGURE 5.5. William Weightman of the pharmaceutical company of Powers and Weightman. Photo courtesy of Merck Archives, Merck & Co., Inc., Whitehouse Station, New Jersey.

Although from a devout Quaker family, young Squibb joined the U.S. Navy as an assistant surgeon. His decision was fortuitous, since his old mentor at the Jefferson Medical College, Franklin Bache, was director of the U.S. Naval Laboratory in New York. Squibb soon got the opportunity to work with his favorite teacher, and made the most of his innovations in ether manufacture while serving as Bache's assistant director.[38] Dissatisfied with the pay and disgruntled over the bureaucratic ineptitude that seemed to typify the prewar Medical Department, Squibb left the Brooklyn Navy Laboratory on September 1, 1857, and struck out on his own. The venture ended in tragedy, as his entire operation burned to the ground due to the careless handling of ether by a young and inexperienced assistant. It was a bitter twist of fate that saw Squibb's first laboratory burn as the result of an ether

TABLE 5.1. Rosengarten and Sons, Manufacturing Chemists Selected Items (March 1862)

Item (Prices Subject to Fluctuation)	Qty.	Price
Antimony chloride (crystals)	lb.	$2.50
Antimony chloride (solution)	lb.	.20
Antimony sulphuret, precip.	lb.	.45
Bark, bruised	lb.	1.20
Bark, Calyisaya	lb.	1.10
Bark, powdered	lb.	1.25
Bromine, chloride	oz.	.50
Bromine, pure	lb.	4.00
Chloroform	lb.	.80
Cinchonia (1 oz. Vials)	oz.	.40
Cinchonia sulphate	oz.	.40
Dover's Powder	lb.	1.35
Ether, acetic	lb.	.32
Ether, butyric	lb.	1.25
Extract of jalap	lb.	3.50
Extract of nux vomica (1 oz. Jars)	oz.	.20
Extract of opium, aqueous	lb.	13.50
Mercury, Ethiops. Mn.	–	–
[calomel]	lb.	.90
Morphine, pure alkaloid	oz.	5.50
Opium, denarcotized	lb.	10.00
Opium, powdered	lb.	8.00
Quinidine sulphate	oz.	1.25
Quinine sulphate	oz.	2.25

Source: Data from flyer in Merck Archives, Merck & Co., Inc., PWR files, R6, 2.5.2.

fire; it was, after all, his improved still apparatus that placed the distillation in sealed and comparatively safe conditions rather than the old procedure of refining the anesthetic crudely over an open fire.[39] Nevertheless, with himself severely scarred for life, Squibb nonetheless forgave his penitent helper and with the aid of some devoted friends,

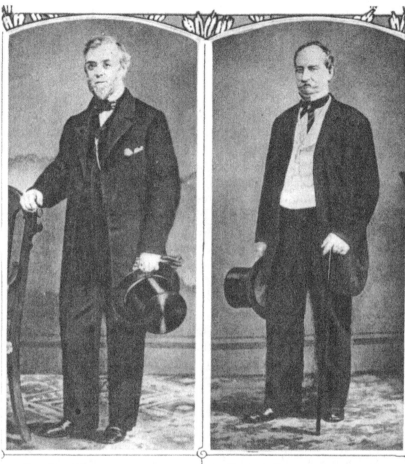

Dr. Squibb in 1864 when his efforts were devoted to supplying the needs of the Medical Department of the Armies in the field.

Surgeon-General R. F. Satterlee, U. S. A., who was chiefly responsible for Dr. Squibb's entrance into commercial life.

FIGURE 5.6. Incorrectly identified as "Surgeon-General R. F. Satterlee" in this clipping of the period, medical purveyor Richard S. Satterlee gave Edward R. Squibb encouragement and professional support in starting his civilian drug manufacturing operations after being impressed with the young physician's work as assistant director of the U.S. Naval Laboratory prior to the war. Illustration courtesy of the American Institute of the History of Pharmacy, Madison, Wisconsin.

rebuilt his laboratory at 149 Furman Street in Brooklyn in the summer of 1859. It was none too soon, for the guns of Charleston Harbor echoed across the country in April 1861. Fortunately, for both Squibb and the U.S. military, the ex-navy man had caught the eye of Richard S. Satterlee (1798-1880) (see Figure 5.6), chief purveyor for the army. Squibb's rebuilt plant was already being fed orders from Satterlee,[40] long impressed with the skill and integrity of the naval lab's former assistant director; with the advent of war the purveyor pleaded for Squibb to expand his facility. At first Squibb hesitated but with the appointment of George B. McClellan to high command, Squibb, the savvy businessman and astute political observer, was finally convinced that this would not be a three-month war.[41]

Not far from his Furman Street plant, Squibb located a lot at Vine and Doughty Streets where an adequate two-story building could be erected, and construction started in May 1862. One year later he had forty-four employees manufacturing virtually all of the standard items listed on the U.S. Army supply table, amounting to one-twelfth of all army medical stores. To give some idea of the scale of his orders, Squibb completed delivery on $40,000 worth of panniers, which were large 88-pound army-issue medicine chests designed to be carried by a pack mule; from these the surgeon's knapsacks and field companions were replenished. After this initial run Squibb anticipated orders for panniers selling at $111 each to flood in at the rate of $5,000 to $10,000 *per week*.[42]

But even this could not meet the pressing demands of the military. Satterlee asked Squibb to expand his operations even further, but this time Squibb hesitated. He did not want to get stuck with a facility too massive for postwar demands. Satterlee had tried to establish a U.S. Army lab earlier, but pressures from private industry and a reluctant Medical Department kept him from realizing this aim.[43] Hammond was a different kind of surgeon general, however, and he grew impatient with the inefficiencies of the Medical Purveying Bureau. Although Satterlee was not in favor of establishing an army lab in New York, Squibb knew that Satterlee's preference for an army lab would be revisited by the new surgeon general. To make matters more complex, surgeon Charles McCormick had recently criticized the quality of Squibb's opium.[44] McCormick's opinion—right or wrong—would carry some weight in Hammond's office. The brash surgeon had shortly before returned from New Orleans, where General Benjamin

F. Butler had called him "the most competent medical director in the matter of yellow fever . . . in the country."[45] Squibb became nervous. Writing to Hammond on February 2, 1863, Squibb made a suggestion: "In order to arrive at a good basis for your final decision I would suggest that one or more sound and judicious medical officers [implying *not* McCormick] be ordered for a month or more, to inspect closely the entire operations of my laboratory."[46]

Hammond took him up on the offer, and detailed assistant surgeon Joseph Howland Bill to report on the Squibb plant. Bill's preliminary report gives an interesting glimpse into the operations of one of the army's chief private drug manufacturers.[47] After describing the physical plant, Bill outlined the functions on each floor. The basement contained an engine and boiler in separated enclosures to reduce the risk of fire and/or explosion to the rest of the building. The first floor held glassware, storage for crude drug materials (roots, barks, and desiccated aerial portions), a delivery room, a room that was under construction for preparing fluidextracts, and a repair shop. The second floor included a metal shop where tins could be prepared for finished goods; a restroom "for the girls;" the pill making, bandage rolling, and labeling operations; a packing room; storeroom; and watchman's room. The third floor held three drying rooms, a bottling area, a laboratory for experiments, a study and library, and a bulk storage area. The top floor had more space for experiments, a compounding room for pharmacopoeial composites, a chemical room with evaporating vats convertible into stills, and other assorted apparatus. The analytical laboratories, styled a "Department of Investigation and Study," examined incoming crude drug product for quality and adulteration, a serious concern at the time. Squibb and his chief assistant John Maisch managed this essential activity. One of the most important departments was designated for "applied chemistry and pharmacy." Employing six workers, this unit made, by Bill's estimate, calomel, adhesive plaster, magnesia wine, and quinine sulfate sufficient to supply 100,000 men in the field. In addition some of the other items processed by this department included arsenic, phosphoric acid, sulfuric acid, alum, ammonia, aromatic spirits of ammonia, tartar emetic (antimony), Fowler's solution, subnitrate of bismuth, chloroform, collodion, sulfate of copper, Monsell's salt, acetate and chlorate of potash, acetate of lead, and extracts of belladonna and colocynth. Ether, because of its volatility, was made in the basement. Overall,

Bill was quite impressed with Squibb's plant and personnel and even suggested to Hammond—a point Squibb was undoubtedly keen that he emphasize—that the facility was operating at only one-fifth to one-sixth of capacity.

Although Hammond must have been pleased to know that the government's contracts were in good hands, it was not sufficient for the military's purpose and on January 12, 1863, Hammond ordered Andrew K. Smith, medical director of transportation in Philadelphia, on a mission to establish a laboratory to help fill the army's needs.[48] Squibb did not think much of the plan, especially of McCormick's efforts to establish a similar lab at Astoria; Squibb thought McCormick was "a great quack."[49] But when the talented and resourceful John Maisch (1831-1893) (Figure 5.7) agreed to head up the U.S. Army

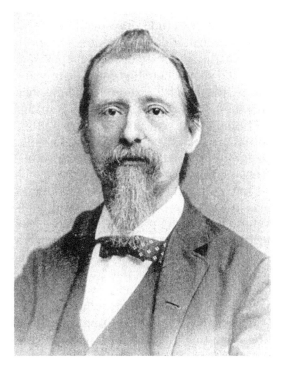

FIGURE 5.7. Serving as chief chemist at the U.S. Army Laboratory in Philadelphia, John M. Maisch managed with skill and ingenuity the first large-scale, government-operated pharmaceutical manufacturing facility. Photo courtesy of the Reynolds Historical Library, Lister Hill Library of the Health Sciences, University of Alabama at Birmingham.

Laboratory at Philadelphia, the project was set for success. The selection of Maisch was an excellent one since he had been, as Dr. Bill already noted, employed as Squibb's chief assistant and had firsthand knowledge of large-scale manufacturing processes for government medicines.[50]

THE LABORATORIES

As one would expect, the notion of a large U.S. Army laboratory was not greeted with universal praise or enthusiasm. The idea of a government drug manufacturing enterprise would have been feared not only by Squibb but also by every other private pharmaceutical business covetous of lucrative army contracts. Besides, government exercises of this type ran counter to the laissez-faire economic system vehemently defended by entrepreneurs and touted loudly by politicians. Fearing resistance from Secretary of War Stanton, Hammond decided not to request formal approval but merely decided to attach his Philadelphia and Astoria labs to their local purveying departments. This was probably wise. When William Procter, professor of pharmacy at the Philadelphia College of Pharmacy (PCP) and editor of its journal, announced Hammond's plans for government labs, he was a bit equivocal.

> Should the war continue, this arrangement may be conducive to economy, if its management falls into able and conscientious hands; yet it may well be doubted whether the result will prove its wisdom as to economy in expenditure. If the same liberal course is pursued that formerly appertained to the Naval Laboratory, these establishments may have a useful influence in controlling the quality of drugs by exposing imposition, whether the result of ignorance or rascality.[51]

"Able and conscientious hands"—that would be the key to success, and it was proving somewhat problematic. This was demonstrated at the small factory established by army storekeeper Robert T. Creamer, the selfsame who had such difficulty getting his appointment. Stationed at the St. Louis purveying depot, Creamer suggested to Hammond that he try some limited manufacturing of necessary medicines. Hammond agreed, thinking that the effort might save

money. Between March and July of 1863 Creamer was producing comparatively small amounts of quinine sulfate, syrup of squills, catechu, and camphor.[52] The attempt might have been a good prototype for the much bigger operations back East, but Creamer's quality control was poor and complaints over his products forced Hammond to order his shop closed, his books liquidated, and all further acquisitions to come strictly through the purveying depot.

Back in Philadelphia, Smith went at his work earnestly and with almost cavalier boldness. Finding a suitable building owned by Powers and Weightman, Smith assured Hammond that if either Powers or Weightman objected he would tell them that it would matter little if they rented the structure to the army or not, since the laboratory was going to be established somewhere, with or without their building.[53] They *did* agree and signed a lease agreement for ten years at $208 per month; after adding another building nearby, Smith had the facility fitted out and ready to deliver finished goods by March 1863.[54]

As mentioned previously, Smith chose John M. Maisch to head the Philadelphia laboratory. Maisch could not have been more different from Creamer. This young German pharmacist held the professorship of materia medica at the PCP, and had an exacting mind with a penchant for detail. Described as "of tall and commanding appearance," Maisch impressed virtually everyone who met him.[55] It was no wonder that Procter's announcement of the laboratory experiment included a delighted mention of the fact that the Philadelphia post would be filled by "our friend Prof. Maisch."[56] Procter was easily won over. Within a few months of its opening, the editor and voice for American pharmacy noted that "great economy has attended the experiments, and all has been done well."[57] Procter warned that it would take time for a final verdict but observed, "there can be but little doubt of the expediency of the measure, and under the care of such earnest workers as A. K. Smith and Prof. Maisch it will receive a fair trial."[58]

Smith was ecstatic over Maisch's work at the lab, and by every indication there was mutual admiration. Working as a team—with Smith as administrator handling the politics and dealing with the military brass, and Maisch as the de facto chief of operations monitoring production and all aspects of quality control—the lab was a success. Indeed, Maisch's lab served as a training ground for some of the nation's most able pharmaceutical chemists. One, C. Lewis Diehl

(1840-1917), would himself rise to prominence in the postwar years, becoming a prominent Louisville druggist and a leading figure within the American Pharmaceutical Association.[59] Diehl had been injured at the Battle of Stones River while serving with the 15th Pennsylvania Cavalry, and found another way to serve his country by becoming Maisch's assistant at his Philadelphia lab. Years later Diehl described his experience working in the facility. As with Dr. Bill's report on the Squibb plant, Diehl's description offers a valuable and close-up tour of the army lab operations:

> More than forty years have elapsed since I entered upon my duties in the United States Army Laboratory at the N. E. corner Sixth and Oxford Streets, Philadelphia (during April, 1863), and I depend altogether on memory, with the slender reminder of several photographic interiors, for what I am about to say. The grounds on which the laboratory was situated occupied a parallelogram of, I should say, about 150 to 175 feet. The main building, three stories high, with a well-lighted basement throughout, faced west on Sixth Street, flush with a pavement, about 100 feet long and adjoining a one-story building on Oxford Street, facing south, about 60 or possibly 75 feet long, and perhaps 60 feet in depth, while on Sixth Street, or the main front, it was separated by a gateway from another one-storied structure, extending eastward about 85 to 100 feet and constituting the northern boundary of the grounds. The remaining portion of the northern and southern boundaries were enclosed by a wooden fence, as was also the rear, or eastern boundary, when the laboratory was first opened, but in time was occupied by a frame structure, running the entire length, and used for washing and storage of bottles, the carpenter-shop and other similar purposes. The only entrance into the laboratory from the street was an ordinary doorway, immediately adjacent to the gateway mentioned, which was for the exclusive use of teams. The doorway opened into a short, rather narrow passage, to the left of which was a small office, and immediately adjoining this the office of the Superintendent Surgeon A. K. Smith, and of the Chief Chemist, Professor Maisch, who, however, used it chiefly as an experimental laboratory. Through the short passage mentioned, leading into the packing room, the employees had to pass on their way to and from work, and consequently under surveil-

lance from the office—those employed on the upper floor of the
main building reaching their stations by a single (and only)
stairway along the east wall of the packing rooms—the latter
occupying about one-half the space of the first floor, minus the
space occupied by the offices and hallway. The remaining half
of the first floor—composing the southwest corner of the main
building—was the mill room, where the drugs used were
ground and pulverized for further treatment or disposition; this
important department being provided with numerous mills,
sieves, etc., of suitable variety, size and construction to meet the
requirement of the time. Immediately adjacent to this mill room,
in the one-story structure on the Oxford Street (south) side of
the building complex, was the laboratory for operations requiring the application of steam, the entire structure being occupied
by this, with the exception of a space in the northeast corner in
which the engine and boilers supplying the necessary steam
were enclosed—a space over the boilers being so constructed as
to form a drying room, which was conveniently reached by a
door from the mill room.[60]

Diehl himself worked in the furnace room, a one-floor building on
the northern end of the grounds. There he prepared mercuric substances, including corrosive sublimate (mercuric chloride); silver nitrate; heavy oil of wine (ethereal oil); solution of chlorinated soda
(Labarraque's solution); potassium carbonate; potassium acetate; citrate of iron and quinine, "of which immense quantities were in constant requisition; various ferric (iron) solutions; syrup of squills; and
a few other items." He concluded with the following summary:

> In the foregoing I have about outlined the work in which I
> was directly concerned. In order to round up, however, it may be
> of interest to mention that the entire second and third floors of
> the main building were occupied almost exclusively for bot-
> tling, labeling and wrapping the medicaments manufactured in
> the different departments; in the manufacture of roller ban-
> dages, the spreading of isinglass plaster, the rolling out of pills,
> and like operations, by a force of probably 150 women and girls,
> under the superintendence of Miss Maggie Davis. From here
> they were turned into the packing rooms, where they were
> boxed, transferred to the warehouse—a large building situated

on the northeast corner of Sixth and Master Streets—from whence they were delivered on the requisition of the Medical Purveyor. The spacious upper floors of this warehouse, extending through to Marshall Street, were used in the manufacture of sheets, pillow slips, and other similar hospital requisites, in which several hundred women and girls were engaged constantly to the end of the war.[61]

The Astoria lab was not nearly so successful. Charles McCormick dawdled while Maisch produced. By May 1863, while the Philadelphia lab was beginning production, the Astoria lab had yet to produce anything. It was not for lack of expenditures; McCormick had spent nearly $10,000 for apparatus, over $1,500 in wages, $5,000 for fixtures, and additional sums for miscellaneous expenses for a total of $17,601.51.[62] Squibb's accusation that the Astoria director was a "quack" turned out to be an apt word for McCormick. When Hammond discovered that his Astoria chief had previously been engaged in selling "Magic Waverly pills," he had had enough and dismissed him on May 25.[63] He was replaced by assistant surgeon Bill, who had earlier visited and reported on Squibb's facilities. But Bill was plagued by lack of support and interest, chiefly from Satterlee, who may have been trying to protect the business interests his old friend Squibb operating in the same city. The Astoria lab would not be fully operational until February 1864, and its production was short-lived when, just a year later, it was destroyed in a fire emanating from an improperly constructed drying room.[64] By 1865 Hammond was gone, replaced by Joseph K. Barnes, and there was little interest in restarting the plant. Even at its demise, the extent of its production capabilities was small. Squibb easily picked up the Astoria orders for twenty-seven cases of powdered opium, thirty-two ceroons (a bale covered in hide) of ipecac, eighteen ceroons of calisaya bark, and 280 bags of cubebs.

Not so with the Philadelphia lab. From its start in March 1863 through September 1865, Maisch produced 160 different items at a cost of $1,422,525.78.[65] Maisch concluded his report on the laboratory thus:

Notwithstanding the opposition to the Government Laboratories and the denunciations which this one had to encounter from private parties and Government officials, it has worked its way through the dark times of civil war, and has a record to show of which it need not be ashamed.[66]

Maisch claimed he had saved the government $766,019.32.[67] Perhaps, but George Winston Smith, historian of the Civil War laboratories, casts doubt on this optimistic figure. His reasons are fourfold: (1) the valuation of goods produced reflected wartime highs and did not reflect the lower postwar market values; (2) the apparatus was run at capacity, causing a more rapid depreciation of the lab's durable property; (3) the valuation of the apparatus was probably high, since Powers and Weightman purchased nearly $22,000 of equipment for a mere $4,000; and (4) many of the lab's costs were expensed out to other government departments, much of it charged to the quartermaster.[68]

Smith is probably right, but that should not be the final verdict. The government laboratories, especially the one managed by Maisch in Philadelphia, had important implications for future pharmaceutical developments in the United States. Far from impeding growth in the private sector, the U.S. government's first effort at pharmaceutical manufacturing actually stimulated entrepreneurial activity after the war. This was borne out in William A. Brewer's postwar report on the drug market to his colleagues in the American Pharmaceutical Association.[69] The New York market could boast a healthy retail trade "and the character of the dispensing establishments," Brewer noted, "has been steadily rising."[70] Likewise, the Philadelphia market witnessed a good supply of drugs with prices "well maintained."[71] Brewer did not have exact figures for Philadelphia drug production, but he confidently stated, "the amount is very large, and the quality good."[72]

All things considered, a fair assessment of the government experiment in pharmaceutical manufacturing is that it adequately supplemented private industry by providing medicines that were in inordinately high demand. Fears that government labs would destroy private initiative and investment in the drug industry proved unfounded. Indeed men such as Diehl and others who had, in effect, cut their pharmaceutical teeth under the watchful eye of the meticulous Professor Maisch, especially the hospital stewards detailed to assist with operations there, formed an important postwar cadre ready to carry mass manufacturing processes and standards into the twentieth century.

Chapter 6

The Medicines:
A Military Materia Medica
and Therapeutics

Thus far the organizational structure and manufacturing of medicines for the U.S. military has been discussed, but little has been said about the medicines themselves. What exactly were these mysterious pills, potions, and powders that the manufacturers labored to put out and for what purposes were the purveyors providing them? In short, much has been said about the medicinal supplies and manufacturing operations but nothing of the medicines themselves. This chapter examines the materia medica of the Union. What were the men taking and why?

THE AILMENTS

Before the materia medica and therapeutics can be understood, the diseases affecting the men in camp and field need to be briefly examined. Although every possible malady recorded during the war cannot be covered in detail, it will be recalled from previous discussion, that diarrhea and dysentery, various fevers, respiratory ailments, and digestive disorders were the chief maladies affecting both Union and Confederate troops. For Union forces alone, the numbers were high: 711 per 1,000 for diarrhea/dysentery; 584 per 1,000 for various camp fevers (the vast majority diagnosed as malarial, at 522 per 1,000); 261 per 1,000 suffered from respiratory ailments (mostly acute bronchitis); and 252 per 1,000 reported digestive complaints. Each of these will be addressed, but it is important to emphasize that disease was a serious and ever-present problem for the medical corps of both sides.[1]

Historian Paul Steiner has argued convincingly that disease played significant roles in major campaigns. First, General Robert E. Lee's failure to reclaim western Virginia in 1861 was due to his troop's debilitating bouts of diarrhea and dysentery, typhoid fever, and pneumonia. Lee wrote home to his wife during this "sickly period"[2] in August 1861, complaining that "soldiers everywhere are sick."[3] Next came the Union's initial campaign in late 1861 and early 1862 along the South Carolina coast, where attempts to seize Charleston and sever the railroad between that city and Savannah were stopped by devastating epidemics, principally yellow fever.[4] About the same time yet another operation, this time in eastern Kentucky, was severely hampered by enteric disorders, and in July and August the Union was robbed of manpower by dysentery, typhoid, and malaria.[5] The Peninsular Campaign was also affected by disease. Despite official claims from the inept Medical Director Charles Tripler that there were no epidemic diseases spreading through the Army of the Potomac, 48,912 cases of diarrhea and dysentery were hard to ignore.[6] Army of the Potomac Commander George B. McClellan was not a leader of action and resolve, but Lincoln's complaint that his general had a bad case of the "slows" was ironically true, in part, because so many of his men had worse cases of "the trots." The first siege of Vicksburg, lasting from May through July 1862, failed largely for two reasons: first, a serious attack of malaria; second, a serious shortage of quinine.[7] Even late in the war, Union troops were decimated by disease in Arkansas from 1863 to 1865. Here debility stemmed again from malaria, statistics showing that 1,287 cases occurred per 1,000 men.[8] In other words, on average every Union soldier in Arkansas could expect an attack of malaria once a year, sometimes twice.[9]

Disease consistently ran nearly twice the mean troop strength throughout the war (see Figure 6.1). So the average soldier could expect to become ill—at least ill enough to report it—about twice a year. The image of surgeons lopping off arms and legs as quickly as possible with the appendages falling into bloody heaps may have lodged itself securely within the popular imagination, but it bears little resemblance to what most Civil War surgeons faced on a daily basis. These men were not cutting half as much as they were prescribing. Moreover, it could be argued that the effectiveness of the U.S. Medical Department in combating disease was at least as important

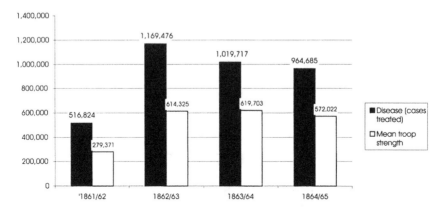

FIGURE 6.1. Union Army mean troop strength and incidents of disease (cases reported). Figures taken from *The Medical and Surgical History of the War of the Rebellion*, Part 1, Volume 1, *Medical Volume* (Washington, DC: GPO, 1875), pp. 147, 297, 453, 605. Incidents of disease were even higher among Confederate troops (see Table XIV in *Med. Surg. Hist.*, Part 3, Volume 1, *Med. Vol.*, p. 32).

as combat in the field and, in fact, more important to the Union side than the Confederate. Although disease was a great leveler to both sides, the nature of the war itself should be kept in mind. It has been pointed out by historians and military strategists that the South could win by simply doing nothing.[10] By waging a defensive war of attrition the South could gain its independence by simple passive obstinacy, testing the adversary's resolve to the point of victory. The North, on the other hand, would have to fight an aggressive war, win decisively, and occupy 750,000 square miles of territory. To be sick and avoid defeat is much easier than it is to be sick and win victories; strange as it may seem, at least early in the war, disease was the South's great ally. With the exception of Lee's loss of West Virginia, most other major campaigns in which disease figured prominently worked to the detriment of Union actions.

All of this underscores the importance of the materia medica in the healing art of the military surgeon and compounding hospital steward. Statistics may give some sense of proportions in the Civil War medical armamentarium. In the course of the war, the Medical Purveying Bureau issued 775,000 ounces of ipecac (an expectorant, diaphoretic [causing sweating], and emetic thought to be beneficial in stomach ailments); more than 1 million ounces of quinine sulfate and its crude drug derivative cinchona (used for fevers); and some 2.3 million ounces of opiates (anodynes and antidiarrheals) among other items on the standard supply table. Even when physicians were doing surgery there was a pharmaceutical component, as seen in the essential anesthetics distributed—almost 3 million ounces of ether and over 1.1 million ounces of chloroform.[11]

THE SUBSTANCES

Despite a poor knowledge of the etiology of disease, an imperfect and crude understanding of infection and contagion, and little appreciation for the pharmacological actions of the drugs they prescribed—other than an empirical (albeit keen) appreciation for dose-response relationships—surgeons had a wide and varied armamentarium at their disposal. The *United States Pharmacopoeia* (fourth decennial revision adopted in 1860 and made official [i.e., published] in 1863) listed a total of 871 different substances, of which 587 (or 67 percent) were botanicals.[12] Confronting such a massive materia medica would be a daunting task were it not for the fact that the U.S. Army pared this down considerably by selecting those thought to be the most essential in military practice. The result was the standard supply table. The original table at the beginning of the war was deemed outdated and virtually useless, forcing surgeons and purveyors to improvise as disease and demand dictated. A committee of revision was called together (Edward R. Squibb was among its members) and the official supply table adopted—sans calomel with Hammond's Circular No. 6 just days before—with Circular No. 7 on May 7, 1863. This circular contained 127 different pharmaceutical substances for hospital use; the supply table for the field service reduced this further to seventy-nine items (see Appendix A). Other substances could be ordered from the medical purveyor's depot by special requisition, but these were the required substances to be on hand at all times. Perhaps the best way to view and understand these substances as a whole is by a summary. Table 6.1 gives the official pharmacopoeial names of the most commonly used items, their names in English, their properties, and uses.[13] To avoid excessive length and redundancy, only the principal substances are listed in the table; those interested in the entire list, with all the variants, should consult Appendix A.

TABLE 6.1. Selected Items of the Standard Supply Table (As Adopted in Circular No. 7, May 7, 1863)

Name	Properties and Uses
1. Acaciæ Pulvis (gum arabic [powdered])	Chiefly a demulcent. Used on inflamed surfaces and catarrhal affection. Can be mixed in water; also used in the formation of pills.
2. Acidum cetum (citric acid)	Used in a variety of other preparations (e.g., Ferri et Quiniæ Citras, etc.). Believed to be of some value in scurvy (though inferior to lemon juice).
3. Æther Fortior (strong ether)	An anesthetic. Inhaled and also used as a topical anesthetic.
4. Alcohol Fortuis (strong alcohol)	Regarded as a stimulant. Its uses were many: anodyn, preservative, solvent, suspension medium, etc.
5. Alumen (alum)	A powerful astringent used in chronic dysentery, bronchial affections, hemorrhage, opthalmia, and toothache.
6. Ammonæ Liquor (ammonia)	Stimulant. Used in chronic catarrh and bronchitis as well as a wide variety of other uses (a wash for ulcers and contusions, etc.).
7. Argenti Nitras (nitrate of silver)	Sometimes referred to as "lunar caustic," it was given topically and internally. Used externally as a counterirritant; used internally for dyspepsia, diarrhea, croup, cough, tonsillitis, and other affections of the throat, ophthalmic conditions, and even reportedly used for gonorrhea.
8. Arsenitis Potassæ Liquor (tasteless ague drops)	A solution of equal parts arsenic acid and bicarbonate of potassa. Possessed variety of uses, but chiefly for fevers.
9. Asafœtide (asafetida)	Its horrible smell earned it the nickname "devil's dung." Used principally as a moderate stimulant, antispasmotic, expectorant, and mild laxative.
10. Bismuthi subcarbonas (subcarbonate of bismuth)	Considered tonic.
11. Camphora (camphor)	Moderate stimulant, anodyne (pain relief), diaphoretic (causing sweating), and used frequently in the treatment of typhoid.
12. Cantharides (Spanish fly)	This beetle, when pulverized, produced a poultice that caused blistering and was considered a counterirritant. Used topically for cutaneous eruptions, obstinate herpes, erysipelas, and other local inflammations.
13. Capsici Pulvis (cayenne pepper powder)	A powerful stimulant used topically for rheumatism and internally for "enfeebled and languid" stomach and palsy or other "lethargic affections."
14. Chloroformum (chloroform)	Anesthetic
15. Cinchonæ Caliayæ Pulvis (powdered yellow cinchona)	A tonic febrifuge, especially antiperiodic (see Chapter 7).
16. Collodium (collodion [a solution of gum in ether and alcohol])	Used chiefly as a vehicle for external medicines, often with cantharides (cantharidal collodion) or tannic acid (styptic collodion).
17. Copiaba (balsam of copaiba)	Considered gentle stimulant, diuretic, laxative, and in large doses purgative. Also used according to Stillé in "protracted and obstinate dysenteries."

TABLE 6.1 *(continued)*

Name	Properties and Uses
18. Creasotum (creasote)	Considered similar to carbolic acid. Used topically for hemorrhages and cutaneous eruptions; used internally as an antiemetic and in some bronchial affections.
19. Cubebæ Oleo resina (oleoresin of cubeb)	Diuretic, stimulant, and carminative (expulsion of flatus).
20. Cupri Sulphas (sulfate of copper)	Externally it was irritant and mildly escharotic (produced sloughing); diluted it was used as an astringent and stimulant.
21. Ext. Aconiti Fuidum (fluidextract of aconite root)	Used in treating rheumatism, gout, and neuralgia. Also used as a basis for other aconite preparations (abstracts, plasters, extracts, liniments, etc.)
22. Ext. Belladonnæ (extract of belladonna)	The active agent is atropine. In neuralgia, it was preferred over opium. Used in cases of whooping cough, scarlet fever, spasmodic asthma, and other instances calling for an antispasmodic.
23. Ext. Buchu Fluidum (fluidextract of Buchu)	Used in urinary tract and bladder inflammations.
24. Ext. Colchici Seminis Fluidum (colchicum seed fluid)	Sedative and anodyne. In higher doses, it was emetic and purgative. Used in gout and rheumatism.
25. Ext. Colocynthidis Comp. (colocynth compound)	A powerful cathartic. The *USD* called this "a favourite preparation with many practitioners" and combined with calomel, extract of jalap, and gamboges, a "safe cathartic."
26. Ext. Conii (hemlock)	Considered a "nervous sedative." Also sometimes used for whooping cough and asthma.
27. Ext. Ergotæ Fluidum (fluidextract of ergot)	A mold from rye used in internal hemorrhages and reportedly used for whooping cough.
28. Ext. Gentianæ Fluidim (fluidextract of gentian)	A tonic classed along with the "simple bitters."
29. Ext. Glycerrhizæ (extract of licorice)	A demulcent (containing a soothing mucilaginous and saccharine nature) used in catarrhal conditions.
30. Ext. Hyoscyami (extract of henbane)	Sedative and anodyne.
31. Ext. Ipecacuanhæ (extract of ipecac)	A powerful emetic. In smaller doses, it was used as a diaphoretic and expectorant.
32. Ext. Nucis Vomicæ (extract of nux)	The seeds of *Strychnos nux vomica* used in a similar manner as its alkaloid strychnine.
33. Ext. Pruni Virginianæ Fluidum (fluidextract of prunes)	A laxative.
34. Ext. Rhei Fluidum (fluidextract of rhubarb)	Prescribed in cases of diarrhea. Stillé considered it "a useful purgative in the bowel-complaint of summer."
35. Ext. Senegæ Fluidum (fluidextract of senega root)	The senega root was considered stimulant, expectorant, diuretic, and in larger doses emetic and cathartic. Beasley stated that it was used in "latter stages of pneumonia" and as a stimulant in "low and typhoid fevers."
36. Ext. Spigeliæ Fluidum (fluidextract of spigelia)	*Spigelia mirilandica,* native to the South, was used as a powerful anthelmintic (vermifuge or worm expeller).
37. Ext. Valerianæ Fluidum (fluidextract of valerian)	An antispasmodic used in epilepsy, hysteria, dyspepsia, spasmodic cough, and neuralgia.

Name	Properties and Uses
38. Ext. Veratri Viridis Fluidum (fluidextract of American hellebore)	An anodyne and used externally as a discutient (an antitumor agent). Stillé reports its use in influenza, jaundice, dysentery, and peritonitis.
39. Ext. Zingiberis Fluidum (fluidextract of ginger)	Ginger was used as a stimulant and carminative, often prescribed for dyspepsia.
40. Ferri Chloridi Tinctura (chloride of iron [tincture])	Used in "pseudo-membranous croup" and in arresting hemorrhages in the throat and gums. Beasley stated that all iron preparations worked as tonics that "raise the pulse, heighten the complexion, and promote the secretions."
41. Ferri Iodidi Syrupus (iodine of iron [syrup])	Used in scrofula (inflammation of the lymph nodes, especially in the neck). Also used in secondary syphilis.
42. Ferri Oxidum Hydratum (hydrated oxide of iron)	With water, it was used as an antidote for arsenic poisoning.
43. Ferri et Persulphatus Liquor (solution of subsuphate of iron [Monsels' solution])	Made by the reaction of sulfate of iron with sulfuric and nitric acids in water. An astringent.
44. Ferri et Quiniæ Citras (citrate of iron and quinine)	A specific tonic that supposedly combined the virtues of iron (a tonic used in chronic diarrhea and dysentery, enlargement of the liver and spleen, anemia, and dyspepsia) and quinine (a tonic febrifuge and antiperiodic).
45. Ferri Sulphas (sulfate of iron [green vitriol])	An astringent.
46. Hydrargyri Chloridum Corrosivum (corrosive sublimate)	Like all the mercurials, mercuric chloride ($HgCl_2$) was regarded as an alterative. A biliary stimulant and cathartic used in a wide range of ailments (see Chapter 7). It was also supplied as yellow iodide of mercury, red oxide of mercury, and in pill and ointment. Not quite the same as calomel (Hydrargyi Chloridum Mite or mercurous chloride [HgCl]). Because it was much harsher than calomel, corrosive sublimate was used far more judiciously by medical staff.
47. Iodinium (iodine)	Considered stimulants. Beasley indicates their use "in simple hypertrophy of any of the organs" and their valuable antiinflammatory action, especially in scrofulous disorders. It was used in combination with many prescriptions; Beasley alone gives fifty-six.
48. Linum (flaxseed)	Used externally as a poultice, it served as an emollient (moistening and soften agent); internally as a laxative.
49. Magnesia Sulphas (sulfate of magnesium)	A cathartic laxative often given with senna.
50. Morphiæ Sulphas (sulfate of morphine)	A powerful anodyne.
51. Olei Menthæ Piperitæ Tinct. (tincture of oil of peppermint)	An aromatic stimulant. Given for nausea and dyspepsia. A carminative and excipient.
52. Oleum Cinnamomi (oil of cinnamon)	Used as a cordial with carminative properties. Often employed with other remedies.
53. Oleum Morrhue (cod liver oil)	An alterative long employed in rheumatic and scrofulous disorders. Also reportedly used in phthisis (tuberculosis).
54. Oleum Olivæ (olive oil)	A mild laxative.

TABLE 6.1 *(continued)*

Name	Properties and Uses
55. Oleum Ricini (castor oil)	A purgative and laxative. Stillé touts its benefits in bowel disorders and asserts that in dysentery "it is generally sufficient for the cure."
56. Oleum Terebinthinæ (oil of turpentine)	Given internally as an anthelmintic, styptic, and stimulant. Used in certain intestinal fluxes (especially in dysentery) and in low fevers (especially typhoid). Used externally as a rubefacient (producing redness) for rheumatic conditions.
57. Oleum Tiglii (croton oil)	A powerful cathartic and, according to Beasley, "in very obstinate constipation, in dropsy, and in apoplexy or paralysis where a speedy irritant action on the intestines is desired." Stillé reported its use to expel tapeworms.
58. Opii Pulvis (powdered opium)	Also available in tincture and camphorated. From the opium poppy *(Papaver somnifera),* a powerful anodyne. Also used in cases of diarrhea.
59. Pilulæ Catharticæ Comp. (compound cathartic pills)	Composed of colocynth, jalap, mild chloride of mercury, and gamboge. The name fairly well describes its use. Prescribed especially in cases of bilious fever.
60. Plumbi Acetas (acetate of lead)	A powerful astringent and sedative. Used externally for astringent lotions; internally for diarrhea and dysentery.
61. Podophylli resina (mayapple)	A slow-acting but powerful cathartic. It was a favorite of botanic practitioners, who used it as a substitute for calomel.
62. Potasii Iodidum (iodide of potassium)	Used in secondary and tertiary syphilis. Also, generally used the same as iodine (see number 47).
63. Potassæ Acetas (acetate of potassa)	A powerful caustic and rubefacient.
64. Quiniæ Sulphas (sulfate of quinine)	During the war this was the most important tonic febrifuge and antiperiodic (see Chapter 7).
65. Scillæ Syrupus (syrup of squills)	From the sea onion *(Urginea martima),* used as an expectorant, diuretic, and emetic purgative. Its most common use was in the treatment of chronic bronchitis. Beasley gives more than thirty different prescriptions.
66. Sodæ Bicarbonas (bicarbonate of soda)	Used as an antacid and in dyspepsia, heartburn, and flatulence.
67. Sodæ [Sodii] Boras (borate of sodium)	A powerful antiseptic.
68. Sodæ et Potassæ Tartras (potassio-tartrate of soda [Rochelle salt])	A mild purgative laxative, used much as a Seidlitz powder. Made by combining cream of tartar with a solution of carbonate of soda.
69. Spiritus Frumenti (whisky)	Probably the most prescribed "stimulant" of the war. In combination with quinine, it was commonly given for prophylaxis of malarial fevers.
70. Spiritus Lavandulæ (spirit of lavender)	Used as an aromatic.
71. Strychnia (strychnine)	Used equivalently to nux vomica. An antispasmodic prescribed in cases of chorea and spasm of the esophagus. Stillé reported its use in epidemic cholera. Calling it "possessed of active and dangerous properties," Beasley gives thirty-six prescriptions for a wide range of conditions.

Name	Properties and Uses
72. Sulphur (sulfur)	Given topically for skin diseases, especially "the itch." Internally it is used in combination with cream of tartar as a laxative. Also sometimes used as a fumigant.
73. Vinum Xericum (sherry)	A stimulant, especially in typhoid fevers.
74. Zinci Acetas (acetate of zinc)	An ophthalmic astringent.
75. Zinci Carbonas (carbonate of zinc)	A topical for excoriated and inflamed surfaces.
76. Zinci Chloridi Liqour (chloride of zinc)	A topical for ulcers and tumors.
77. Zinci Sulphas (sulfate of zinc)	A tonic and astringent. Stillé reports it "to have been very efficient in curing epidemic diphtheria."

It can be seen from Table 6.1 that the armamentarium was wide and varied, applying both mineral and vegetable substances to a variety of complaints. These substances had attained their therapeutic status not by experimentation and double-blind study but by empirically established dose-response relationships acquired over time and handed down didactically to each successive generation of practitioners. Modern analysis of the supply table suggests that for its day it reflected "a judicious and thoughtful selection of galenicals [botanicals] as well as good judgment in their quantitative allowances."[14] It should be pointed out that besides the hospital and field service supply tables, portability was achieved with panniers. These medicine chests (88 pounds when full) had been developed by Edward R. Squibb for field use. Designed to be carried by pack animals and holding essential medical materials, panniers were much-used items.[15] In addition to the panniers, medical personnel could carry a regulation knapsack to the front. Initially, the knapsack was made of wicker and weighed 18 pounds when full. In 1862 the knapsack was modified by a slight reduction in size and the addition of drawers. Almost 20 pounds when full, it was found to be too cumbersome for its purpose and was abandoned early in 1863, when Medical Inspector R. H. Coolidge developed a smaller field case (or "surgeon's companion") that had convenient shoulder and waist straps.[16]

Nonetheless, the summary of the supply table above does not do justice to pharmaceutical therapeutics as it was actually practiced. Although we know a great deal about the materia medica from various compendia and texts, we know much less about what the typical physician and surgeon really did, what one able historian has called "the gap which . . . exists between the medicine preached and the medicine generally practiced."[17] Here the historian is presented with a rare opportunity. If the medical corps of both sides did anything, they kept careful notes and records of what they did. The massive *Medical and Surgical History of the War of the Rebellion* is a detailed chronicle of diseases, incidents of diseases, and case-by-case treatments. Add to this the published accounts of Civil War surgeons and hospital stewards and the numerous regimental prescription books still extant in archives across the country, and a fairly clear picture of treatment behaviors emerges.

PRESCRIBING AND DISPENSING
IN CAMP AND HOSPITAL

Scores of diseases were reported during the Civil War, but the chief maladies for which the surgeon's armamentarium was put to use reduce the number to only a few that need be extensively considered from a therapeutic standpoint. The compendious statistics compiled by the surgeon general's office show that only four broad categories of disease were persistent problems throughout the war: diarrhea/dysentery; camp and malarial fevers; respiratory ailments such as bronchitis and pneumonia; and a variety of digestive complaints. Although the incidents of all these diseases per 1,000 soldiers were quite high for whites, among black troops the rate was considerably worse (see Figure 6.2).

On a comparative basis there is little question that the single greatest medical complaint of the war was diarrhea and dysentery. It is not known from today's perspective of differential diagnosis precisely what diseases these reports of diarrhea and dysentery were. In the 1860s there was a tendency to view these symptoms as distinct disease entities within themselves. Yet it is probably a safe conjecture that most complaints represented bacterial, amebic, and parasitic infections from tainted water and food supplies.[18] Of course none of this was known to any of the personnel who were trying to treat it, since the microbial basis for disease was still on the horizon. Still, the symptoms were so marked and unmistakable that surgeons in both the eastern and western theaters of the war duly noted its persistence. Acting assistant surgeon James P. DeBruler of Hospital No. 2 in

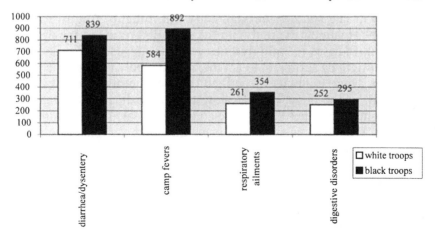

FIGURE 6.2. Incidents of Illness per 1,000: White and Black Troops, Union Army (*Source: The Medical and Surgical History of the War of the Rebellion*, Part 3, Volume 1, *Medical Volume* [Washington: GPO, 1888], pp. 6-77 passim. The figure for "camp fevers" is a compilation of "continued, typho-malaria, and malarial" fevers. See George Worthington Adams, *Doctors in Blue*, p. 240).

Evansville, Indiana, for example, noted, "Chronic diarrhea has been extremely common in this hospital, and in many instances so rebellious as to defy all modes of treatment that we could devise."[19] Similarly, assistant surgeon Samuel A. Storrow of Eckington Hospital in Washington, DC, called it "the most common disease with which the medical staff of this hospital has to deal."[20] The extent of the problem is manifested in the coverage devoted to it in *The Medical and Surgical History:* the entire 842 pages of Part 2, Volume 1 contain more than 900 case studies reported and summarized.

The types of diarrhea and dysentery as they were understood at the time were varied. First of all, surgeons were careful to distinguish between cases of acute and chronic diarrhea and dysentery, the latter more often accompanied by fever, "colicky abdominal pain," frequent and loose stools, and perhaps its hallmark feature, "scanty mucous and bloody discharges."[21] These "bloody fluxes," as they were sometimes called, were divided by their symptoms and alleged types as: mild acute, chronic, sthenic (acute and severe), bilious, and malignant dysenteries. There was a seasonal component to dysentery, with the Sanitary Commission noting that the vast majority of epidemics

occurred in late summer through early fall, roughly August to November.[22] Treatments varied with the so-called forms of the disease
presented. In cases of mild dysentery it was suggested that bed rest
and diet might be sufficient to get the patient safely through the bout.
However, a cure might be "expedited" by the administration of castor
oil in half- to one-ounce doses followed by 10 to 20 grains of calomel
six to eight hours later. Either dose could be repeated on the third day
so that it may evacuate the system by day, and at night "five to 15
drops of laudanum [opium] or wine of opium, or from five to ten
grains of Dover's powder [ipecac and opium], may be administered
to promote rather than enforce sleep, to allay tenesmus [painful
bowel cramps], and moderate the frequency of the stools."[23] With
this treatment a "cure" could be expected in three to six days. In
sthenic cases Epsom salts and Rochelle salts were recommended, followed by three to five grains of Dover's powder every three hours:
"Two or three such courses are generally sufficient . . . for the speedi-
est cure of the disease."[24] The other forms of dysentery called for
similar purgative, emetic, and sedative regimens. Even for cases of
chronic dysentery, vegetable laxatives such as rhubarb and castor oil
along with five grains of blue mass or mercury were recommended.[25]

Given these harsh therapeutics, it is no wonder that medical staffs
had difficulty in combating these disorders. Nevertheless, the fact
that many cases were self-resolving within three to six days caused
many surgeons and hospital stewards to make the error (post hoc,
ergo propter hoc) that their remedies had effected the cure. In other
cases, however, it was recognized that the offending diarrheas and
dysenteries were the result of poor environmental conditions, situations that corrected themselves with or without medical treatment
once the unit moved. Typical were the fairly accurate observations of
surgeon David Little of the 13th New York Volunteers writing from
Fort Corcoran, Virginia, early in the war about the factors affecting
incidents of diarrhea/dysentery:

> It will be observed that diarrhea and dysentery have been very
> prevalent, as well as intermittent fever. Several points might be
> enumerated in explanation of the origin of the first-named dis-
> eases: viz: First, the men are raw troops, unused to the hardships
> and exposures of camp life [more likely, camp conditions], and
> unlearned in the arts that tend to the health and comfort of the
> soldier, more especially in that of properly preparing their food;

second, change of water. Since their arrival in Virginia they have drunk soft water exclusively, whereas they have lived hitherto in the limestone region and are accustomed to hard water [perhaps not technically correct, but mineral content cannot be dismissed as a factor influencing diarrhea]. It may, moreover, be mentioned that while at Camp Lincoln, near the Georgetown ferry and at the foot of the hill from Fort Corcoran, the water used was very foul, with exactly what impurity I was unable to determine. At any rate there is a significant fact in this connection, namely, that these intestinal disorders originated here, and so rapid was their progress that, within a week after their first appearance, sixty-four of the men were ill at one time. Immediately upon our removal to our present encampment, Camp Union, situated about one mile and a half beyond Fort Corcoran on the Fairfax road, diarrhea began to disappear and has been steadily decreasing, so that now only a few mild cases remain.[26]

From this perspective there is a temptation to dismiss the surgeon's treatments as either irrelevant or perhaps even harmful. Other regimens reported similar alterations between cathartics and sedatives such as sulfate of magnesia and morphine; this probably did more to exacerbate the condition than no treatment at all.[27] It should be pointed out, however, that the use of mineral and vegetable astringents might have had some therapeutic value. Subnitrate of bismuth, a combination of nitrate of bismuth and carbonate of soda, was used frequently in cases of diarrhea and dysentery for its tendency to relieve stomach and bowel cramps.[28] Alfred Stillé noted its "marked advantage" when used in cases of chronic diarrhea and indeed whenever astringents and "relaxation of the bowels" were called for.[29] Well into the twentieth century, bismuth and its various preparations were prescribed "as astringents and sedatives to mucous membranes and as gastrointestinal antiseptics."[30] In addition to astringent salts, a variety of vegetable astringents high in tannic acid were also utilized and probably gave some symptomatic relief.

The distinction as to whether one was treating a case of simple diarrhea or dysentery can easily be exaggerated. Charles Beneulyn Johnson noted that pathologists' postmortem examinations suggested that most cases were dysentery, but that the majority of surgeons in the field had diagnosed diarrhea.[31] Interestingly, he recalled few actual cases of dysentery but admitted that "scores and scores" of his Illinois regiment died from chronic diarrhea.[32] Whatever the particular diagnosis, actual treatment often varied little. Dr. S. Carbee prescribed rhubarb (a laxative) and opium for diarrhea patients of the 12th New Hampshire Infantry Volunteers.[33] In one New York unit, Private James P. Smith received two "cathartic pills" for his diarrhea, and Private Andrew Smith was prescribed 10 grains of calomel (essentially the same thing), followed in four hours by two aperient pills (an undisclosed laxative).[34]

Besides these official accounts, considerable evidence suggests that hospital stewards and entrepreneurs made their own remedies and distributed them to the afflicted. One particular favorite was a blackberry-based preparation. One hospital steward, Jonathan Wood, noting the prevalence of diarrhea in his Ohio unit, routinely gathered the root, cleaned and steeped it in hot water, added sugar and spirits "enough to keep from souring," and touted it as a medicine that "usually done [sic] better than other remedies."[35] The popularity of blackberry root as an antidiarrheal prompted George M. Dixon to attempt larger-scale manufacturing of a more elegant and presumably more marketable Dixon's Blackberry Carminative. The complexity of this polypharmacy concoction was nothing if not impressive in its preparation:

Blackberry root crushed	100 lbs.
African Ginger	15 lbs.
Rhubard Root	15 lbs.
Cinnamon Bark	6 lbs.
Caraway Seed	6 lbs.
Nutmegs	6 lbs.
Alcohol 76%	30 galls.
Water	30 galls.

Digest the above for 14 days or more, draw off the clean liquor add

| Refined Sugar | 500 lbs. |
| Ext. Logwood | 20 lbs. |

Dissolve the Ext. Logwood in 6 galls. Water—Cut the following Ess. [essential] Oils in 3 galls. of 92% alcohol

Oil [of] Anise	12 ozs.
Oil [of] Caraway	16 ozs.
Oil [of] Cassia	2 ozs.
Oil [of] Sassafras	½ oz.

Add 60 grains Sulph. Morphine to ea. 10 galls when ready to bottle.[36]

For all of the surgeons' and hospital stewards' efforts to combat diarrhea and dysentery, it remained a serious ailment, increasing throughout the war years as new recruits, poor nutrition, and sources of bacterial and amebic infection continued.[37]

From July 1863 through 1865, the Federal Department of Arkansas saw seven out of every ten soldiers reporting some enteric disorder. By July 1864 there were 698 cases of diarrhea and dysentery per 1,000 in Arkansas; one year later the number rose to 804 per 1,000 soldiers.[38]

Diarrhea and dysentery were not the only afflictions with which the military had to contend—fever seemed ever present and ever deadly. Among black troops it ranked as the single most prevalent disease, although differences in reporting methods may suggest a lowering of total incidents of fever (especially malaria) among African-American soldiers.[39] The concept of fever as a distinct disease entity, rather than a symptom as commonly understood today, made specific diagnoses difficult and the classification of the various fevers vague and subject to change. Early in the war "irritative" fevers along with typhoid and typhus (very different diseases from today's perspective) were all classed as continued fevers.[40] On June 30, 1862, the surgeon general's office made two changes in reporting what it called "idiopathic febrile diseases." First, the term *continued fever* was abandoned, with most cases formerly classed under that heading reported as typhoid fever or "other miasmatic diseases."[41] The second change saw the addition of the term typho-malarial fever, but the absence of instructions on the use of this term simply added to the diagnostic and nosological confusions.[42] What *can* be said of the fevers is that there were no clear demarcations between terms. The surgeon general's office admitted that it was no more possible to distinguish between malarial and typhoid fevers than it was to separate the typhus from the typhoid cases.[43] Camp fevers might include typhus and typhoid, "common continued" fevers, "remittent" fevers, and "intermitting" fevers; paroxymal fevers might embrace malarial fevers that were themselves "remittent" or "intermitting"; and even measles was referred to as an "eruptive" fever. Matters were further complicated by the common practice of identifying fevers by their respective symptomatic cycles. Thus, fevers that recurred every third day were often called tertian fevers, those making their appearance every four days were called quartan fevers, those that recurred every five days were quintan fevers, and so on.

It was a situation that would not soon resolve itself. Well after the war Robley Dunglison, nineteenth-century medicine's great lexicographer, listed more than one hundred different fevers in his dictionary.[44] Indeed the inability of the medical profession to accurately distinguish between symptoms and causes, viewing them as somehow synonymous, affords a clear example of what historian Lester King has called "a continuous dialectic between the rational and empirical view points."[45] As conservative traditionalists rooted in eighteenth-century rationalism contended with early-nineteenth-century empiricists, "there was no complete assurance, no cogency, regarding the nature of the disease."[46] The fascination with symptoms that so intrigued the empiricists proved no better at providing sound therapeutic modalities than had the elaborate theories of the rationalists. Until distinctions in the causative bacteria could be demonstrated and Koch's postulates rigorously applied, it mattered little whether one was labeling a fever as typhoid, typho-malarial, tertian, quatran, quintan, septan, remittment, intermittent, or what have you.

Nevertheless, nosological confusion did not prevent therapeutic recommendations from being made. Charles Beneulyn Johnson observed that "turpentine was the sheet-anchor in the treatment of typhoid,"[47] a medicinal mainstay that was generally and widely followed.[48] Stillé referred to oil of turpentine as "a genial stimulant to the entire economy" and noted its use not only in typhoid fevers but also in yellow fever and "intestinal fluxes."[49] When diarrhea was present, as it often was in cases of fever, Dover's powder and a variety of laxatives were often employed.[50] In so-called simple fevers, sulfate of magnesia and senna were often given; if liver involvement was suspected (jaundice often accompanies yellow fever and other fevers), compound cathartic pills and other "biliary stimulants" might be added to the treatment regimen.[51] In typhoid cases, the Sanitary Commission recommended (in addition to the standard cathartics) camphorated water, Hoffman's anodyne (an alcohol and ether preparation), and opiates in small quantities.[52] For typhus "such hygienic measures, the use of mild evacuents, of diaphoretics, nervous, and arterial sedatives or stimulants, as the case may require, together with the usual means to mitigate febrile action, constitute the whole of the general plan of treatment."[53] The Sanitary Commission concluded its report with two British prescriptions generically titled mild fever mixture (two drachms of ammonia acetate solution "Spirit of Mindererus" in camphor water, each in a half troy ounce of distilled water as a draught) and strong fever mixture (five grains of carbonate of ammonium in camphor water taken each hour).[54] For yellow fever a number of therapeutic regimens were employed: small doses of morphine, prussic acid, and creosote (often combined with an alkali or chalk thought to allay vomiting) taken a drop or two every hour; one ounce of camphor in an ounce of chloroform given in hourly two-drop doses; acetate of lead, carbolic acid, minim doses (one-sixtieth of a fluidrachm) of muriatic or nitro-muriatic acid; rubefacients and opiates might be given as symptoms or "stages" of the disease dictated.[55] The single most prescribed article for all fevers, particularly malaria, was quinine and its derivative cinchona. The importance of these remedial agents was unequivocal. "In the treatment of the miasmatic fevers," stated John T. Metcalfe of the Sanitary Commission, "our main and great reliance is placed on cinchona and its preparations. There is no substitute for these."[56] Furthermore, he added: "The preparation of cinchona, almost universally employed, is the sulphate of quinine."[57] The importance of quinine was best summarized in the surgeon general's report:

> During the War of the Rebellion quinine was the *sine qua non* of treatment for malarial disease. Other drugs and remedial measures were used as called for by particular conditions of the system, but other antiperiodics were seldom employed except in cases in which quinine after fair trial failed to eradicate the disease.[58]

In fact, this one item was so frequently prescribed and so important to the general health of the troops that its full treatment is discussed in detail in for Chapter 7.

The category of ailment most encountered after fever was an assortment of respiratory complaints. Although we know today that most acute respiratory illnesses are the result of streptococcal or pneumococcal infections, surgeons of that day were convinced that the majority of respiratory diseases were due to weather and exposure.[59] Broadly considered, most respiratory problems can be placed into four broad categories: catarrh and epidemic catarrh (upper respiratory and sinus congestion, such as that experienced with the common cold); acute and chronic bronchitis; inflammation of the larynx (laryngitis and membranous laryngitis); and most serious of all, pneumonia.[60] Catarrh was typically treated with expectorants such as syrup of squills; sometimes quinine and Dover's powder were utilized. Bronchitis was treated with cupping, cod liver oil, stimulants, expectorants, and iodide of potassium and liniment when accompanied by rheumatic complaints. Inflammation of the larynx was treated by keeping the airway open, warm/moist inhalations and gargles, hot fomentations, or counterirritants such as cantharidal collodion applications.

The most life-threatening respiratory disease was pneumonia, sometimes referred to as inflammation of the lungs. The treatment of choice throughout the war was tartar emetic early in an attack, given in small doses of one-quarter to one-sixteenth of a grain every two to three hours.[61] If pneumonia persisted, mercurials were used in order to

> allay fever, subdue inflammatory action and promote absorption in the probably now consolidated lung. Small doses of blue-pill [mercury] and opium, calomel and opium, or calomel and Dover's powder, with or without nitre and ipecacuanha, were administered; rarely the iodine employed.[62]

The administration of mercurials met with the emphatic approval of the surgeon general's office (*not* Hammond's administration), which declared "this plan of treatment as of greater value than any other in relieving symptoms and removing the disease."[63] Interestingly, the Sanitary Commission disagreed. Austin Flint and the members of his committee investigating the treatment of pneumonia showed a marked preference for a less heroic and more progressive therapeutics. They dubbed bleeding "not warranted . . . and likely in many cases to do harm."[64] Chiding their colleagues for blistering their pneumonia patients "to hasten resolution," they insisted there is no evidence that they contribute to this object, and they are highly objectionable on account of the annoyance and irritation which they are likely to occasion. Moreover, they [the blisters] interfere with the daily examination of the chest, by means of which alone accurate information respecting the condition of the lung is to be obtained.[65]

Instead they recommended a more supportive treatment that included "tonic remedies, alcoholic stimulants, and nutritious diet."[66]

The final category of disease was the various digestive disorders. Most of these were probably manifestations of amoebic infections from bad water or parasitic infestations of intestinal worms. Also, the standard army rations did not help. The regulation diet of hardtack (a petrified cracker usually barely edible) and salt meats—and the absence of fresh green vegetables—promoted gastroenteritis, nausea, and bowel complaints. Soldiers' indigestion was aided and abetted by profiteering sutlers (civilian provisioners to an army) who sold hungry men overpriced "villainous" pies and other questionable fare, which one brigade surgeon blamed for 10 percent of the illness in his unit.[67] The idea that much of the digestive troubles were secondary to other physical ailments is also undoubtedly true. Treatments for simple digestive disorders, such as nausea, might include the use of creosote drops, liquid diet, and other palliative measures including the administration of bicarbonate of soda.

One important disease for which the materia medica was pressed into service early in the war was measles. As mentioned previously, this was classed as an "eruptive fever." Measles were a special problem for newly formed regiments. Young boys living far apart in rural America often had not been exposed to the usual childhood diseases. Once mustered into a regiment and confined to camp, one case of measles quickly became many. Many developed secondary infections such as bronchitis and pneumonia or lost their hearing. In October 1861 four Indiana and Ohio regiments had to discontinue drills due to measles epidemics.[68] Moreover, simultaneous outbreaks of measles were the norm early in the war, and recurrences and other complications due to poor nursing, diet, and hygiene were frequent.[69] Assistant surgeon for the 92nd Illinois Volunteer Infantry, Dr. Thomas Winston, encamped near Falmouth, Kentucky, wrote to his wife and son that he was worried that measles "will cause us much trouble" and that he received permission "to take a house in the village and use it for our measles cases."[70] By December he wrote nervously, "Many of our boys are taking measles."[71]

Treatment of measles largely revolved around hygienic measures. Pharmaceutical regimens were used chiefly to manage secondary infections.[72] Interestingly, the army surgeons did not seem to have systematically practiced quarantine or isolation to restrict the disease.[73] Nevertheless, it is undeniable that the hospital steward was kept busy compounding prescriptions for the various secondary complaints accompanying the measles.

A final consideration for the military materia medica of the Union army is so-called hospital gangrene (i.e., bacteremia, pyemia, and purulent wound infections) and erysipelas (an acute inflammatory disease caused by hemolytic streptococcus). Although the Civil War medical staffs were clueless as to the etiology of these postsurgical problems, efforts to combat them were relentless. Hospital gangrene generally followed wounds (surgical or otherwise) of the extremities.[74] Of the 2,642 cases, reported mortality was high at 45.6 percent.[75] The surgeon general's office noted the "judicious and successful" treatment of hospital gangrene at the Annapolis Hospital, which consisted principally of applying

> fuming nitric acid to the edges of the sore, to its surface, and especially to the healthy integument beyond the line of diseased action. In some cases nitrate of silver had been successfully applied. The cleansing means employed during the separation of the slough were chiefly "Labarraque's solution," creasote [sic] and vinegar washes, yeast, cinchona, and charcoal poultices, etc.[76]

Treating erysipelas and hospital gangrene was essentially the same, due largely to conditions of overcrowding and poorly ventilated wards. The Sanitary Commission recommended various hygienic measures and "empirical remedies addressed to the constitutional state," namely, tincture of chloride of iron, quinine, alcohol, and antiseptics.[77] Apparently, Goldsmith, who authored the Sanitary Commission's report on gangrene and erysipelas, thought highly of bromine (a nonmetallic element obtained from seawater and saline springs, similar to iodine in its therapeutic properties). This he applied to the affected area either full strength or dissolved in water. Similarly, he applied bromine masks to patients who had erysipelas of the face.[78]

As helpful as it is to know the nature and extent of the materia medica and the diseases for which it was utilized, this armamentarium's true character emerges only in the real-life interfaces between health, sickness, surgical, and pharmaceutical care. These can best come to light in a review of some specific case studies seen from four vantage points: first, a summary of the army's health and therapeutics as revealed in the hospital records, prescription books, and reports of surgeons; second, a careful examination of one particular regiment through the same means; third, a review of pharmaceutical care in naval operations; and fourth, a couple of individual case studies and their therapeutic outcomes.

UNIT AND PATIENT CASE STUDIES

The Register and Prescription Book for Dr. S. Carbee of the New Hampshire Infantry Volunteers, 12th Regiment, gives a fairly typical picture of health late in the war.[79] During the months of January and February 1865 there was an average of twenty-two sick soldiers per day, most with acute diarrhea and intermittent fever. Since a lot of diarrhea was ascribed to "biliousness," mercurials—deemed biliary stimulants—were prescribed frequently. Most common were blue mass, calomel, and compound cathartic pills. Treatments varied, however. A cough might receive Dover's powder, a cold "Blue mass et C.C.P [compound cathartic pills]," or a cold and fever might receive "Quinin et iron" or "colocynth et ipecac." Diarrhea might receive "Rhei sodae et opii" (a favorite of Carbee's), an unofficial preparation that consisted of a laxative/sedative combination of rhubarb and opium in a soda base ("cinchona et iron" for debility or "opii et iron"). All of this was very symptom-based treatment.

Hospitals, such as the one at Fort Sumner, Maryland, utilized a wider array of substances, but familiar items appear with predictable regularity.[80] Mercurials, opium, ipecac, quinine sulfate, morphine, and Dover's powder predominate. Less frequent, but by no means rare, were syrup of squills, zingiber (ginger), buchu, iron, Seidlitz powder, cinchona, castor oil, and copaiba.

One particularly detailed record is available for the 152nd Regiment Ohio Volunteer Infantry, a unit that was formed at Camp Dennison, Ohio, on May 11, 1864, and performed guard and picket duty at New Creek, West Virginia. It later headed for the front, arriving at Beverly, Virginia, on June 4, and was twice attacked by Confederate forces while on the march. By July the regiment was stationed at Cumberland, Maryland.[81]

Surgeon John C. Williamson and assistant surgeon J. A. Jobes looked after the health of the 152nd Ohio Volunteers. Their Register and Prescription Book comprised fifty pages from June 5 to August 31 of 1864 and included about 1,000 entries.[82] Common prescriptions listed were: cinchona, opium, Rochelle salts, and Dover's powders (often in combination with cinchona). Cinchona predominates the book. Standard treatment for "biliousness" (occasionally listed) was mercery (i.e., hydrarg.) followed by "salts." Some specific examples include Private C. Banin, who was given "whisky and water" for measles. On August 2, E. Cassell was treated for rheumatism with Rochelle salts. Alden H. Gillett of Company K was treated for diarrhea with opium. He was first listed in the prescription book on June 5, 1864, and he continued treatment at least through June 30. It is doubtful that Williamson or Jobes could do much for the soldier. When Gillett's company was mustered out on September 2, 1864, he was listed as "absent, sick at Springfield, Ohio, no further record found."[83]

The 152nd Ohio Volunteers had their share of illness. On August 1, Williamson and Jobes struggled with a particularly obstinate wave of typhoid and intermittent fevers accompanied by diarrhea.[84] Some were "sent to general hospital," while others were treated with "opium and antiperiodics." D. Ault, a private in Company B, for example, was treated for diarrhea and fever with cinchona and Dover's powder. Throughout the prescription book, in fact, a lot of typhoid and intermittent fevers appear in the entries; most of the afflicted were sent to their quarters rather than to the hospital.

The navy had its difficulties as well. Secretary of the Navy Gideon Welles (1802-1878), a bewigged and white-bearded fussbudget dubbed "Father Neptune," warned the commander of the North Atlantic Blockading Squadron, L. M. Goldsborough, in the spring of 1862: "The approach of the hot and sickly season upon the Southern coast of the United States renders it imperative that every precaution should be used by the officers commanding vessels to continue the excellent sanitary conditions of their crews."[85] Welles had cause for concern; problems with hygiene were not confined to camp life. Typical was the commander of the U.S.S. *Vermont* at Port Royal Harbor, South Carolina, who found a batch of naval recruits "so overrun with vermin" that he was forced to go ashore to have them wash and disinfect their clothing.[86] Despite the fact that simple hygienic measures could do little against most of the diseases, it could help. Welles had other reasons to be nervous as well. The attempt to put a stranglehold on the South with a blockade stretched his navy from the Potomac to the Texas coast. The flagship of the Eastern Gulf Blockading Squadron, the *St. Lawrence,* reported an outbreak of yellow fever that in September 1862 was "still on the increase."[87] The commander reported to Welles that his ship had eighty-eight cases and twenty deaths but that others were not unaffected: the *Huntsville* had twenty cases and six deaths; the *Magnolia* and an accompanying schooner, the *Eugenie,* both had four cases and one death.[88] Indeed, yellow fever was a particular plague of the navy, with outbreaks reported throughout the war; it was especially severe in the West Gulf Blockading Squadron.[89] The disease was undoubtedly spread to the ship by sailors who visited ports infested with the vector for the virus—the *Aedes aegypti or Haemogogus* spp. mosquito.[90]

The problem occurred not just at sea. Riverboats reported considerable sickness, as when assistant surgeon Penrose aboard the U.S. steamer *Harriet Lane* reported the unwelcome visitation of diarrhea to his commander:

> I would respectfully call your attention to the condition of the water used for drinking purposes on board this ship. Doubtless, you have noticed in the morning reports made to you, that a great number of those reported as sick were suffering from diarrhea; and I am well convinced the principle [sic] cause of it has been from the free use of Mississippi River water drank in its impure condition. I think I can safely say that nearly every officer and man on board has suffered to a greater or lesser extent from the disease since being in the river. I have been led to believe that it has been produced in a great measure from the above cause from the fact that it existed all the time we were in the river before, and disappeared shortly after leaving it and ceasing to use the water taken from it.

Since we have again returned and are again using the water, the diarrhea has also returned; and in some cases so excessive is it as to totally disable the sufferer from the slightest exertion.

I do not attribute the disease entirely to the water, but believe it is the principle cause, and I am sustained in this opinion by the other Assistant Surgeon with whom I have convinced upon the subject.

An attempt was made by me to purify the water, but . . . it was entirely unsatisfactory. I would therefore respectfully suggest that *condensed* water be used for drinking purposes.[91]

Penrose's suggestion that he be permitted to use "condensed water" might have indeed worked. Since this water would have been drawn from the outer steam jacket of the engine, it would essentially have been distilled and therefore germ-free.[92]

As with diarrhea and dysentery among soldiers on land, fevers on ship were a constant medical problem and even affected operations. L. R. Boyce, surgeon on the U.S. steamer *Underwriter* wrote to his commander that he was required to send nine men to the naval hospital at New Bern, North Carolina, and "exclusive of those nine, seventeen (17) on board [are] under treatment with intermittent and remittent fevers, and my sick list is increasing daily."[93] Boyce also told his commander that, "it is my opinion it is actually necessary for the health of the crew of this vessel, that they go to [Cape] Hatteras or some other healthy station for change of air and climate."[94] By November 1863 fevers became so severe that Gideon Welles, on recommendation of the fleet surgeon, directed Rear Admiral David D. Porter, who was commanding the Mississippi Squadron, to send all affected vessels north to Cairo or St. Louis.[95]

Apart from the yellow fever afflicting the Gulf squadrons, calling perhaps for higher uses of oil of turpentine and other therapeutic agents previously described for that disease, there does not appear to be anything distinctive in naval pharmacy care. Support for this conclusion would seem borne out in the diary accounts of Samuel P. Boyer, who provided posterity with a rare and intimate glimpse into the medical practice and daily routine of a Union naval surgeon. Boyer rarely complains of drug shortages, and freely treats a wide array of complaints with the standard materia medica of the day. Fortunately, Dr. Boyer appears to have been spared the horrors of epidemic yellow fever while aboard the U.S. bark *Fernandina,* but he did see fever, diarrhea, catarrh, and stomach complaint. For George Thompson suffering from intermittent fever, for example, he prescribed a "tonic mixture" containing 32 grains of quinine sulfate, one fluid dram of aromatic sulfuric acid, one-half fluid dram of ginger, a wineglass of whisky (60 cc.), and water (180 cc.) taken in a tablespoonful three times a day.[96] For diarrhea, Boyer prescribed castor oil and opium in either purgative or carminative doses.[97] Catarrh and bronchitis cases received the predictable expectorants.[98] When two "contrabands" (ex-slaves seeking asylum under the United States flag) on Sapelo Island asked for some "belly drops to stop the pain and make you sleep," Boyer gave them each a bottled preparation containing tincture of cayenne pepper, ginger, tincture of opium, and oil of peppermint in water.[99]

Boyer's third quarter report for 1863 shows a fairly busy sick bay: fifty-four diseases treated for an average of three patients reporting ill per day over ninety-two days. He saw intermittent fever, dyspepsia, cholera, constipation, acute dysentery, colic, acute bronchitis, catarrh, rheumatism, syphilis, gonorrhea, conjunctivitis, and others. In making out his quarterly requisition for medical stores, he ordered $15.20 worth of medicines and had the lot delivered by 6 p.m., ending his report with, "I have a good supply of drugs on hand."[100]

That surgeons and surgeon stewards were kept busy aboard ships throughout the war is a certainty. Instances of extremely high rates of disease occurred among some ships while others leveled off or even declined; in no case was any Union vessel illness-free or even approximately so.[101] The reasons for this are several: varying attention to onboard hygiene (poor sanitation could exacerbate epidemic diseases and breed pestilence); different ports of call (some ports, as we have seen, harbored yellow fever and other diseases); and varying levels of medical expertise (the caliber of ship surgeons was generally higher than that of army surgeons but incompetents and drunks were not unheard of aboard ship).

Perhaps the success or failure of treatment is best seen in individual case studies that follow treatment from beginning to end. The first is the postoperative treatment of Joseph Leavitt. John Leavitt of Portland, Maine, outlines the case and follows his son's progress for his wife—Joseph's mother—in a series of letters dated from June 6 to July 11, 1864.[102] Joseph was brought into the Mansion House Hospital in Alexandria, Virginia, after having his foot amputated. The operative site itself seemed to be improving, and his father writes on

June 18 that Joseph is "fifty percent better." By June 28 trouble looms as Joseph develops a bad cough. John then asks for some patent medicine cough wafers he seemed to think highly of, but the attending physician dismissed the suggestion and writes his own prescription for expectorants. The next day Joseph develops diarrhea, and he complains on June 30 that the medicine for the diarrhea has done him no good. The son's condition steadily declines despite the ministrations of the physician. By July 8 the exhausted father, who has been keeping a constant vigil, writes home, resigned to his son's fate: "I want to rest very much, when anything happens I will let you know immediately. Keep up the good spirits for we are almost at our journey's end & let us meet the misfortunes of life like true Christians."

At virtually the same time, and about ten miles away, Dr. William F. Norris serving at the Douglas Hospital in Washington, DC, offers a more positive but still uncertain picture of recovery. There a twenty-two-year-old Private John Rial of Company B of the 4th Ohio Volunteer Infantry is admitted on June 12, 1864, with a gunshot wound in his right leg.[103] "General condition [is] good," noted Norris, "though there was much pain in the knee and some irritative fever, which was increasing. Water dressing applied." The next day the patient was restless and his knee swollen; assistant surgeon William Thomson performed an amputation, the stump being sutured closed and wet dressings applied to the wound. Iron, whisky, and beef tea were "freely administered." By June 27 Norris notes "profuse perspiration but no chills" and fears pyemia. To counteract these ominous symptoms he orders an increase in whisky and a tonic preparation consisting of quinine sulfate and aromatic sulfuric acid in water to be taken three times a day. "The perspiration continued for several nights," Norris observed, "but with evident abatement and finally ceased altogether to be replaced however by a diarrhea, which was checked by pills of tannin and opium." On July 4 Norris substitutes sherry for whisky due to his patient's irritable stomach. The recovery is slow and not without recurrence of fever. To counteract night sweats, which apparently developed by July 29, Norris ordered compound tincture of cinchona added to the wine and aromatic sulfuric acid. After this bout with fever Private Rial makes good improvement and is walking with crutches by the end of August. All seems well until October 1, when erysipelas develops in the stump. Tincture of iodine is topically applied, and tincture of iron given internally. By October 3 the inflammation had increased and extended; more tincture of iodine is applied. The next day Norris observed that the inflammation was receding and the patient regaining his appetite. On October 10 the patient was transferred to another hospital.

Both of these cases show the importance of pharmaceutical care, even in postoperative cases. Both cases also demonstrate that even the simplest amputations were rarely without their life-threatening complications. Joseph Leavitt almost certainly succumbed to double pneumonia, whereas John Rial probably survived with a partial leg that would give him health problems the rest of his life. At best, Rial's symptoms would subside and the wound would completely heal; at worst he would live a life of constant misery with recurrent bouts of erysipelas or osteomyelitis.

This does not quite complete the examination of the Civil War materia medica. Although only some mention has been made of quinine and calomel, these two items ranked so high in relative importance in the surgeon's armamentarium that separate discussion is necessary to place them in context. A great many substances have been mentioned, but these two remedies may be justly considered as reigning supreme among the vast vegetable and mineral drugs used in the field. So powerful were both of these medicines that the failure of the surgeon general to take heed of one would cost him his job, and the other would transform a mere business into an industry giant. We next consider calomel and quinine.

Chapter 7

The Remedies of Choice:
Calomel and Quinine

The top remedial agents of the Civil War were alcohol (the ubiquitous "stimulant"), opium (the reliable if potentially addictive narcotic of choice), calomel (the time-honored biliary stimulant), and quinine (an antimalarial that did more than just manage symptoms). Of those four, none carried the political volatility of calomel or the demonstrable efficacy of quinine. These two unique qualities require an extended analysis of both.

By the time of the Civil War neither calomel nor quinine (or more broadly, the febrifugal properties of cinchona bark) was new to the materia medica. Mercury, in its various forms, was of ancient origin; its medical administration can be traced to the dispensing of mercurial ointments by the Persian physician Rhazes (860-932 A.D.). Calomel—or mercurous chloride (HgCl)—as a distinct therapeutic entity dates from about 1595, but the term was definitely first applied by Sir Theodore Turquet de Mayerne (1573-1655), who referred to *mercurous dulcis* sublimated (i.e., the process of separating a volatile solid substance from a nonvolatile substance by the application of heat) six times as *calomelanos turqueti* in his posthumously published *Medicinal Advices* in 1677.[1]

Although the therapeutic benefits of the mercurials are by today's standards doubtful, and more likely outright harmful, quinine really is effective against malaria. In order to understand quinine, one must understand malaria. Malaria is a tropical and subtropical disease transferred to humans from the bite of the *Anopheles* mosquito, which carries the *Plasmodium* protozoa. Once in the bloodstream these parasites cause intermittent or remittent fevers, violent chills, headache, vomiting, and in severe cases coma and death. More often the malaria attacks are so debilitating that the sufferer succumbs to some secondary

infection.[2] Quinine ([6-methoxycinchonine] $C_{20}H_{24}N_2O_2$) and its related alkaloids all work by depressing the ability of the plasmodia to
multiply and by causing the infecting protozoa to transform from
their asexual form to a benign sexual form. When given prophylactically, quinine does not prevent infection but rather keeps the protozoa
level so low that no clinical symptoms develop.[3] Although this was
not known until the twentieth century, the benefits of quinine were
long ago observed at the bedside. Quinine, the principal alkaloid of
Cinchona spp., is sometimes referred to as Jesuits' bark because it
was discovered by Jesuit missionaries who brought the drug to Europe in 1631; is a derivative of the Peruvian name *Quina-quina* ("bark
of barks").[4] Because malaria has been demonstrated to be a disease
introduced into the Americas by European contact,[5] the idea that Peruvian native populations knew of the medicinal properties of cinchona bark is doubtful and, in fact, some evidence supports that they
considered cinchona bark a poison.[6] More important, the pharmacological basis for quinine's mode of action was not clearly understood
until the work of S. W. Hardiker, P. Mühlens, W. E. Dixon, P. De, and
others in the 1920s. In the mid-nineteenth century quinine and its derivatives were being used not only for malarial fevers but also for erysipelas, rheumatic fever, scarlet fever, enervating tonics, stomach
remedies, and uterine stimulants.[7] By the 1860s every physician had
employed it for something. Only calomel rivaled it in therapeutic es-
teem as a specific in combating certain diseases.

Whatever the real or imagined benefits of these substances, one
thing is certain: in the Civil War, surgeons' armamentaria and on the
hospital stewards' supply tables, calomel and quinine reigned as the
remedies of choice. But, as we shall see, calomel was not without its
challengers.

THE MASTODON UNHARNESSED

In 1845 Alexander Means (1801-1883) launched a spirited defense of calomel, asking rhetorically

> [should physicians] consent to cower at the outcry of blind prej-
> udice, or ignorant and interested empiricism, and, before the
> eyes of the living myriads whom it has rescued from the jaws of
> the grave, deliberately pronounce the blistering curse of Science

upon its head, and consign it to the reproach and maledictions of posterity?

For Means, calomel was a mighty remedy—tried and true. It was, for him, "THE MASTODON IN HARNESS . . . [able] to do the work of an age in a year."[8]

Others disagreed. Groups of botanic physicians had risen up against the therapeutic excesses of the "learned" regulars (dubbed allopaths). Men such as Samuel Thomson (1769-1843), Alva Curtis (1797-1881), Wooster Beach (1794-1868), and John King (1813-1893) challenged the "heroic" doctors with their debilitating bleeding and massive doses of calomel and antimony. For them, this behemoth was unharnessed and running amuck across the therapeutic landscape, leaving in its wake a populace robbed very often not only of their livelihoods but of their lives by the very masters of this much-praised and prescribed "pachyderm."[9]

By the Civil War this movement of therapeutic iconoclasm had evolved from the Thomsonians into the physio-medicals under Curtis. Beach had long since faded away into obscurity in favor of John King, who had assumed the mantle of leadership for the Eclectic Medical Institute (EMI) of Cincinnati, chartered in 1845, the mecca of botanicism that would last well into the twentieth century. Arrayed with the botanics in their opposition to the heroic bleeding and purging of the regulars were the homeopaths. Their elegant minuscule-dose preparations and sophisticated-if-recondite like-cures-like doctrines appealed to some of America's wealthiest and most influential citizens.[10] Homeopathy, founded by German physician Samuel Hahnemann (1755-1843), was exported to New York City by Hans Gram, when he began his medical practice there in 1825. Homeopathy flourished and spread throughout the city. By 1844 the homeopaths of that city, and others such as Constantine Hering (1800-1880) of Pennsylvania, helped found a national institute. "After its initial period of spectacular growth in the 1840s and 50s," writes Francesco Cordasco, "homeopathy continued to compete with the orthodox profession both in terms of personnel and institutional activity."[11]

Thus by the mid-nineteenth century, American medicine had become an arena of professional animosity and therapeutic contention. Far from representing a hegemonic force in health and healing, regular practitioners were being challenged on almost every front—schools, societies and associations, and theory and practice had become emblematic of one's professional affiliations; all of these competing forces were vying for scientific respectability.[12]

Nowhere was this more evident than in therapeutics. The deleterious effects of persistent bleeding and massive dosing with toxic minerals such as mercury (most commonly in the form of calomel) and antimony (usually prescribed as tartar emetic) became matters around which all sectarians could agree. The *Eclectic Medical Journal,* official mouthpiece of the EMI, voiced the protests of many when it declared,

> Among all the absurd, irrational and fatal means made use of to restore the sick to health, there is none to compare with bloodletting. . . . In sickness we need all the strength and vital forces it is possible to command, and yet blood-letting is resorted to as a rapid method of depletion. Again, it is in violation of every law of physiology, and is never indicated by the natural efforts of the system to throw off disease.[13]

Although the regulars could argue that the practice of bleeding was in definite decline by the mid-nineteenth century, the same could not be claimed for mercury. "Of the poisons, among which the most injurious is mercury," charged eclectic physician G. Price Smith in 1855. "There is scarcely a disease now treated by Allopathic physicians," he added, "in which some preparation of mercury is not given; and what is worse, their text-books sanction this malpractice."[14] In contrast, Charles Wilkins Short (1794-1863), faculty member at Transylvania University's allopathic medical school, told his materia medica students that "none others equal in utility, excellence and universal employment the preparations of Mercury and Antimony, for without the aid derived from these giant remedies, our art would be stripped of its main resources."[15] William H. Cook (1832-1899), intellectual leader of the physio-medicals, explained in partisan terms the reasons for the regulars' preference for mercurous chloride:

> Probably no agent, whether of simple remedies or admitted poisons has ever received from the [allopathic] profession such universal and unqualified praise as calomel—subchloride of mercury. Among many admirable qualities ascribed to it, is that of inducing freer action of the liver, and thus securing a more abundant flow of bile and more regular movements of the bow-

els. We will admit that calomel favors such results. . . . But when it is claimed and admitted that calomel will induce these very advantageous results, only a *part* of the truth is stated. The *whole* truth includes the additional facts, that weariness of the liver always follows its stimulation by calomel; that congestion of it, with chronic enlargement and tenderness, *very* frequently ensues; and that hardening and abscesses, rather extensive abscesses, and even cancer of this organ, have often been found as ultimate consequences of the exhibition of this article.[16]

Cook essentially agreed with the diagnosis—torpid liver or biliousness was the source of most chronic disease. His argument was with the remedy. So physio-medicals, eclectics, and other sectarians attempted to adjust biliary secretions through the use of alternative cholagogues. Instead of calomel, many botanics prescribed Culver's root *(Leptandra virginica)* and mayapple *(Podophyllum peltatum)* to do the same thing. In fact, mayapple was so frequently used by eclectics where calomel was indicated that it received the dubious distinction of being called "vegetable calomel." Dr. Charles Hempel of the Homeopathic Medical College of Philadelphia recommended chamomile in numerous bilious complaints.[17]

Both the sectarians and the regulars were proceeding from two fundamental errors. The first error was diagnostic: the belief that improper liver function caused many diseases. This had a long tradition in medicine, a notion that was in some measure little more than a continuation of Galen's ancient concept of humoral imbalance.[18] Galen suggested that the liver was the source of veins and that it was the organ responsible for the manufacture of blood, thus making it a central feature of his humoral theory. William Harvey's 1628 work on the circulation of blood, *De motu cordis,* challenged this idea; however, this refined knowledge of liver function did not reduce the importance of that organ in the etiology of disease. Dr. James Johnson gave the conventional wisdom of the day in noting,

> The liver is the largest gland, or organ of any kind, in the human fabric. . . . Now, as the organ exists in almost every class of animals, even where other important viscera are very imperfectly developed, we may fairly conclude, that it answers some great purpose in the animal economy."[19]

This idea that the liver was the source of many illnesses led to the second fundamental error, which was therapeutic: the notion that an imbalance of biliary secretion was the root of the problem and that this could be manipulated through the administration of calomel or some vegetable substitute.[20] After recounting the many afflictions to which biliary imbalances could be ascribed, Johnson spoke for the regulars by declaring, "As an internal medicine, there is none which so steadily increases and meliorates the hepatic secretion as some of the mild preparations of mercury."[21]

This concept had been tested in animal experiments during the 1850s. The mounting evidence suggested that calomel, in fact, did *not* have any influence over biliary secretions, and in 1868 the Edinburgh Committee's report published by Dr. J. Hughes Bennett in *The British Medical Journal* thoroughly refuted the idea of calomel as a biliary stimulant. Nonetheless, the medical community's faith in calomel as a valuable cholagogue remained unshaken.[22] The persistence of this stubborn adherence to calomel derived from physicians' attachment to tradition and overreliance on empirical observation. The stools evacuated by a patient dosed with calomel were greenish in color due to the presence of biliverdin. This alone suggested increased hepatic activity, but what the nineteenth-century physicians did not know was that this greenish color resulted not from more bile production but rather from the antiseptic action of mercury, which did not allow the normal conversion of the bile pigment in the bowel due to its violent cathartic action. In short, the intestinal contents were discharged too rapidly for the biliverdin to convert normally into bilirubin.[23]

Unswervingly faithful to their medical forebears in bestowing the liver with major powers over the human constitution, and convinced that their eyes were not deceiving them, regulars remained steadfastly devoted to mercurous chloride as a significant weapon in their armamentarium.[24] The sectarians on the other hand often agreed with the diagnosis only to argue over the specific agents to be employed to achieve the desired result.

Specific lines of therapeutic demarcation between allopaths and sectarians were often distinguished by only *one* ingredient, such as mercury, with additional substances blurring into a sea of commonly prescribed plant-based drugs. The standard American pharmaceutical text for the period, Edward Parrish's *Introduction to Practical*

Pharmacy, recommended a compound cathartic pill made up of 1 grain of calomel augmented by some plant cathartics commonly used by eclectics: 1½ grain of colocynth, 1 grain of jalap or podophyllum (whichever was available), and one-fifth grain of gamboge. Parrish declared,

> Under the name of *anti-bilious pills,* this preparation is vended in great quantities over the country, and by its admirable combination of cathartic properties, is well adapted to supersede as a popular remedy, the numerous nostrums advertised and sold for similar purposes.[25]

It was within this context that therapeutic matters came to a head during the Civil War. Sectarians were clamoring for recognition of their "gentler" therapies; regulars were earnestly defending their "proven" remedies; *everyone* was convinced that the liver was of considerable importance as a source of systemic disease. Moreover, these convictions were not divided by region. Just as Northern physicians were convinced of the preeminence of the liver in the human constitution, so too were their Southern colleagues. It is no mistake that the longest article in the relatively short fourteen-issue history of the *Confederate States Medical and Surgical Journal* was a two-part essay by H. D. Schmidt titled "On the Microscopic Anatomy, Physiology, and Pathology of the Human Liver."[26] Schmidt believed the liver took on added importance in hot summer months, declaring,

> This organ, notwithstanding its participation with the other organs in the general relaxation of the system, and with scarcely sufficient ability to perform properly its own functions, is called on to assist the lungs in the elimination of carbon. In some cases it may succeed in performing the additional function, but in others a congestion of its blood vessels is the result. . . . Such a congestion, if persistent, gives rise to various complaints, as hemorrhoids, pain in the bowels, stomach, & c., and will even keep up an existing diarrhea or dysentery. The pain in the stomach or bowels is not acute, but, on the contrary, dull and heavy, resembling very closely the pain experienced in dyspepsia. A number of these cases has come under my observation, and I have cured them by relieving the congestion in the portal circulation.[27]

Undoubtedly, that "relief" came in the form of calomel.

Despite the long-standing tradition of these agents in the regulars' armamentarium, some members of the allopathic community had already reacted against the abuse of these substances and against heroic therapeutics in general. The medical elite of Massachusetts consisted of leading figures such as James Jackson, Oliver Wendell Holmes, and Jacob Bigelow—all of whom placed great faith in nature's ability to heal and became vocal proponents of therapeutic moderation. Indeed, Bigelow, echoing Molière more than 200 years earlier, suggested that most disease left alone without treatment of any kind was self-limited and would resolve itself.[28] During the war years some forward-thinking physicians such as James L. Brown were beginning to take the Bennett studies seriously and doubting the value of mercurials as biliary stimulants.[29]

But most practitioners remained steadfast in their use of mercurials and antimony.[30] All during the Civil War they remained important articles of allopathic practice and faith. Even so, noted authorities Charles S. Tripler and George C. Blackman recommended tartar emetic in treating dysentery in their *Handbook for the Military Surgeon*. Faced with a case of dysentery, they gave "at once a purgative dose of sulphate of magnesia ℥ j combined with ¼ to ½ a grain of tartar emetic."[31] Well after the war physicians continued to vehemently defend the use calomel in a variety of disorders.[32]

Calomel's War Casualty: William Hammond

The young, ambitious, and progressive Surgeon General William A. Hammond (1828-1900) had his own doubts about these heroic approaches to therapeutics. By spring of 1863, he had seen enough. Reacting to what he felt was the unbridled use of these substances among his medical corps surgeons, Hammond made a fateful decision to remove calomel and antimony from the standard supply table. In an order that was issued as Circular No. 6 on May 4, the Surgeon General "struck from the Supply Table" calomel and antimony because of their being "pushed to excess" and concluded that to keep either item available to the medical staff would be "a tacit invitation to its use" (see Appendix B).

The response of the sectarians and the regulars was swift. For the botanics, Hammond's order was heralded as a great leap forward for the healing arts. John King of the Eclectic Medical Institute spoke for many irregulars when he declared,

> For our part we are glad to see that our old school friends are advancing in the right direction, and feel satisfied that the order of the Surgeon General will hasten the day when mercurials will be entirely discarded in the treatment of disease.[33]

John King hit an especially sensitive professional nerve when he pointed out, "If the Old School discarded their poisonous minerals entirely, what will be the difference between them and the Eclectics . . . ?"[34]

King had made an important point, and the allopaths knew it. Dr. E. P. Bennett of Danbury, Connecticut, fumed,

> If I were an army surgeon, I should consider such an order as a direct impeachment of my capabilities, and offer my resignation at once. Besides, this order is calculated to bring these two important remedies into great disrepute with the public, and give aid and comfort to our enemies, the quacks.[35]

Calls for Hammond's removal from office soon followed. The committee formed by the American Medical Association to investigate Hammond concluded that Circular No. 6 was "entirely unwarranted" and constituted an "unmerited *insult*" that "this Association condemns, as unwise and unnecessary."[36]

Hammond was a bright and talented administrative reformer, but many of his reforms (needed though they were) incurred the wrath of his colleagues. In addition, Hammond had increasing disagreements with his superior, Secretary of War Edwin M. Stanton. Thus by 1864 Hammond had lost valuable support both within the Union medical corps and Lincoln's cabinet. The issuance of Circular No. 6 represented nothing short of professional treason. For most of his allopathic colleagues this was the last straw. On January 17, 1864, Hammond was arrested to face court-martial. The court preferred three charges against Hammond: (1) "Disorders and neglects to the prejudice of good order and military discipline"; (2) "Conduct unbecoming an officer"; and (3) "Conduct to the prejudice of good order and military discipline."[37] The chief complaint was that Hammond had "wrongfully and unlawfully, and with intent to favor private persons," ordered blankets from one Christopher C. Cox, an acting purveyor in

Baltimore, to receive blankets from William A. Stevens from New York.[38] In addition, he was charged with purchasing from John Wyeth, a Philadelphia College of Pharmacy graduate who—along with his brother F. H. Wyeth—ran a large and successful drugstore on Walnut Street in that city,[39] medical supplies allegedly "inferior in quality, deficient in quantity, and excessive in price."[40] The charges themselves were groundless and ably defended by the surgeon general, who pointed out that the "facts" of the case were "not set out or in any way shadowed forth by specifications."[41] Unfortunately, Hammond's energetic reforms, especially removing the old seniority system of promotion within the medical corps in favor of advancement based on merit, had lost him the support of his colleagues.

By summer, a weak and compliant review board found Hammond guilty, and he bid a reluctant farewell to the medical corps on August 22, 1864. He was succeeded by Joseph K. Barnes (1817-1883), who continued most of Hammond's programs, a tacit admission that his predecessor's troubles were due more to personality conflicts and political machinations than job performance.[42] Great Britain's medical community, which could assess the Hammond controversy objectively, gave a noteworthy response:

> Of course all the charges relating to purchases imply a fraudulent intent on Dr. Hammond's part, but when the prosecution failed in proving this it charged him with exceeding his authority. It appears to us that every one of the acts laid to his charge . . . comes within the ordinary duties of the head of the Army Medical Department. But Dr. Hammond was unlucky enough to fall out with Secretary Stanton.[43]

An official inquiry would later substantiate this observation. In 1878, a Senate Military Committee reviewed Hammond's court-martial and found that the charges stemmed largely from personal conflicts with Secretary of War Stanton and not from any dereliction of duty or improper conduct. It fully exonerated him, restored him to the U.S. Army, and appointed him to the rank of Brigadier General (retired).[44] But the damage had been done. "The old-guard's victory had long-lasting effects," writes historian George Worthington Adams. "As the older men began to get the important posts the best young men tended to leave the service. There was an end of new ideas, and after 1865 a partial relapse into ante-bellum lethargy."[45]

Hammond lost because his removal of calomel and antimony placed him directly in the therapeutic cross fire that persistently raged between allopaths and sectarians. But was Hammond's order even necessary? At least one historian sees Hammond's action as precipitous, arguing that Circular No. 6 failed to establish that calomel was so widely abused as to warrant its immediate removal.[46] Circular No. 6 also seems excessive given the conventional historical wisdom that the use of calomel and antimony was on the wane by the mid-nineteenth century.[47] Both these assertions, however, are questionable.

The evidence that calomel was not widely used and that neither calomel nor tartar emetic was viewed as indispensable by the army medical staff is based on the replies of sixty surgeons to a questionnaire circulated by Hammond concerning the use of these agents. The responses of this extremely limited sample are hardly unanimous in this regard, and it is unlikely that physicians were going to collectively admit to widespread therapeutic abuse. Whatever the value of the questionnaire, the results did not persuade the Surgeon General to rescind Circular No. 6.

Others in the medical corps substantiated the widespread use of calomel and antimony. Joseph Janvier Woodward stated that mercury was recommended "in purgative and in small repeated doses" and that "calomel figured prominently in the treatment of dysentery [one of the soldiers' chief complaints] both in the field and in general hospitals."[48] Dr. John Allard Jeancon (1836-1903), a fellow of London's Royal College of Surgeons of England and assistant surgeon in the 32nd Regiment Indiana Volunteers, investigated Hammond's charges of calomel abuse and gave an "elaborate representation of the evils resulting from the indiscriminate use of the drug" in a report supporting the circular.[49] Jeancon's observations may have been enough to cause his abandonment of regular practice, for in 1874 he joined the Eclectic Medical Institute (EMI) as chair of physiology and chemistry. Others concurred with Jeancon. "I may with no impropriety remark," wrote surgeon Charles H. Hughes of the Missouri First Infantry,

> that the melancholy results of the unrestricted administration of *calomel,* as complained of by the Surgeon General, are familiar to every army surgeon, or, at least, to such surgeons as were in the service any considerable length of time previous to the appearance of this order.[50]

It is interesting to note that although Hammond's most vocal opponents adamantly denied widespread abuse of calomel, the crux of their dispute was based on professional rather than therapeutic grounds, suggesting that perhaps the charges issued in the order had more than an air of truth.

The second question related to Circular No. 6 is even more interesting: Was the infamous "calomel circular" removing an agent already dying a natural death among physicians? One historian has made reference to "the marked diminution in its [calomel's] use during the first two-thirds of the century" and has conducted an elaborate discussion of this transformation on the medical profession.[51]

Reliable data suggests, however, that the therapeutic use of mercury was not declining. David Cowen and Donald Kent compared 958 prescriptions written by Burlington, New Jersey, physicians in 1854 with 800 prescriptions written by Kentucky physicians in 1887. The results were surprising: despite a dramatic falling off in the use of ipecac, virtually all other agents remained unchanged. In particular, from 1854 to 1887 mercury still ranked second only to opium and morphine in total number of prescriptions written, dropping a mere 3 percent throughout the period.[52] The Gathercoal study, one of the most extensive compilations of prescription behaviors, also supports the widespread use of calomel well past the Civil War. The Ebert survey, an Illinois-based study in 1885, shows that in 15,734 prescriptions, calomel was prescribed 450.7 times per 10,000 occurrences, ranking behind only quinine, morphine, potassium iodide, opium, and phenol out of over 1,000 ingredients examined.[53] In fact, the prescribing of calomel rose considerably from Ebert's 1895 figures to those in the Hallberg-Snow survey of 1907. Not until the Charters survey of 1926 and thereafter does calomel show a significant and sustained decline.[54]

The assumption of this agent's decreased importance in the allopathic armamentarium is based on records compiled by hospitals (most notably the Commercial Hospital of Cincinnati and Massachusetts General Hospital) and journal literature of that period. But if one physician in the 1840s was right, hospital practice in large cities, influenced very often by progressive faculty from nearby medical schools, did not reflect everyday practice. A Professor Webster of Geneva College warned those trained in big-city hospitals, let him [the newly trained physician] go home and commence practice among the yeomanry of his native town and he will soon find that he has a set of very different patients a different class of diseases and that [they] require a very different course of treatment from those he found in the hospitals.[55]

Even without Gathercoal's statistics this seems almost intuitively correct. Hospital practice was by its collectivist nature a higher-profile therapeutics, and the journal literature tended to reflect the cosmopolitan practices of a small elite rather than the care delivered by the "village Doc" who *may have* read the medical journals but had neither the time nor the inclination to contribute to them. Cowen and Kent's evidence and the Gathercoal study represent compelling benchmarks of what *really* went on in terms of therapeutics.

The point is that if Hammond's circular was an attack on allopathy's badges of professional practice, they were also badges with very real therapeutic meaning. Allopathic physicians called for Hammond's removal not on the basis of some theoretical abstraction and vague challenge to their professionalism; Hammond's order was stripping them of therapeutic agents that held a prominent place in their materia medica. What angered them most was that Circular No. 6 played into the hands of their enemies.

The calomel controversy was the "cathartic" climax to allopathic/sectarian contentions during the Civil War. Although the allopaths held the upper hand throughout the conflict, the one casualty of this professional rivalry was one of their own: William A. Hammond. Hammond had seriously miscalculated the lengths to which allopaths would defend their therapeutic faith, especially when it represented agents that so clearly defined their professional practice. It cost him his job, and it cost the Union Medical Department an able and progressive administrator.

But while calomel was working its mischief among the medical corps ranks, another medicinal substance, quinine, was taking hold like wildfire in field, camp, and hospital armamentaria. Physicians might argue over the virtues—real, imagined, or discounted—of calomel, but in the Civil War nearly every medical professional had elevated quinine to "most favored" remedy status.

QUININE: "ALWAYS AND EVERYWHERE"

John D. Billings, author of a stunningly detailed firsthand account of a soldier's life with the Army of the Potomac, wrote, "Quinine was always and everywhere prescribed with a confidence and freedom which left all other medicines far in the rear. Making all due allowances for exaggerations, that drug was unquestionably the popular dose with the doctors."[56] In hospital records, field prescription books, and therapeutic manuals and guides, quinine or cinchona (sometimes both) was doled out as a matter of course, whether on land or sea.

Sulfate and extract of cinchona were used essentially where quinine was indicated. Dr. William M. McPheeters had compared both sulfates in ninety cases of remittent and intermittent fevers and found cinchona "very little, if any, inferior to sulphate of quinia."[57] This, plus the unrelenting demand for quinine sulfate, suggested that preparations of cinchona might serve as a useful substitute or perhaps even as a coequal febrifuge with quinine. The board of revision for the U.S. Army supply table recommended that fluidextract of cinchona be made a standard item. Edward R. Squibb, who had served on the board, considered the preparation of red cinchona bark, calamus, sugar, and alcohol a tonic remedy "well adapted to the convalescence from typhoid and miasmatic diseases."[58] At the U.S. Army Laboratory in Philadelphia John Maisch manufactured 12,305 pounds of the product throughout the war.[59] This notwithstanding, the surgeon general's office reported that "sulphate of cinchonia was occasionally used during the war," but that the "opinion formed was unfavorable to its use."[60]

For most surgeons and hospital stewards, quinine sulfate was considered superior in strength and purity to other cinchona derivatives. In fact, the medicinal virtues of quinine hardly knew any therapeutic bounds. Quinine was used not only as a cure for fever and as a general enervating tonic—similar to but often regarded as more powerful and effective than stomach "bitters"—it was also used as prophylaxis for fever (see Figure 7.1). This came early in the war in the form of a recommendation by the U.S. Sanitary Commission. As a test, the commission issued to regimental surgeons, upon request, 220 gallons of solution of quinine sulfate in alcohol (quinine "bitters"), from which they reported "a marked improvement in the health and efficiency of the men."[61] Based on the recommendation of the Committee of In-

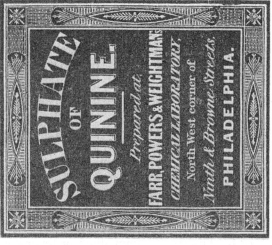

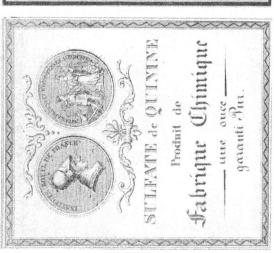

FIGURE 7.1. The discovery of quinine sulfate from cinchona bark in 1820 by the French chemists Pierre-Joseph Pelletier (1788-1842) and Joseph-Bienamé Caventou (1795-1877) became one of the therapeutic sensations of the century. Quinine sulfate was one of the few demonstrably effective drugs of the Civil War. Efficacious against malaria, it was often used indiscriminately for all fevers. By 1827 Pelletier and Caventou proudly announced that the use of quinine was sweeping Europe, with French manufacturers producing about 90,000 ounces annually. Although the French article was first preferred in the United States (above left), William Farr, along with Powers and Weightman, soon gave Americans a reliable domestic source for the much-prized medicine (above right), with Rosengarten and Sons soon to follow. Civil War demands would have Rosengarten and Sons and Powers and Weightman producing some nineteen tons of quinine sulfate from 1861 to 1865. Illustrations courtesy of Merck Archives, Merck & Co., Inc., Whitehouse Station, New Jersey.

quiry chaired by William H. Van Buren, the surgeon general ordered
that quinine and alcohol be distributed generally in the field, particularly where the miasmatic fevers where most feared (see Figure
7.2).[62] Soon, just about every hospital steward quickly became familiar with the bitter draught of quinine and alcohol (usually whisky but
sometimes wine or whatever "stimulant" could be had). Typical was
Edwin Witherby Brown, steward for his 81st Ohio Volunteer Infantry
unit, who noted in his diary while encamped near Corinth, Mississippi: "This was a malarial section and as a preventive I had to fix two
barrels of whiskey with quinine—take myself as well as give every
man in camp a dose every morning. In this way we prevented ague,
chills, etc."[63] Similarly, assistant surgeon George Martin Towbridge
of the 19th Michigan Volunteer Infantry noted the daily "Quinine call
which must be attended by Drs. as by men."[64]

Of course, fever and its prevention was not quinine's only use.
Charles Beneulyn Johnson mixed up whisky and quinine and administered the concoction to his Illinois comrades "for exhaustion."[65]
Billings observed that the "proverbial prescription of the average
army surgeon was quinine, whether for stomach or bowels, headache
or toothache, for a cough or for lameness, rheumatism or fever and

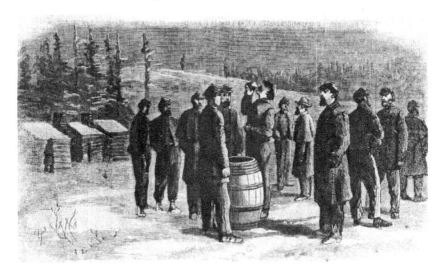

FIGURE 7.2. "Quinine call" was a familiar camp routine for the boys in blue, as
shown in this sketch from *Harper's Weekly* from March 15, 1865. Illustration
courtesy of the National Library of Medicine, History of Medicine Division.

ague."[66] Surgeon William Watson's affinity for quinine earned him the nickname "Old Quin" among the soldiers of the 105th Pennsylvania Volunteers.[67] The Seminole Wars in Florida that flared up between 1817 and 1855 with the intermittent regularity of the fevers to which its participants were prone was an excellent—and successful—proving ground for the army's use of quinine.[68] But quinine's demonstrable benefits in malarial conditions held an implicit danger in a medical era that could claim few genuine and consistent remedies. The real merits of quinine in malarial fevers undoubtedly caused many medical men to extrapolate rather wildly and assume that quinine and its derivatives of cinchona were a veritable panacea. Indeed, Dr. John W. Churchman pointed out that after calomel and whisky, the remedy most missed from the dispensary was quinine.[69] Churchman admitted "that a generation of practitioners had sprung up trained to transform their patient's mouths into funnels gapping for quinine."[70]

By the 1850s and 1860s quinine had reached its apex in the physician's armamentarium. *Cinchona* spp. were mentioned thirteen times among the primary list of substances in the *United States Pharmacopoeia* of 1850, twelve times in 1860, and thirteen times again in 1870.[71] *Cinchona* spp. covered nearly fifty pages in the 1858 edition of the *United States Dispensatory,* and ten pages were spent discussing three different preparations of quinine.[72] Never before or since were cinchona and quinine so prominently featured in the pharmaceutical compendia.

The therapeutic importance of quinine and cinchona forced the medical profession to explain its expansive therapeutic properties within the existing corpus of knowledge regarding health and healing. Here Dr. Frederick William Headland stepped up confidently to offer his opinion of quinine:

> It appears from the character and results of its medicinal influence, that it is exerted primarily in the blood, and not on the nerves [as Sir J. Martin and others had asserted]. It is included in the Restorative group of Haematics, and the general results of its action differ widely from those of a Catalytic Haematic. It produces no marked effect on the system in health [i.e., a healthy person]. Its operation consists in the cure of general debility, however produced, and in the prevention of periodic disorders in the blood. Debility depends on a want in the blood, and

not on any active morbid process; and there are circumstances which render it likely that Ague may be curable by the supply of a similar want.

Quinine is also serviceable in Gout, Srufula, Dyspepsia, and other disorders; in all of which other medicines, which stimulate the secretion of the bile, are more or less applicable. Torpidity of the liver is likewise a usual accompaniment of the various forms of debility, and occurs in intermittent, remittent, typhoid, and yellow fevers; in each of which this medicine has been recommended, and used with advantage. In fact it may be said, that in all diseases in which Quinine is used there is a failure in the secretion of bile; and in all diseases in which there is a failure in the secretion of bile, Quinine is serviceable.[73]

It was a view that undoubtedly caught the attention of the American medical community for several reasons. First, it accorded with what they already believed: namely, that biliary imbalance was the cause of most disease. To suggest that quinine corrected a disorder by adjusting bile secretion not only made sense to most practitioners, it had the additional benefit of seemingly substantiating the premise of bile's primacy in health. Second, it supported the notion that quinine was not only a specific in malarial fevers but was also a "restorative hæmatic" for a whole range of diseases only vaguely understood. Third, by wartime Headland had an established reputation on both sides of the Atlantic. He was a member of the Royal Society of Physicians and the London Medical Society, whose treatise on the action of medicines had received award-winning acclaim. The American pharmaceutical leader William Procter greeted the fourth edition of Headland's *Action of Medicines in the System* with considerable enthusiasm, stating that "few writers on this subject have kept closer to the inductive path that leads to ultimate success, and shown more acuteness in observation, than has our author."[74]

Of course it was the inductive method—the penchant for rationalism—that was the problem. Extending therapeutic benefits based on false premises, though logical in itself, had been the source of diagnostic and therapeutic error for centuries. The march of scientific empiricism, whereby hypotheses based on selected theories were checked by systematic observation under controlled conditions, was slow in coming and by the 1860s had not quite arrived.[75] Of course, Headland was correct about one thing: as explained earlier, quinine *does* work on blood (more accurately on the plasmodia invading the bloodstream). But since there was no clear understanding of microbial disease at that time, the rest of his ideas were theories built on the foundations of tradition rather than empirical demonstration. The only thing more absurd than Headland's notions concerning quinine would be to chide him for these notions. He and all of his colleagues were struggling to understand problems that had vexed humankind since time began. Galen sought to answer this problem of pathology and therapeutics in Roman times, and by Headland's writing the medical profession was on the brink of casting off the last vestiges his time-honored but flawed notions.[76] To consider nineteenth-century physicians naves, fools, or charlatans because they did not possess *our* knowledge of disease is the folly of twenty-twenty hindsight—unhistorical and unfair.

Yet the Civil War had an unintended benefit: it could serve as a practical proving ground for quinine just as the Seminole Wars had done. The experience with this remedy during those protracted but much smaller engagements in Florida was suggestive of certain dose-response relationships with fevers. The Civil War would be the *real* test. The problem of dosage was a difficult one. Even prophylactically, recommendations varied widely.[77] Since many physicians regarded quinine and cinchona as a tonic, they tended to keep doses relatively low but repeated. Dr. Thomas Fearn (1789-1863) of Huntsville, Alabama, on the other hand, had treated his fever patients successfully with large doses (twenty grains of quinine sulfate or more) and had advocated such during the Seminole Wars. The typical therapeutic dose of quinine sulfate came to be established at ten to twenty grains for intermittent fevers, and fifteen to twenty grains for remittent fevers.[78] The "typical" dose for intermittent fevers—three to five grains, four times per day—would suggest that the higher end of the scale probably produced the best results.[79]

Yet individual physicians undoubtedly adopted their own favored doses. In revisiting William F. Norris's case of Private Rial, it will be recalled that the surgeon fought his patient's postoperative fever with a prescription that contained quinine sulfate; the dosage he gave was thirty grains, three time per day.[80] Surgeon Ezra Read of the 21st Indiana Volunteers established twenty to forty grains as a "full dose" of quinine sulfate.[81] "I have frequently given quinine in twenty-grain doses since arriving at this place with the effect of a speedy arrest of the intermittent paroxysm," reported surgeon David Merritt of the 55th Pennsylvania Volunteers while stationed at Beaufort, South Carolina, "and then, by continuing the remedy in smaller doses, have been much gratified with the result."[82] Even in the so-called continued fevers, quinine was employed. Surgeon W. H. Thayer of the 14th New Hampshire Infantry gave daily doses of quinine sulfate in twelve, twenty, or sixty grains for cases of typhoid fever, depending on the severity of the attack.[83] Surgeon R. N. Barr, while in Summerville, Virginia, found the cases of fever in his Ohio unit especially obstinate. He complained:

> There has been a comparatively large number of fever cases, and what is peculiar, every case of illness of whatever character took . . . a typhoid form and yielded slowly to treatment. In most cases my reliance is on quinine, [with] whiskey or brandy in large and repeated doses.[84]

The problem of dosage was certain to be complicated by the mixed results obtained from such generalized use of the drug under so many different conditions of fever. A fatal dose of quinine is approximately eight grams (or 123.456 grains), so it can be seen from some of the previous examples that many soldiers received exceedingly high doses of the substance. Spread out over a period of time these doses might not produce death, but symptoms of cinchonism would likely have appeared (ringing in the ears, headache, nausea, and blurred vision). But even where dosages were within sound limits, the therapeutic results would be highly variable.[85] In genuine cases of malaria the drug would be very effective, working as a specific against the invading plasmodia and—in continued moderate doses—acting to prevent recurrence. In other fevers there might be some modest antipyretic action and some analgesic action but no cure.[86] Given all the problems associated with quinine, in the end it was clearly the one medicinal agent that worked against a known disease. In the words of historian Dale C. Smith, "Probably the Civil War helped remove any lingering doubts of American physicians concerning effective quinine dosage."[87]

Whatever the effects of quinine in practice, it was in much demand. A total of nineteen tons of quinine sulfate and nine-and-a-half tons of sulfate of cinchona in their various dosage forms were distributed by the Purveyor's Department.[88] A product of such high demand could net manufacturers sizeable profits. Where fortunes are to be made, an interesting story is always to be told.

THE QUININE MARKET

The single best historical barometer for the drug market of the Civil War era is the Market Report, issued annually by the American Pharmaceutical Association. Unfortunately, the Committee on the Drug Market was not formed until the association's tenth annual meeting in Philadelphia in 1862, after widespread dissatisfaction with its predecessor, the Committee on Adulterations.[89] The first report on the drug market would not be issued until 1863, with Edward R. Squibb as chair. Thus, we have no good source of information on market factors early in the war. But Squibb's report was predictably thorough and intriguing with regard to the quinine market:

> This appears above all others to be *the* "fancy" article of the market to which it belongs. The speculations and "corners" into which it has entered, and the amount of capital employed in its market management during the past two years would doubtless make a most curious history. Beyond all other articles, this has tempted outside persons to invest in it for speculation, and as such are generally easily frightened, they get "weak kneed," as it is called, and by selling out in a falling market, aid to depress it often to extremes upon which opposite extremes find surest basis. It is a curious circumstance alleged to be true, particularly with outside speculators, that they commonly overstand [sic] a rising market and miss the highest point, but will rarely pass through a depression without selling near the lowest point.[90]

Squibb's comments give an interesting glimpse into the volatile market conditions of a highly viable product, which quinine had become.

With a high-demand product such as quinine, Squibb's indications of speculation should not be surprising. But in 1906 John W. Churchman, a young clinical assistant at Johns Hopkins Hospital studying under Dr. Hugh Hampton Young, wrote an interesting—albeit scathing—analysis of the quinine market during the Civil War. The article is unfortunately not referenced, but the fact that the essay was issued at a time when many of the participants in those events were still alive also gives his essay added force. Churchman's accusations are so pointed and potentially damning that they require some in-depth investigation.

Churchman begins his review of quinine use by tracing the story of its development and rise in popularity as a virtual cure-all drug, topics that have been previously discussed and need not be recounted here. Churchman's record adds interesting detail to the story, but nothing new. His treatment of quinine's wartime market conditions, however, is another matter. He points out that during the war there were only two manufacturers of quinine: Powers and Weightman and Rosengarten and Sons. As we have seen, the process of making quinine sulfate came to both firms independently. John Farr (1791-1847) was the first to manufacture quinine sulfate in America, which he did under the firm name Farr and Kunzie in 1823. Thomas H. Powers and William Weightman became heirs to Farr's quinine sulfate process when they formed a partnership with him in 1837. The firm Farr, Powers, and Weightman lasted until the death of the senior partner ten years later. Quinine came to George D. Rosengarten through a Frenchman, N. F. H. Denis, who had studied under Robiquet, a chemist who, in turn, had undoubtedly learned of the process discovered by his colleagues Caventou and Pelletier in 1820. Rosengarten, with Denis heading his manufacturing department, was making quinine sulfate one year after Farr. Careful to guard the precise processes by which they made the product, Powers and Weightman and Rosengarten and Sons were the only two domestic firms to manufacture quinine sulfate commercially throughout the war.[91]

Armed with this fact, Churchman smells a conspiracy. He implies (without any hard evidence) that the two firms worked in collusion, "[a]nd before long the price of the drug ($2.10 per ounce at the outbreak of the war) was, by reason of this monopoly aided by certain economic conditions, soaring heavenward."[92] For Churchman, the 40 percent duty went beyond reasonable domestic protection. Only when the quinine tariff was lifted with the Dingley Bill in 1897 was this alleged "oppression" removed. Chief among villains was Weightman. William Weightman died on August 29, 1904, "the richest man in Pennsylvania."[93] In true Progessivist style, Churchman paints the portrait of a robber baron, finding little to praise in the industrial giant:

He was a singularly reserved man, a captain of industry, a practical scientist of rank; a man of sagacity, energy, and thrift, who amassed a fortune of at least $50,000,000 and died in the harness. Eminently fitted to serve the community he had little in common with it, finding his chief interests in the making of a fortune and the raising of chrysanthemums to a variety of which his name became attached. He owned more property in Philadelphia than the Pennsylvania or the Reading Railroads. The Garrick Theatre and the Hale Building—assessed at $2,000,000—were two of his holdings. He made it a point never to sell any of his properties—the only exception to this rule being the sale of the Bingham House, which brought him $1,000,000. The store of Darlington and Co. belonged to him; whole blocks in Philadelphia were his; and his personal property tax return for 1903-04 was over $5,000,000. Here we find, then, the resting place of the dollars that went for those 19 odd tons of quinine and of the many thousands of dollars that followed them when the monopoly established during the war lived on and grew fat . . .

But in estimating the price [of the Civil War], do not think only or chiefly of the life lost in the four unfortunate years. Remember as well the disability and debility they left behind them: and in considering the vast financial perplexities which came when reconstruction days began, do not overlook the quinine monopoly which the war had made possible but which a suffering people overthrew.[94]

Looking at the matter as a whole, some circumstantial evidence supports Churchman's allegations. First, two firms holding all domestic production of one high-demand drug during a time of war set the stage for all kinds of potential business chicanery. Second, it *is* known that Powers and Weightman, along with Millinckrodt and others, engaged in a bromine cartel in the late nineteenth century.[95] Third, it is suspicious that with all the demand for quinine sulfate, the U.S. Army Laboratory never produced a drop. Even historian George Winston Smith wondered about this "singular fact."[96] Yet Smith could find no "clandestine arrangements" between the two firms and the Army Medical Department. Hammond seriously considered having the Philadelphia plant try its hand at producing the precious article; as soon as word got out that the government might start production, the price plummeted 33 percent.[97]

Yet allegations of corruption—even in the historical bar of jus-tice—need more than circumstance for proof. Maisch examined the problem of quinine sulfate manufacture in a report submitted on April 17, 1863, and decided against the proposal because of unreli-able cinchona bark supplies and the fact that it would not be economi-cally advantageous for the government to pay the existing manufac-turers higher prices for bark already in their hands. In addition, Maisch noted the start-up costs of machinery and equipment in order to begin production, which might even include the necessity of con-structing or at least procuring another building.[98]

Maisch's analysis seems reasonable on the face of it, and there is no reason to assume any undue outside pressures (financial or other-wise) for him to have rendered it. But there are other reasons to argue against a conspiratorial oligopoly such as the one described by Church-man. Although it is true that Powers and Weightman made huge sums of money in the manufacture of wartime quinine, being uniquely well positioned during a particularly advantageous time and making a profit is not a crime. If Powers and Weightman and Rosengarten and Sons engaged in business practices that would be considered illegal by today's standards (and there is no evidence of that), the historian is still hard-pressed to indict them on rules and regulations unknown and unpracticed in their day. Yet Churchman's assertions suggest a certain degree of price-gouging unacceptable by even nineteenth-century standards. It should be noted in this regard that Squibb, him-self a manufacturer and one who had little financial interest in quinine, did not chide his colleagues for gouging. In fact, Squibb states in his Market Report of 1863 that "manufacturers cannot sell it [quinine sulfate] at fair profit below $2.87" and that the item's high- and low-end prices were due to speculators.[99]

Furthermore, it will be recalled that Squibb attributed this specula-tion to "outside persons," meaning no doubt persons *not* associated with drug manufacturing. Price alone does not determine conclu-sively that there was no collusion on the part of the principal manu-facturers, but it surely is one indicator. Figure 7.3 shows the highest annual quinine sulfate prices per ounce for the period. It can readily be seen that although there is a modest rise during the war years, this can easily be attributed to normal wartime demands. Whatever else may be said about prices, they certainly were *not* "soaring heaven-ward."

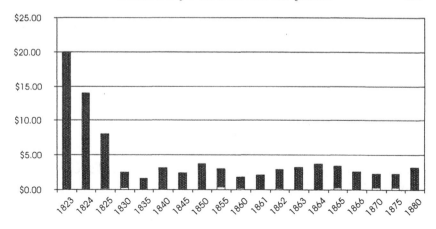

FIGURE 7.3. Quinine Market by Highest Annual Prices, 1823-1880 (*Source:* "Table of Prices of Quinine Since 1823," *Pharmaceutical Era* [October 15, 1891]: 238, and Joseph W. England, "The American Manufacture of Quinine Sulphate," *American Journal of Pharmacy* 102 [1930]: 707).

One final piece to this puzzle is worth mentioning. In 1907 Rene Leon de Milhau presented a paper for the American Pharmaceutical Association in which he provided a biography of his pharmacist grandfather, John Milhau. Described by his grandson as a "public-spirited man of the highest type," Milhau rose to become director of a large New York bank and was therefore in a position to thwart "a band of speculators who were demanding, with good prospects of getting, 33 percent. During the entire war, he kept close watch over the quinine market, defeating every attempt to corner the drug."[100]

The final word may not have been written on the quinine story during the Civil War. Evidence yet to be discovered may bring new light to the subject. But the present conclusion must be against any machinations on the part of Powers and Weightman or Rosengarten and Sons in manipulating the prices of quinine sulfate during or even after the war. In order for them to have effectively controlled (much less *manipulated*) prices as suggested by Churchman, they would have had to been able to dominate the supplies of South American cinchona bark. With plenty of international competition from Britain, France, and Germany, this assumes power neither firm possessed. Both companies were probably content to supply burgeoning domestic needs with the protective duty in place and prices relatively stable; their greatest enemies were the outside speculators who, left unchecked, could make the crude drug prices highly unpredictable. Conditions do not always equal crime, and the imputation of impropriety does not make it so.

SUMMARY

Calomel and quinine are representative of medicinal agents at two extremes. On the one hand, calomel, an age-old remedy, came to epitomize the regular profession so much that to remove it from the standard supply table was viewed as an attack on the profession itself. The fact that it cost the career of so enterprising a surgeon general as William A. Hammond shows how ossified and tradition-bound the medical profession and military had become. On the other hand, quinine sulfate was the very opposite of calomel. Although cinchona had been around for quite a while, its sulfate cousin was comparatively new and really seemed to work in reducing fevers. As a result, quinine helped create industry giants and encouraged production on an unprecedented scale.

Yet quinine, perhaps more than any other medicinal substance, showed the power of Northern industry over the South. Without any assistance from government laboratories or foreign imports, two firms supplied the most prescribed drug for a huge standing army. The South could not have hoped to duplicate this feat of mass manufacturing. When it received quinine it was largely through smuggling or the capture of Northern supplies.

The Confederacy had its own standing army to provide for, and it had its own administrative structure and system in place to answer those medicinal needs. But it had its own special problems too. Lacking the industrial infrastructure of the North, and saddled with a stifling blockade of its coast and port cities, the drug story in the South is one of ingenuity and even daring.

PART III:
PHARMACY IN THE CONFEDERACY

Chapter 8

Administration

The record of Confederate medical administration is a mixed one. Unlike the old, tradition-bound Medical Department of the Union army, the Confederacy had an advantage in being able to start from scratch. Surgeon General Samuel Preston Moore could be overbearing, officious, and obsessive over details, regulations, and protocols, but at the same time he had all those attributes essential to an able administrator: focused, methodical, confident, innovative, and doggedly determined in the face of adversity. With Moore at the helm, an administrative structure was established to provide and distribute medicines to large and widely disbursed forces; this structure was copied largely from that of the North, without the latter's ossified adherence to tradition and a system of promotion based on seniority rather than merit. Despite poor transportation, a blockade of every major Southern port that placed a stranglehold on foreign imports, and an inflationary spiral in medical supply prices, the Confederacy attempted to meet these formidable challenges with improvisation and resolve. At times, however, the administrative structure itself impeded the process of getting medicines to the troops by requiring needless paperwork and protocols. Given all the challenges facing Moore's department, it is a wonder that it could maintain service as well and as long as it did.

CIVILIAN ASPECTS OF CONFEDERATE PHARMACY ADMINISTRATION

Before discussing the military aspects of pharmaceutical care, it is a significant fact that the Southern war for independence would tax the resources of the region to its limit and beyond. The Confederacy understood that it had a dual responsibility to care not only for its large standing army and smaller but crucial navy but also its civilian population. The larger and richer economies of the North permitted civilian health care to proceed independently of the war effort; not so in the South. In recognition of this fact, the Confederate War Department, through an Exemption Act, permitted certain pharmacists to remain in their communities as druggists and primary caregivers. A provision of the 1862 Conscription Act exempted from military service "in each apothecary store now established and doing business, one apothecary in good standing, who is a practical druggist."[1] The law was designed to keep some modicum of health care available to civilians whose towns and villages found themselves without physicians or druggists of any kind. Yet abuses occurred, as men seeking to avoid military duty set up bogus stores with some bottles of castor oil and a few boxes of patent medicines.[2] In 1864 the law was changed to snare these draft dodgers by stipulating that applicants for exemption as pharmacists had to have been "doing business as such apothecary on the tenth day of October, 1862, and had continued said business, without intermission, since that period."[3]

Yet there were other pharmacists who did *not* use the exemption clause to avoid military service and asked for it only as a last resort. Consider the case of pharmacist William E. Besson of Eufaula, Alabama. The Secretary of War appointed Besson hospital steward of the Eufaula Light Artillery late in 1862.[4] By 1864, however, Besson received word that his drugstore could no longer be managed by his partner, curiously "an invalid widow [his mother?]" who had become ill.[5] The townspeople pleaded as hard for Besson's case as Besson himself.

> We . . . certify that the said W. E. Besson volunteered in the Confederate Service before the passage of the Act, exempting apothecaries, and has been in said service ever since. That his partner in the Drug business is a widow lady of feeble health, whose only son is, and has been in the service since the commencement of the War, and that it is almost a physical impossibility to get any one suitable to carry on the said Drug business.

Seven Eufaula citizens signed the letter; two of them, interestingly enough, were physicians.[6] Besson, and undoubtedly many others like him, received the discharge.

Many other situations were to affect civilian pharmacy throughout the war: poor and deteriorating transportation, increasing inflation, and worsening drug shortages. These, however, are best handled separate from administrative issues, since they were primarily part of the exigencies of war. But as pharmacists sought to deal with these difficulties, many more of their colleagues were struggling to provide pharmacy care in military camps and hospitals under even more trying circumstances; these were the medical purveyors and hospital stewards of the Confederacy.

MEDICAL PURVEYORS AND HOSPITAL STEWARDS

The Medical Department of the Confederacy was enacted by law on February 26, 1861, and grew, in historian H. H. Cunningham's words, into "[a] rather impressive medical organization" that included a surgeon general's staff of six officers, eighteen medical directors in the field, eight medical directors of hospitals, seven hospital inspectors, and five medical boards charged with examining candidates for appointments as assistant surgeons and for promotions from assistant to full surgeon.[7] It has been estimated that 834 surgeons and 1,668 assistant surgeons cared for 673 regiments; at sea, the entire Confederate navy had a total of seventy-three medical officers.[8] When the 154 principal hospitals serving the Confederate army are added to these numbers in the field, a survey of the United Confederate Veterans in 1892 determined that the entire medical corps comprised less than 3,000.[9] Despite the many challenges posed by a system cobbled together out of necessity on comparatively short notice (and the many difficulties of supply and distribution that plagued the department as the war lengthened), the surgeons and assistant surgeons of the Confederacy, according to one historian, "met the demands imposed upon them as courageously and as effectively as could have been expected."[10]

In terms of pharmacy, the backbone of supply, distribution, and compounding of medicines resided, as with the U.S. Army, with the purveying department and hospital stewards. Stewards were the foot soldiers of pharmaceutical care, compounding prescriptions and delivering medicines directly to the men under their charge. They were authorized by act of Confederate Congress on May 16, 1861, to be employed "as the service may require"[11] and had comparable rank and pay to Union stewards. Hospital storekeepers, "not to exceed six," were established with duties and responsibilities also similar to their Northern counterparts.[12] It should be pointed out that the structure, requirements, duties, responsibilities, and character of the Confederate medical supply and distribution system mirrored that of the North. Just as its Union counterpart, the position of storekeeper never gained much standing or importance in the overall Medical Department organization. And as for hospital stewards, although they held the rank of sergeant and were expected to have a sound knowledge of the apothecary art just as those of the North, many found themselves in the position merely as the commanding officer's most expedient choice under the prevailing circumstances.

Whereas the steward provided the most immediate pharmacy care to the men in the field, it was the medical purveyor's responsibility to acquire and maintain adequate supplies at the depot, from which field and hospital supply tables were filled and replenished. This was no small job. The Medical Department earnestly tried to set down clear guidelines for an efficient purveying system. Circular No. 3 laid out the administrative structure for the medical purveyors.[13] It consisted of nine districts, with Edward W. Johns assuming an unofficial role as lead purveyor in Richmond, Virginia. Below these were another nine field purveyors stationed throughout the South (for details, see Appendix D). The "undersigned" signature is absent in the original holographic transcript, but presumably it was issued by Edward W. Johns and endorsed by Samuel Preston Moore.

This circular not only speaks to the general structure of the purveyor's department but also to the urgency felt by the medical leadership in terms of drug scarcity and the viability of native plant substitutes for medicines increasingly difficult to obtain from foreign sources. Much more about this will be said in Chapter 10, but suffice it to say that at least on paper a working purveying system was put into place.

The number of purveying depots continued to expand as the war prolonged; by November 1864 a total of thirty-two depots and field purveyors stretched from Richmond to San Antonio.[14] The purveyors were important not only because they had to purchase and distribute all medical stores but also because they were the men through which virtually *all* Confederate appropriations for the Medical Department passed. Purveyors were required to write quarterly, and later monthly, reports indicating the funds necessary for their purchasing activities. Once reviewed and approved by the surgeon general's office, these reports (essentially requests for funds) went on to the Treasury Department.[15] That large Treasury warrants were needed for this all-important medical function can be seen in a sampling of requisitions placed by an assortment of purveyors. Surgeon Potts of Jackson, Mississippi, asked for $300,000 for the third quarter of 1862, and by April 1864 he asked for twice that amount; surgeon Prioleau in Savannah asked for $150,000 to cover fourth-quarter expenses in 1862, and, as with Potts, wartime inflation and drug scarcity had him quadrupling the amount requested in 1864; in Columbia, South Carolina, surgeon J. Julian Chisolm (1830-1903) (Figure 8.1) asked for and received the single-largest Confederate warrant for medical supplies, over $850,000, issued on April 13, 1864.[16] Naval records are sketchier, but from July 1861 to September 1863, the Treasury Department issued forty-two warrants totaling about $200,500 for navy medical supplies.[17]

These sums, coming as they did out of a limited Confederate war chest, speak to the central role of the medical purveyors in the South's military economy. The entire nation itself could collapse under an inefficient administration of the Purveyor's Department, or worse, un-

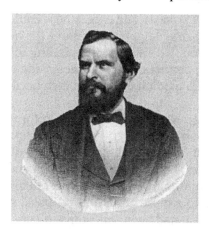

FIGURE 8.1. Surgeon J. Julian Chisolm ran a Confederate laboratory at Columbia, South Carolina, and was one of the South's most important medical purveyors. Photo courtesy of the National Library of Medicine, History of Medicine Division.

der a system prone to corruption and malfeasance. Fortunately, there were few examples of the latter. Although examples of speculation and profiteering can be found, they were not epidemic. A congressional investigation early in the war into the operations of the Medical Department commended the surgeon general and his staff.[18] The committee found "no want of power for its efficiency, and, except in a few particulars, no necessity for a change in the regulations which control it."[19] Committee Chair T. N. Waul also noted, however, that the supply of medical stores were generally "incomplete and insufficient in many of the leading and necessary articles for the prevailing diseases"[20] but that this was due to the admittedly stifling effects of the Union blockade and the utter inability of the department to obtain reliable imported medicine supplies.[21] Nevertheless, the committee's findings were not completely glowing. It concluded, "The health, comfort, and efficiency of the Army results less from defects in legislation than in the proper enforcement of the Regulations and regular and thorough system of inspection."[22] The report serves to show that the huge and far-flung purveying network was even more than the officious Moore could always handle, and these summary comments probably did little to ameliorate that side of his character. Still, Moore did unquestionably instill and inspire a sense of loyalty and self-sacrifice to The Cause.

But no amount of honesty and earnestness could satisfy the relentless need for steady drug supplies or relieve the heavy burden on the public coffers. Table 8.1 illustrates the spiraling inflation that plagued the South as the war continued and the increasing costs of the medical corps, particularly in medicines and the men needed to maintain and dispense them.

These escalating costs brought system-reforming efforts by the Confederate leadership who recognized the importance of the Purveyor's Department. A proposal for the closure of the purveyor's office caused Jefferson Davis to "fear the unfortunate consequences" of such an act, and on March 7, 1863, he referred his Secretary of War, James A. Seddon, to a more ambitious proposal suggested in an unsigned document that had been sent some months before to the Confederate president. In outlining the deficiencies of the purveyor's office as then constructed, it made three main points:[23] (1) the functions of the Medical Department and the purveyors were really separate and distinct; (2) a "unity of plan and action" regarding medical sup-

TABLE 8.1. Confederate Appropriations for Medical Supplies and Pharmacy Personnel

Appropriation	1862	1863	1864	1865	Hospital Stewards
Fiscal year ending February 18, 1862	$350,000	–	–	–	–
February 18 to April 1, 1862	$120,000	–	–	–	–
April 1 to November 30, 1862	$2,400,000	–	–	–	–
December 1 to December 31, 1862	$400,000	–	–	–	–
January 1 to January 31, 1863	–	$400,000	–	–	$12,000
February 1 to June 30, 1863	–	$3,500,000	–	–	$60,000
Fiscal year ending June 30, 1864	–	$15,420,000	–	–	$100,000
July 1 to December 31, 1864	–	–	$14,820,000	–	$100,000
Estimates of funds required for 1865	–	–	–	$16,000,000	$200,000
Totals	$3,270,000	$19,320,000	$14,820,000	$16,000,000	$472,000
Grand total	–	–	–	–	$53,882,000

Source: The War of the Rebellion: A Compilation of the Official Records of the Union and Confederate Armies (Washington: GPO, 1900), Series 4, Volume 1: pp. 339, 939, 1045; Series 4, Volume 2: pp. 112, 120, 392; Series 4, Volume 3: pp. 139, 480, 1111. *Note:* Changes in reporting methods make much of the data incomplete. Hospital steward allocations, for example, are probably included in the report for April-November 1862, and the figure (though not stated) for the month of December 1862 was likely $12,000 as in the following month. Although these figures undoubtedly include some nonpharmaceutical items (e.g., hospital bedding, surgical equipment, etc.), much of these reflect the manufacture and procurement costs of the materia medica. Figures are exclusive of funds for the establishment and maintenance of hospitals, physician's salaries, and ancillary personnel (e.g., laundresses, cooks, nurses, etc.).

ply is prevented by requiring the surgeon general to be responsible for a function he knows little about; and (3) purveyors at principal depots have "but limited control over the other purveyors" and the "interference of a third party [i.e., the surgeon general] cannot but lead to confusion."[24] The solution was to be found in the establishment of a purveyor general and an assistant to oversee all purveying operations.[25] Because the vast majority of medical stores in both quantity and value had to deal with pharmaceuticals, the proposal is not unlike one suggested after the war in the North for an apothecary general. The idea, intriguing as it seems, was apparently never adopted. As difficulties in procuring supplies and transporting them became increasingly severe and the resources of the Confederacy strained, administrative experiments no matter how justifiable were just too impractical and costly to implement. Besides, the suggestion was very likely to incur the wrath of Moore, who would certainly have viewed the new position as an unwelcome intrusion over areas of his administrative domain.

It is *not* that some such or similar position was not needed. The administrative structure of the purveyor's office could be rigid and counterproductive. Surgeons were required to order their drug supplies on forms designed for that purpose and then submit them in duplicate—one copy going to the purveyor and the other to the surgeon general's office—and woe to the surgeon who failed to comply or properly fill out the requisite paperwork.[26]

Problems could particularly arise when rules were changed. For example, when Surgeon General Moore issued an order in March 1862 requiring that medical supplies be requisitioned in one-month instead of three-month quantities, confusion reigned and real suffering ensued.[27] Writing desperately to William H. Prioleau in Savannah, surgeon W. S. Lawton of the 2nd Georgia Cavalry called the purveyor's attention to

> a requisition for medicines sent in by me nearly a month ago and recently corrected and returned to you. The supply of medicines at the post is almost gone on account of this delay and I must urgently call your attention to the matter as my patients have already suffered for the want of medicines. Lt. Moore, our quarter master, will take charge of the transportation of these supplies.[28]

Four months later things had not improved. Surgeon I. L. Harris Jr. of the 55th Georgia Volunteers complained on August 7, 1862, that for a whole week he had "not a grain" of quinine because his supply form was returned to him unfilled. The reason stated on the returned form was that Harris requisitioned a three-month quantity instead of the one-month quantity mandated back in March. The purveyor also noted that there was no accompanying duplicate. But forms distribution apparently did not keep pace with the surgeon general's new orders. Harris, obviously angered over an incident that could have easily been corrected by the purveyor's adjusting the quantity and pointing out the procedure to be followed in the future, pleaded his case:

> I sent the duplicate. I sent the duplicate as I have been directed heretofore by the next mail. . . . Had I been furnished with a supply table for one month or been notified that I could obtain only

a month's supply I would have used it, instead of the three month's furnished me and the sick would not have been suffering for want of some of the articles.[29]

These were not the only ones to complain. Even Samuel H. Stout, medical director of the Army of the Tennessee, admitted, "that [because of] the want of prompt action by purveyors, quartermasters, and commissaries unnecessary suffering was experienced by the soldiers in consequence of their rigid adherence to the *red tape* routine of the regulations."[30]

ADMINISTRATIVE ASPECTS
OF SUPPLY AND DRUG PROVISION

The previous example illustrates one important fact in regard to drug supply and provision: the ability of the surgeon in the field to minister to sick and wounded men in the field and hospital was directly dependent on the administrative effectiveness of the supply and provisioning system. Although considerable praise has been heaped on Moore and his Medical Department,[31] much of which is deserved, experiences such as those of surgeons Lawton and Harris lowers the estimation of the South's purveying system.[32] Confusion as to the proper requisitioning of supplies was not uncommon, as demonstrated in this plaintive report to surgeon Joseph P. Logan, medical officer in charge of the Atlanta hospitals:

> Sir.—I am entirely out of medicine and made a requisition yesterday on the Quartermaster for a supply. When he was about to purchase it some one came up and said he was a Medical Purveyor and that the Government would not pay for medicines bought by a Qr. Master [sic] when there was a Purveyor near. Is there a Purveyor in Savannah? If there is, why does he keep it a secret from us? I made a requisition on the Purveyor on the 19th Jan. on the Purveyor of this department in Charleston and did not have it filled until the 9th of March, and then there was not one-third of the articles required. If the government has prohibited Q. Masters from purchasing please inform me that I may try

the Savannah Purveyor. Be kind enough to give me the name that I may get a supply at once.

Respectfully yours,

L. H. Lansar
Asst. Surgeon of Ga. Battalion[33]

It was not just procedural confusion that plagued the purveying system; there could even be some question as to who exactly was in charge. As mentioned previously, Edward W. Johns assumed the position of "chief purveyor," and when Prioleau questioned some orders issued therefrom, he was told to comply by the assistant adjutant general, who confirmed both the rank and authority of Johns.[34] When Prioleau appealed to the surgeon general, he was told that a chief purveyor's position did not exist and that the final word on all orders were to come from his office.[35] Six months later Moore would officially assume this status for himself.[36]

Sometimes evidence of gross incompetence surfaced, as when assistant surgeon and field purveyor John C. Stickney complained to the purveyor in Atlanta,

> I assure you it is as disagreeable to me to be compelled to note these differences as it is unpleasant for you to hear of them. I do wish sincerely I could say "All right," but there will be mistakes with the best. I found the Morphine in 28 gr. bottles, and one tin box (Gray's Ointment) marked 32 grs. of Morphine. I weighted contents. I found only 16 grs. there was but one box. The ink I found was in (7) seven store bottles, each labled 16 oz. and two vials with 2 oz. in each. I measured two of the store bottles which were full; in one I found 12½ ozs. in the other there were 11½ ozs. so I averaged them 12 ozs.—according to the labels there would have been 116 oz. in all. I tend to these things myself.[37]

By late 1863 there are clear indications that serious drug shortages were beginning to be felt. This, coupled with administrative bungling earlier in the war, led Lafayette Guild (1826-1870), the medical director of the Army of Northern Virginia, to adopt a defensive posture with his medical staff:

The supply of medl. [sic] & Hspl. [sic] Stores in the Confederacy is very limited. Medical Purveyors fully appreciate the importance of not wastfully using these supplies, and are strictly governed by order and regulations from higher authority as well as by the imperative necessity of economizing and justly apportioning the cause.

The present Field Supply Table, chanced to regulate the monthly allowance of medicines to a Regiment [illegible], therefore, in all cases [must] be rigidly adhered to without great detriment to the Public service.

Another great embarrassment under which the Medical Purveyor's Office labors results from the extreme scarcity of proper vessels in which to transmit medical supplies, such as jars, vials & glass stoppered bottles, for lack of which, articles called for are sometimes withheld, although on hand at the Purveying Depot. Medical Officers are, therefore, directed to turn over to the Medical Purveyor such empty vials, bottles, jars, jugs, etc. in their possession for which they may have no use.

Various complaints have been made to this office against the Medical Purveyors, which upon investigation have proved groundless and frivolous in their character. All officers in this army are responsible for any dereliction of duty and there is always a way to punish the delinquent.

Hereafter where complaints are made they should be placed in some tangible form. The officer preferring charges against a brother officer should at the same time recollect that if the charges be frivolous and malicious he himself can be subjected to punishment.

In order to enable the Med. Purveyor to apportion firmly the Medical supplies among the different Regiments, attention is called to the "Letter of Instructions" issued from this office on the 19th of January 1863, a non compliance with which has probably given rise to the disaffection among the complaining Surgeons.

Medical Officers are instructed to economize the Stimulants, Chloroform, Morphine, Dressings, etc. issued to their monthly requisitions in order to avoid encroachment upon the supply reserved for the use of the Field Infirmaries.

> The harmonious cooperation of Medical Officers with the Medical Purveyor in his efforts to meet the arduous duties resting upon him will greatly increase the efficiency of his Department and of our whole Corps.[38]

Guild was trying to soften the criticism by ascribing the complaint to a single order, but the record shows that problems with filling orders in a timely and efficient manner were problematic from the beginning. Drug shortages only exacerbated the problem *and* exasperated the surgeons, assistant surgeons, and hospital stewards who had to watch their men suffer for it.

The problems did not entirely reside with the purveyors. Difficulty also came from the nature of the Confederate government itself. The lessons learned by the delegates at Philadelphia's Constitutional Convention about a weak and ineffective confederacy of states were not impressed upon the Southern leadership. As if the South did not have enough handicaps, interstate cooperation that was assumed as a matter of course in the Union war effort was a constant challenge south of the Mason-Dixon. As one recent historian of the Confederacy has pointed out,

> the crisis of being a nation at war for its life, especially a new nation lacking many of the inertial traditions of custom and habit in federal-state relations, led to one contention after another. . . . Overwhelmingly, the occasions grew out of national military policy, chiefly enlistments and conscription, and procurement of supplies, and they began early and escalated.[39]

Medical supplies were not immune. Of all the medicinal substances, probably the single most prescribed was alcohol, which was useful not only as a "stimulant" remedy but also as a solvent and suspension medium for other drugs. The inability to obtain alcohol could have disastrous results, since no tincture or fluidextract could be compounded without it. Yet the war brought an even more urgent need for alcohol. Our guide to the materia medica, Dr. Alfred Stillé, stated the conventional wisdom of his colleagues when he insisted that alcohol

> is frequently required to relieve *temporary debility* of the system. This is strikingly the case after grave accidents, particularly where the tissues are crushed, and also during severe

surgical operations; under such circumstances these liquors eminently deserve the name of *cordials,* and prevent that sinking of the courage which may end in fatal syncope.[40]

There were a lot of "grave accidents" to attend to in the field. Add to this the general notion that alcohol could serve as a stimulating tonic, and there was in an assortment of liquors a virtual panacea of the medicine chest and supply table.[41] Imagine, then, the consternation of T. C. Howard, who found his efforts to obtain the much-needed article for Richmond blocked by his very own state of Georgia. Writing in exasperation to George Blackie in Atlanta, Howard stated that he had already informed purveyor Johns in Richmond that the governor and legislature of Georgia

> had by the most stringent and occatious [audacious?] hindrances made a compliance on my part with the terms of my contract to deliver the one thousand btls. of Whiskey or any part thereof an utter impossibility. Of this fact I gave the proper department due notice in a letter to Dr. Johns enclosing the Govt. Proclamation and the law of the Gen'l Assembly.[42]

Howard sent an agent to plead the harm this decision was doing to the Confederacy but was told he could argue his case in court. Howard further stated that the law passed by the Georgia legislature

> practically annulled any outstanding contract, changing the pay, etc. It stipulated for *an oath* on the part of the contractor, that the grain used by him in supplying the Govt. should *not be raised short of 20 miles of a Rail Road* [emphasis in the original], besides much foolery of the same sort.[43]

Howard, in disgust, turned the contract over to E. M. Bruce of Chattanooga, Tennessee, apparently giving up all hope of making any profit in the matter.

Problems with state governments and the procurement of alcohol for medicinal purposes reared up again early in 1864, when Moore had to remind Governor Vance of North Carolina that the distillery operating in that state belonged not to the Governor but to the Confederate Medical Department. Vance's insistence that North Carolina could provide liquor to Moore's office under contract brought an angry reply of clarification to the secretary of war:

> [T]he Medical Department has no contract for alcoholic stimu-lants in the State of North Carolina. The distillery at Salisbury referred to by Governor Vance is owned by the Medical Depart-ment and is engaged in the manufacture of whisky and alcohol for the sole use of the sick and wounded of the Army. This dis-tillery was purchased by this department for the purpose of dis-pensing with the system of contracting for alcoholic stimulants, as it has been found that a large quantity of whisky manufac-tured by contractors is of an inferior quality, and their contracts were not in other respects faithfully complied with. It is also be-lieved that a large quantity of the whisky made by contractors has been sold to private parties when it should have been deliv-ered to the Government. . . .
>
> The Attorney-General has decided that the Confederate Gov-ernment has the express power to support armies; that any means may be used which are necessary and proper to obtain supplies for that support. . . . In conclusion I would state that it is absolutely necessary for the comfort and welfare of the sick and wounded of our Army that the Government distillery at Salis-bury should not be interfered with or the supply of grain cut off.[44]

These incidents show a fatal flaw in the Confederacy itself. States, concerned for their own supplies, could essentially legislate away any national need, no matter how pressing. The law described by Howard was clearly designed to do precisely what it did, namely, "annul any outstanding contract." The administrative battle between Governor Vance and Surgeon General Moore shows that state interests were not always one with national requirements. In a bitter twist of irony that echoed Lincoln's 1858 speech, the South had become its own "house divided against itself," and it was most apparent in its procurement of medical supplies.

Lacking funds, a manufacturing infrastructure, reliable outlets for procurement, even a unified government through which they could operate, the accomplishments of the purveyors were remarkable and, at times, ingenious. The operations of the Confederate laboratories will be examined in Chapter 9, but it should be stated here that the purveyors' skills were most noteworthy in their efforts at manufacturing certain medicinal items. On the eve of Gettysburg, for example, the surgeon general announced that J. Julian Chisolm had commenced the manufacture of blue mass, mercurial ointment, and sweet spirit of nitre at his purveying depot in Columbia, South Carolina.[45] Dr. Milo Smith of Chattanooga made up his own Epsom salts and told the War Department that a supply "ample for the needs of the army can readily be manufactured and at very little cost."[46] George Blackie reported that he had discovered a large deposit of black oxide of manganese (dioxide of manganese, a popular tonic and alterative usually given in three to twenty grains in pill form) "of extreme purity" in a nearby Georgia County.[47] In these and many other ways, purveyors attempted to provide for a beleaguered Confederate Medical Department. That they had difficulties is to be expected; that they succeeded as well as they did is a testimony to their diligence and ability to innovate.

But, as in the North, the heart of pharmacy lay not in its administration but rather in its materia medica and the ability of hospital stewards in the field and in hospitals to provide care. From the drug supply table to the drug manufacturing laboratories to the men who prescribed and dispensed the drugs, the materia medica was the foundation of all nonsurgical and postoperative care in the Civil War. In the South, however, all of this took place under conditions of serious disease and severe drug shortages caused by a steadily tightening Union blockade. Indeed, before the Confederate materia medica can be understood, the conditions of privation under which it labored must be explained. The story of how precisely the South managed to provide pharmacy care amidst these obstacles rivals even the most quintessential Yankee ingenuity.

Chapter 9

Fighting More with Less

In terms of disease and the armamentarium to combat it, the South was clearly fighting more with less. The blockade that has been mentioned repeatedly throughout this book was an essential context through which drug supply, provision, and dispensing took place. The wartime shortages thus created forced the South to respond in unique ways that transformed its supply table and dictated the manner in which that table was filled and sustained through a network of small-scale but active laboratories that dotted the Confederacy. The need for an efficient and effective drug supply was made all the more urgent by the pressing demands of disease in camp and field and at sea.

DISEASE IN THE CONFEDERACY

It has been explained earlier that disease rather than battlefield injury was the principal challenge to medical departments, North and South. Yet poorer rations and greater exposure left the Confederates more susceptible to illness than their Union rivals. Although the North clearly suffered more severely from disease in the Peninsular Campaign from April to July of 1862, mainly because it was forced to occupy unhealthier ground and was equally devastated by disease in its first siege of Vicksburg (a problem intensified by a critical shortage of quinine),[1] it was the South that suffered proportionately higher incidents of disease. A comparative analysis of malaria conducted by the Union surgeon general's office, for example, found three times the reported cases of the fever among Confederates (41,539, compared with 14,842 Union cases).[2]

Clear and reliable information on the incidents of disease among Confederate forces is not easy to find. The burning of Richmond at

the end of the war destroyed many of the Confederate Medical Department's records, and nothing is comparable to the massive compilation *The Medical and Surgical History of the War of the Rebellion,*
completed by the surgeon general's office detailing disease among
Federal troops. Some data worth noting does exist. Figure 9.1 illustrates in unequivocal terms the preponderance of disease over combat
injury and how most were treated in the camp and field rather than in
hospitals. The chief culprits, diarrhea/dysentery and fevers, were
fairly evenly divided at 313,332 and 319,233, respectively. If a soldier was able to avoid these two primary scourges, he might still suc-
cumb to bronchitis, pneumonia, or any number of other maladies
(from intestinal parasites to rheumatism).

One category of disease that was largely unreported because it was
not well understood at the time was that caused by various nutritional
deficiencies. Both sides recognized some correlation between diet
and certain diseases—that had been demonstrated by British naval
surgeon James Lind with the introduction of orange and lemon juice
to prevent scurvy in 1753—but the role of vitamins would not be

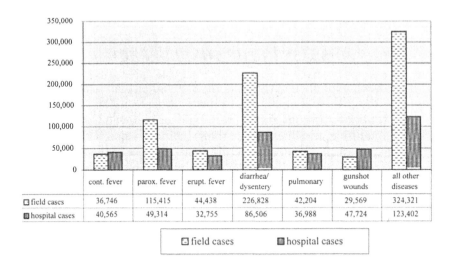

	cont. fever	parox. fever	erupt. fever	diarrhea/ dysentery	pulmonary	gunshot wounds	all other diseases
☐ field cases	36,746	115,415	44,438	226,828	42,204	29,569	324,321
▨ hospital cases	40,565	49,314	32,755	86,506	36,988	47,724	123,402

☐ field cases   ▨ hospital cases

FIGURE 9.1. Confederate Sick and Wounded: Reports on File in the Surgeon-
General's Office, 1861-1862 (*Source:* From "Grand Summary of the Sick and
Wounded of the Confederate States Army Under Treatment During the Years
1861 and 1862," *Confederate States Medical and Surgical Journal* 1, No. 9 [Sep-
tember 1864]: 139-140).

known until nutritionist Casimir Funk's landmark paper on the subject in 1912. Medical staffs on both sides tended to lump nutritional deficiencies as "scorbutic diathesis." In this regard the South seemed to have a more enlightened approach. The Union commissary and medical staff sought to relieve these "scorbutics" with potatoes and desiccated vegetables (which destroyed the very vitamin C the men so desperately needed). However, leading Confederate surgeons such as J. Julian Chisolm and Medical Director William A. Carrington were recommending fresh vegetables and fruits for their men.[3] Dr. Samuel H. Stout ordered his Army of the Tennessee hospital stewards to purchase "abundant supplies of vegetables, butter, eggs and other articles for the sick and convalescent."[4] Nevertheless, nutritional deficiencies are especially important to discuss in terms of Confederate health because there is reason to believe their more spartan diets left them more vulnerable to scurvy, rickets, and other diseases.

Late in the war the Army of Northern Virginia was beset with widespread nyctalopia (night blindness), and one observer recalled witnessing "men led by the hand all night . . . [only] to go into battle with the command in the morning."[5] Likely due to a lack of vitamin A, dietary deficiencies such as this could lead from one medical problem to another. Not only would these men have suffered night blindness but also increased susceptibility to infectious diseases.[6] Although the surgeons and stewards did not recognize the specific correlation, the problem could have been quickly resolved with a regimen of cod liver oil (itself rich in vitamin A); but more likely than not, the men just suffered until a better diet could be obtained. It is possible, however, that some of the vision problems experienced were due to excessive dosages of quinine given to patients along with diets poor in vitamins A and B complex and ascorbic acid.[7]

One disease, pellagra, deserves special attention. Before Joseph Goldberger discovered in the 1920s that pellagra was the result of poor diet, the characteristic weight loss, ulceration on the arms and legs, and general debility was usually ascribed to some vaguely defined "infection."[8] The monotonous Southern "3-M/2-H" diet—meat, meal, and molasses or otherwise referred to as hogs and hominy— would make Confederates more prone to pellagra than their Northern counterparts. Though likely recorded by Civil War surgeons as perhaps an "eruptive fever" or some other infectious or "miasmic" disorder, there is every reason to believe that genuine cases of pellagra plagued Confederate camps. The disease was endemic to Kentucky, Tennessee, Alabama, Mississippi, Louisiana, Texas, Arkansas, both Carolinas, and Georgia. Efforts to understand the nature of pellagra were made by the medical community in the early twentieth century, with one researcher identifying 10,663 fatal cases of the disease in 1915.[9] It would strain credulity to believe that pellagra was nonexistent among the often ill-fed troops of the Confederacy. Despite the inability of the surgeons of the day to diagnose—much less treat—pellagra and similar nutritional deficiency diseases, many more diseases were all too familiar to the Southern medical staff. The epidemiology of measles was well understood. Often called an "eruptive fever," almost every surgeon had to deal with this potentially dangerous disease, especially early in the war. Medical Director Stout observed that his 3rd Regiment, almost wholly composed of rural young men never before exposed to measles, rose to about 650 cases of measels and spread "before it was possible to perfect adequate accommodations for the sick in the regimental or general hospitals."[10] The epidemic nature of measles, fevers, and dysenteries probably explains, at least in part, the preponderance of cases treated in the field as opposed to hospital cases, since that latter would not normally have been able to accommodate such numbers anyway.

Nevertheless, the image of busy and bloody hospitals with butcher-like surgeons lopping off arms and legs as fast as their saws would sever them is just grossly inaccurate. Even the large and important Chimborazo Hospital near Richmond, Virginia, saw far more diseases than wounds and still managed to maintain a remarkably low overall mortality rate of 6.42 pecent (see Figure 9.2).[11]

These disease statistics are borne out by the men who treated them. Assistant surgeon for the 19th Virginia Infantry, William H. Taylor, for example, recalled, "The prevailing diseases were intestinal disorders [i.e., diarrhea and dysentery], though we had a share of almost every malady."[12] Likewise, John Samuel Apperson, hospital steward in Company D of the 1st Virginia Brigade, noted while camped near Manassas on July 28, 1861: "This morning 105 men were up to be examined, prescribed for and administered to. I am very busily engaged until 10 o'clock."[13] Just a few days later he wearily observed, "Sickness seems to threaten a great many of our boys—many are becoming ill every day."[14] By May 1862 things were not much better. Marching through Brown's Gap toward the Blue Ridge Mountains, Apperson

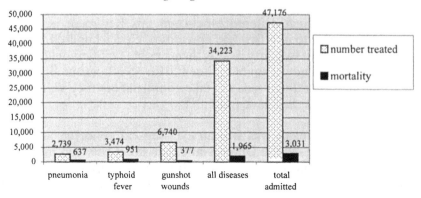

FIGURE 9.2 Confederate Injury/Disease/Mortality Rates: Chimborazo Hospital November 1861 to November 1863 (*Source:* "Confederate States Hospital Reports," *Confederate States Medical and Surgical Journal* Vol. 1, No. 1 [January 1864]: 8).

writes that thirty-eight of his regiment were ordered to fall to the rear to join an ever-growing number of men suffering from rheumatism, bronchitis, diarrhea, dysentery, and just about "all other diseases."[15] The hospital steward remarked in half-pity, and half-disgust what a "dilapidated set they were."[16]

One might be inclined to conclude that since both sides were suffering from essentially the same diseases (save for pellagra) that all these diseases canceled themselves out as an important factor in the war. However, the South's medical staff had a more difficult task in dealing with diseases. No better example of this can be seen than in the letters of George E. Waller, hospital steward for the 24th Virginia Regiment. On June 8, 1862, Waller bemoaned the condition of his unit:

> We have a good deal of sickness now in camp. A good many are taking fever now. I sent off Hainston Payne with it yesterday and Tom Stone today. Stone is very sick and I do not think he will live—good many cases of same from other companies.[17]

Indeed in just one year following the regiment's formation, Waller recounted the devastation that disease and suicidal charges had wrought upon the regiment.

There is a great difference between this Regiment now and when I came to it. It first had upwards of eleven hundred, it now musters about two fifty. It was then a noble regiment with good officers, it is now a small regiment with no officers at all. Capt. Gardner went down today to take command but they will never fight again as they have fought.[18]

By March 1864 health was still an ever-present concern, but only then could Waller see the Union Navy that stood between him and much-needed supplies. Camped near Smithfield, North Carolina, he wrote to his sister, "I fear if we stay here long we will have plenty of sickness. There is small pox here now & in the fall they have yellow fever and cholera."[19] But he added ominously, "I could see the billows on the ocean rising like mountains & looking as white as cotton & away in the distance the masts of ships were visable [sic], supposed to be the [Union] blockading fleet."[20]

THE BLOCKADE

By 1864 the Union blockading squadrons had a death grip on the South. Lincoln's declaration of a naval blockade, an operation that Winfield Scott took and incorporated into a larger strategy designed to bring the South to its knees, was by then having its intended effect. Although derisively dubbed "Scott's Anaconda" by the old warhorse's opponents, the term was more apt than Scott's detractors would care to admit, as the life was slowly squeezed out of the Confederacy's supply lines.

The blockade of all Southern ports really had its beginning with Jefferson Davis. One of the Confederate president's first acts was to call for privateering in order to assist in the effort to "repel the threatened invasion."[21] On April 19, 1861, President Lincoln responded with a blockade.[22] The U.S. action would seem to have been a logical extension of quelling what it saw as an open rebellion anyway, but the issuance of a blockade would have at least two potentially lethal effects on Federal diplomacy: (1) it would give tacit recognition to the rebels; and (2) it might cause Great Britain to officially recognize the Confederacy. The first consequence could be answered by the general acceptance of a blockading strategy as a means of dealing with a hostile power, and would give the U.S. Navy considerable powers to search and seize vessels. The second consequence was avoided with some rather adroit diplomacy on the part of William Seward, who carefully broached the matter to British Ambassador Lord Richard Lyons before the official announcement. The upshot of this meeting was that the United States would have to be careful not to overstep its bounds; but Lyons assured Lincoln's secretary of state that Britain was quite familiar with the practice and would not embroil itself in this matter. Predictably, Britain declared its neutrality on May 13, 1861.

The Confederacy never quite accepted that its old trading partner could live without its precious cotton, and it continued to hope for British aid in its war for independence. Thus, in the face of Lincoln's application of naval pressure, Davis remained unimpressed. On May 28 he even upped the stakes and added enticements to Southern vessels' seizure of enemy cargoes by reducing by one-third the normal duties on captured goods and granting 5 percent on all such "good and lawful prizes of war."[23]

The point-counterpoint political maneuvering would, in the long run, be less significant than the protracted effects of virtual closure of Southern ports. Although the aged and ailing Winfield Scott was often caricatured as "old fuss and feathers," he understood this important point. As politicians and newspaper editors continued the pipe dream of a ninety-day war, Scott put in place a general strategy that set the stage for long-term naval operations. It was a plan that would not change substantively throughout the war: (1) strengthen the blockade; (2) split the Confederacy by gaining and maintaining control over the Mississippi; and (3) use the navy in support of ground troops.[24] This was, in historian Stephen R. Wise's words, "the first modern blockade. Its focal points were the Southern ports, and its power would come from steam engines."[25] The blockade would have a profound effect on drug supplies for the Confederacy. John W. Mallett of Virginia noted that of the many drugs listed on the supply table, four were principally needed at all times: quinine for fever, opium (or morphine) for pain, and ether and chloroform for anesthesia.[26] The Confederacy partly answered the need for general anesthetics by manufacturing sulfuric ether at J. Julian Chisolm's laboratory in Columbia, South Carolina.[27] Morphine, however, was "almost entirely brought in by means of the blockade runners."[28] The South lacked anything like the North's industrial capacity for large-scale pharmaceutical manufacturing. Even if they could match their rivals, much of the crude drugs (plant products from South America such as cinchona bark, ipecac, and copaiba; opium from Turkey and the Far East; and camphor from China and Japan) would have to come through open seaports. Moore recognized the importance of maintaining overseas drug supplies, and he took measures to try to ensure it by working with the Ordnance Department in London to obtain medicines for blockade runners in exchange for cotton on their return trips.[29] In effect, it became an arrangement for smuggled medicines purchased partly in cotton currency. Indeed, this operation was so essential to the medical corps that a Confederate Medical Bureau was established at Nassau.[30]

Of course, drugs could be acquired without access to naval supply lines. Items could be obtained through overland smuggling and/or capture. Writing from Memphis, General Cadwallader Washburn was so worried about the smuggling and illicit trade occurring under his watch that he closed all egress from the city by land, allowing only departure by river and then only with a special pass. His General Order issued on May 10, 1864, gives an interesting picture of conditions in occupied Memphis:

> The practical operation of commercial intercourse from this city with the States in rebellion has been to help largely feed, clothe, arm and equip [he might have added, medicate] our enemies. Memphis has been of more value to the Southern Confederacy since it fell into Federal hands than Nassau. To take cotton belonging to the rebel government to Nassau, or any foreign port, is a hazardous proceeding. To take it to Memphis and convert it into supplies and greenbacks and return to the lines of the enemy, or place the proceeds to the credit of the rebel Government in Europe, without passing again into rebel lines, is safe and easy. I have undoubted evidence that large amounts of cotton have been, and are being, brought here to be sold, belonging to the rebel government.[31]

Washburn's concerns were real. Memphis did indeed serve as a focal point for overland smuggling operations for the Confederates' western theater.[32] It was men such as a Mr. Berg who had Washburn worried. Berg, a so-called Alabama merchant, decided to make his wartime profits by running drug contraband out of Memphis. Transportation was the problem until he discovered the perfect convey-ance—an abandoned hospital wagon sporting the well-known yellow hospital flag and identified with the large painted words SMALL-POX. Loading up his perfectly disguised two-horse vehicle with morphine, quinine, ether, and an even riskier cargo of rye whisky, he set out for Alabama. For four days all went well. Then Berg, unable to resist the temptation of sampling from his keg, arrived at a farmhouse reeking of liquor. Berg stopped in hopes of some food; the woman there hoped to obtain her own stash of the precious alcohol. The woman in-sisted that Berg provide a portion of his whisky in exchange for a meal, and he complied. However, he had little time to enjoy his chicken dinner. Four Federal bluecoats soon arrived, and noticing the unmistakable odor of whisky decided to commandeer their newfound treasure. They were about to kill Berg and steal his wagon when Con-federates busted up their party. The errant entrepreneur lost his inven-tory to his Southern compatriots, but the price of his life probably seemed a fair one. Berg undoubtedly left with a new appreciation for the evils of alcohol. [33]

The pressing need for medicines caused incredible risks to be taken elsewhere. One particularly noteworthy instance was the acqui-sition of desperately needed quinine, calomel, and opium for Wright's Arkansas cavalry during Grant's siege of Vicksburg. In order to ob-tain these supplies, the unit's surgeon—a Dr. Edwards—had to use much ingenuity and resourcefulness. Crossing the Mississippi at Greenville, Edwards proceeded by horse and buggy to Canton, where he obtained the medicines. On his return trip, however, he found his way blocked by a Union gunboat. Searching for another place to cross the river, Edwards found an old dugout barely capable of float-ing. Loading the questionable craft with the drugs, Edwards rowed under cover of darkness back across the river and deposited his pre-cious cargo safely with his unit.[34]

These daring exploits make for exciting tales, but they never be-came a significant factor in overall drug supplies for the Confederacy. Although such methods of acquisition could yield good quantities of much-needed drugs at times, they were simply too unreliable and variable to be counted on. The occasional seizure of Union medical stores was no better. Though on the eve of open war there were some notable Confederate drug seizures, as when surgeon D. Camden deLeon wrote to the secretary of war in Montgomery that he had no need to make significant purchases of articles for his dispensary due to the capture of "a large supply of medicines, instruments, & c.,"[35] acquisition by direct seizure of Union supplies during the course of the war never became an important means of drug acquisition for the South. Purveyors and medical staff could become elated over the unexpected windfall of a Confederate capture of enemy supplies,[36] but actual quantities and specific items might or might not match the real needs and their occurrence was infrequent enough to be ascribed to mere chance or luck. Atlanta pharmacist Joseph Jacobs recalled that "while the army frequently captured the wagon trains of the enemy, thus obtaining some supplies of medicines and surgical appliances, these were barely sufficient to supply the most distressing needs of the army."[37] All things considered, historians seem justified who have argued that blockade-running netted far more reliable drug supplies than either overland smuggling or capture.[38]

The economics also support this conclusion. The sums expended on foreign purchases of drug supplies were not insignificant, especially considering that the dollars in Confederate currency represent only partial payments for goods provided (the rest came from cotton on the Confederate carrier's return). In 1862, for example, Captain Caleb Huse was asked to purchase £20,000 worth of "drugs and medicinal supplies" through a London agent, Mr. A. C. Evans.[39] The escalating costs of supplies can easily be seen in the financial reports of the Confederacy: by October 1863 the Medical Department was requisitioning £30,000 for supplies;[40] by 1864 the amount rose to £50,000.[41] Estimates for further purchases of medicines climb to £113,000, with one contract already reaching £22,500.[42] If currency was not enough, the rather inflated price of cotton at fifty cents per pound in England (remarkable, given the fact that it could fetch only pennies in the South itself) did little to bring down the overall cost of drugs for the Confederacy. Quartermaster R. W. Sanders of the Bureau of Cotton Exchange for Alabama, Mississippi, and East Louisiana complained in November 1864 that quinine was costing his office $100 per ounce in cotton.[43]

Despite the costs to the Confederate government, the absolute necessity of obtaining reliable drug supplies and the promise of handsome rewards caused Confederate blockade-runners to risk life and limb in getting foreign goods into Southern hands. The value of drugs coming into Southern ports during the war shows that prices were variable but always high. This fact enticed mariners interested in adventure and profit: prices (in U.S. currency) of blue mass (mercury) could range from $7 to $20 per pound; casks of wine as much as $72 per gallon; calomel from $8 to $20 per pound; camphor was valued from $16.50 to $20 per pound; ether from $7.25 to $17.50 per pound; morphine from $10 to $100 per ounce; and precious quinine sold for as little as $17 to as much as $100 per ounce.[44] Prices in Confederate dollars show the increasing devaluation of Southern currency. By the fall of 1864 calomel cost $102 per pound in Confederate money; quinine, $80 per pound; and morphine, a whopping $180 per ounce.[45] Confederate currency by the end of 1864 was worthless.

The extent of blockade-running is difficult to assess, since records on such activity are understandably sketchy, but one knowledgeable investigator has estimated that 1,300 attempts were made by vessels to enter blockaded Southern ports, of which 1,000 were successful.[46] Still, the efforts of the U.S. Navy proved increasingly effective. In 1861 only one in ten runners were captured; in 1862 the Union success rate rose to one in eight; the next two years the number of seized vessels climbed to one in three; and by war's end only one in two were getting through.[47]

The turning point in the blockade came in 1863. According to Virginia Surgeon Herbert Nash, "Until the latter part of 1863 the supplies of quinine, chloroform, and other medicines were quite sufficient, and only subsequently, when blockade running had become irregular and finally suppressed, did our sick and wounded really suffer for the proper supplies."[48] The illustrious career of the *Ella and Annie* (Figure 9.3), a 747-ton side-wheeler known to carry medicinal supplies,[49] illustrates the changing fortunes of the blockade-runners. Operated not by the Confederate government but by the Importing and Exporting Company of South Carolina, the *Ella and Annie* netted her owners fantastic profits. Under the command of dashing and bold Frank N. Bonneau (Figure 9.4), this steam-powered vessel made eight successful runs through the Union blockade, accounting for a total profit of around $800,000 in cotton, medical stores, and assorted cargo.[50] The beginning of the end for the Confederacy's blockade-runners occurred on November 5, 1863, when the *Ella and Annie,* along with two sister ships, the *Cornubia* and the *Robert E. Lee,* were departing St. George's Harbor in Bermuda. These three ships alone had made forty-one successful runs through the Union fleet.[51] Head-

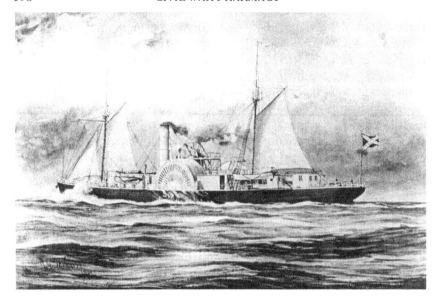

FIGURE 9.3. Built at Wilmington, Delaware, in 1860, this 747-ton side-wheeler was originally used for commercial purposes. Seized by Louisiana when war broke out in April 1861, the *Ella and Annie* was known to carry pharmaceutical cargoes and became one of the Confederacy's most successful blockade-runners until her capture on November 9, 1863. Photo courtesy of the Naval Historical Center, Department of the Navy, Washington Navy Yard.

ing for New Inlet, North Carolina, the *Cornubia* reached her destination first (on November 7), where she was spotted by the Union gunboat *James Adger*. The *James Adger* immediately sent up a flare attracting the blockader *Niphon*. Soon the *Cornubia* was trapped and ran aground. The next day the *Robert E. Lee* was observed near Bogue Inlet. Pursued by the *James Adger*, the heavy-laden *Robert E. Lee* quickly surrendered. When the *Ella and Annie* appeared shortly thereafter, Bonneau refused to give in and challenged the *Niphon* to a test of seamanship. But the *Niphon* was a smaller and more maneuverable vessel. Turning his ship to avoid a direct impact with the Confederate blockade-runner, the Union captain was able to open with canister fire and quickly board the ship. By November 9 it was all over.[52] Blockade historian Stephen Wise has called the capture of these vessels "a devastating blow to Confederate blockade running.

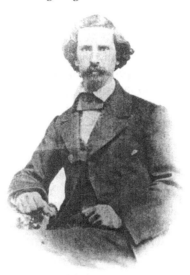

FIGURE 9.4. Confederate blockade-runners were commanded by daring seamen such as Frank N. Bonneau. Bonneau was appointed acting master of the *Ella and Annie* and skippered the ship until her capture late in 1863. Though he sailed under letters of marque issued by the Confederate Congress on May 6, 1861 (technically making him a legal privateer), one nation's privateer is another nation's pirate. He was convicted of piracy, but the sentence was subsequently suspended and Bonneau was paroled in September 1864. Photo courtesy of the Naval Historical Center, Department of the Navy, Washington Navy Yard.

In less than forty-eight hours three of the best blockade runners had been lost."[53] In terms of Confederate imports, this three-ship capture represented at sea what Gettysburg had represented for the Confederate army earlier that summer.

This was particularly serious for Confederate supply prospects because successful round-trips for blockade-runners were rare; the important port city of Charleston recorded only 115 for the entire war.[54] If the Confederacy's success rate in sneaking through the blockade steadily declined, so did the number of cities in which they could unload their cargoes. Sometimes it was not so much a matter of getting materials *into* the South as getting cotton *out of* it. By summer of 1864, for example, when cotton was serving as de facto currency, Thomas Bayne had to tell the secretary of the treasury, G. A. Trenholm, that even if the cotton necessary to procure needed supplies from Europe could be obtained, only Wilmington, North Carolina, and Charleston, South Carolina, remained available ports for their loading and that the "tonnage at present commanded by the Government is entirely inadequate to so large an export."[55]

Meanwhile, the Union blockade was netting returns that would total $10 million in prize money by war's end.[56] How much of this booty was composed of medicines can be ascertained from the availability of goods seized and sold at auction by order of secretary of the navy, Gideon Welles, from the prize court records. Based on his examination of the records of the New York Prize Court, Norman Franke estimated that about half of all blockade-runners carried sizable cargoes of medicines.[57] An investigation of the naval records at the National Archives would suggest a rate of nearly 70 percent, and perhaps even higher.[58]

An idea of the nature and value of those drug supplies can be ascertained by looking at specific auction lists of captured blockade-running vessels. The steamer *Ella Warley*, for example, had its store of fifty bottles of castor oil, one case of magnesia, two cases of quinine, two cases of potassium iodide, one case of ipecac, one case of opium, and other assorted medicines auctioned for $5,652.47 ($74,273.45 in current U.S. dollars)[59] The *Anglia*, captured by the *Flag* on October 27, 1862, carried an especially precious cargo of 1,600 ounces of "Pelletier's Quinine" and 315½ ounces of opium that auctioned for $9.25 per ounce.[60] The total of both netted nearly $7,500 for the two items alone. In one very early and notable Union blockade success, the U.S.S. *Mercedita* captured the *Bermuda* on April 27, 1862, and found much of its cargo consisting of medicines, mortars and pestles, and pillboxes.[61] The total sold for $4,715.64 ($61,963.50 in current U.S. dollars) One of the proportionately largest pharmaceutical seizures occurred with the capture of the steamer *Alabama* by the *Eugenie* on September 12, 1863.[62] When auctioned in New Orleans the following month its medicinal stores sold for $7,754.31 ($101,893.63 in current U.S. dollars) out of a total cargo worth $11,316.81.[63] It should be kept in mind that these auction prices reflect "normal" market values, not necessarily their worth within the Confederacy, where inflated dollars and needs might dictate sale prices many times what could be obtained in the Union. Summaries of the auction sales suggest that the entire standard supply table was aboard these blockade-runners. The aforementioned *Alabama* alone carried rum, wine, anisette, molasses, cream of tartar, carbonate of ammonium, sal soda, alum, Epsom salts, borax, linseed, gum arabic, sublimed sulfur, castor oil, copaiba, carbonate of soda, copperas (sulfate of iron), turpentine, adhesive plaster, essence of thyme, mustard, tannin, hydrargyrum cum creta (mercury with chalk), aqua ammonia, logwood, liquorice, gum camphor, cantharides, calomel, quinine, chloroform, opium, iodide of potassium, benzoic acid, creosote, ipecac, flax, assorted phials and pillboxes, and one medicine chest.[64] Besides those medicinal substances, cinchona, antimony (tartar emetic), and many others commonly appeared on the sales lists.

These examples were, of course, all medicines and pharmaceutical apparatus that did *not* get into Confederate hands. By 1864, drained Confederate finances and a trickling of supplies were having serious consequences for the medical corps. Captain Graybill at the commissary of Columbus, Georgia, had to tell surgeon Terry that he had "no funds for hospitals or for any other purposes."[65] The ensuing exchange went up the ladder to Surgeon General Moore. A distraught Moore wrote: "Respectfully referred to the Secretary of War requesting his perusal of these indorsements [sic.] and urging that measures be adopted to enable surgeons in charge of hospitals to feed the sick and wounded. The evils resulting from a failure to supply cannot be exaggerated."[66] The money simply was not there to be supplied; the commissary general admitted to being $30,000,000 in arrears.[67] Even the usually optimistic chief naval surgeon, W. Spottswood, had to admit in November of 1864 that

> owing to the strict blockade of the seacoast and harbors of the Confederacy, rendering it impossible now to procure medical supplies from abroad, I fear that there will necessarily be much difficulty in procuring many valuable articles soon required for the use of the sick.[68]

As the Union's "anaconda" tightened, the South desperately sought alternatives to foreign drug supplies that were always chancy at best. The South did so by establishing a supply table of indigenous Southern plants. Readily at hand and bountiful in supply, these botanicals would be the proposed mainstay of the Confederacy's medicines.

THE SUPPLY TABLE

Moore had anticipated the problem of the blockade early on. He sought to remedy the situation with a call to utilizing indigenous plants for medicinal purposes. With the war not quite a year old, the surgeon general called for an effort "to diminish its [the South's] tribute to foreigners" by "the appropriation of our indigenous medicinal substances of the vegetable kingdom."[69] Moore instructed the medical corps to comb their districts and collect and forward to the purveyors "the enumerated remedial agents, or others found valuable."[70]

And comb they did. Surgeon W. A. Carrington suggested that "wheat straw is an excellent substitute for oak-wood ashes for the manufacture of soap,"[71] and surgeon Potts, medical purveyor in Montgomery, recommended sorghum seed as a substitute for grain in the manufacture of whisky.[72] The medical purveyor in Atlanta, George Blackie, recommended dittany *(Cunila mariana)* in place of black tea.[73] Dr. M. B. Beck proposed that boneset *(Eupatorium perfoliatum)* and snakeroot *(Aristolochia serpentaria)* be administered in cases of fever. At the same time he issued a call "for all our valuable *indigenous medicines,* [that] a more extended and general use [be made], especially when other remedies are difficult to be obtained, and command so high a price."[74] Throughout the South, old remedies were being resurrected, new ones tried, and even some foreign medicinals cultivated. Women were growing poppies domestically for processing into opium. Homemade preparations came to the fore, such as: astringent teas made of raspberry or whortleberry leaves; dysentery remedies of blackberry roots and persimmons made in a decoction; and simple homely ointments for "the itch" were made from poke root or even more complicated ones made from elder bark, lard, water, sweet-gum, olive oil, and sulfur powder.[75]

Although these random sources of drug substitutes were often tried and abandoned, the one quasi-official source was Francis Peyre Porcher's (1824-1895) *Resources of the Southern Fields and Forests.* Moore actually commissioned the South Carolina physician to prepare a work of indigenous plant-drug substitutes, and even years later hailed its use in the Confederate medical corps. "This book was of so much importance, containing a great deal of valuable and useful information," proclaimed the former surgeon general in an address delivered in Richmond on October 19, 1875, "that a large edition was published, and the volumes distributed free to those who desired them."[76]

Porcher's *Resources* was a monumental work. Listing some 35,000 native plants, Porcher believed that 410 had medicinal value. Moreover, he gave an exhaustive list of native substitutes for imported drugs. For gum arabic (acacia), for example, he recommended slippery elm.[77] Citing McKeown, Porcher suggested that "a teaspoonful of the powdered [pleurisy] root in hot water, often repeated, acts as a safe and useful substitute for the preparations of antimony."[78] Porcher had particular favorites and tended to give them in running lists. A typical commentary ran as follows:

> The plants just mentioned, the blackberry, chinquapin, *(Castanea)* and dogwood to be used as astringents, the gentians, pipsissewa, *Sabbatia,* etc., as bitter tonics, can easily be obtained by our soldiers while in camp, and they will be found to fulfill all the indications required in most cases of fever, dysentery, diarrhea, catarrhs, etc. In the formation of demulcent drinks, as substitutes for flaxseed and gum-arabic, the roots and leaves of the sassafras, and the leaves of the *Bené (Sesamum)* will suffice. The *Podophyllum* (wild jalap [i.e., mayapple]) will supply the purgative; therefore, with the possession of opium and calomel, the surgeon *in the field* can himself obtain almost everything desired, and with comparatively little aid from the Medical Purveyors. Our chief desiderata now are the preparations of potash, viz: nitrate chlorate and bicarbonate, and sup. carb. of soda. We may procure soda from our *Salsola kali* [saltwort].[79]

Porcher was being a bit disingenuous when he suggested that native medicinal plants would liberate the medical corps from the medical purveyor. True, a simple decoction, infusion, or poultice could be made easily enough, and some plants needed no further processing whatsoever, but fluidextracts and genuine tinctures took some processing. Also, as we shall see, the surgeon general went to great lengths to establish medical laboratories to process these indigenous plants into finished pharmaceuticals. There is a sense that Porcher considers these woodland remedies too much like panaceas, ready for use and virtually within arms' reach. The other problem with Porcher's *Resources* is its sheer breadth and many unanswered questions. With hundreds of suggested substitutes, which were the easiest to work with? Which were the most readily obtainable, and which were the most reliable?

Surgeon General Moore sought to answer these questions. In the spring of 1863, Moore issued an indigenous supply table (see Appendix A). Comprising ninety-three different items, the table featured plants of the Southeast commonly used for medicinal purposes. It would be wrong, however, to conclude that this list contained only novel or new medicinal plants. Nearly a third of the botanicals were already on the primary list of the *United States Pharmacopoeia*.[80] Others, such as Indian turnip *(Arum triphyllum),* pleurisy root *(Asclepias tuberosa),* persimmon *(Diospyros virginiana),* Sumach *(Rhus glabrum)* were among the secondary list of pharmacopoeial substances. The table was designed to be a ready reference guide to the prescribing surgeon and hospital steward, and include not only the name of the plant but also its uses, dosage, and dosage form information.

Moore's commitment to indigenous remedies was strong and steadfast. He sincerely believed that indigenous remedies could sustain the medical corps' needs. One hospital steward called it "a nightmare that sits upon the brain of the Surgeon-General."[81] But botanicals were hardly new to the materia medica. When Simon Baruch, surgeon for the 7th South Carolina Battalion for just two weeks, was asked by a Charleston woman exactly what herbs to gather, he could name five common plants off the top of his head without even referring to Moore's table.[82] Many of his colleagues could certainly do the same.

THE LABORATORIES

No matter how many indigenous herbs could be collected, this crude drug supply needed to be made into medicine, and thus the accumulation of plant stores did not remove the necessity for an infrastructure of manufacture. Medicinal substances, whether botanical or chemical, usually needed some processing from their natural state. Without anything near the industrial capacity of Tilden and Company, Rosengarten and Sons, Powers and Weightman, Edward R.

Squibb, or the U.S. Army Laboratory in Philadelphia, the South sought to cobble together its own makeshift drug-processing network.

Two general methods were employed in drug manufacture in the Confederacy. First was the establishment of main depot laboratories at Lincolnton and Charlotte, North Carolina; Columbia, South Carolina; Macon and Atlanta, Georgia; and Mobile and Montgomery, Alabama.[83] Moore was proud of his medical laboratories and felt that their uninterrupted operations were essential to his medical corps. Calling the directors and employees of these labs "expert chemists, druggists, and distillers," the surgeon general hailed them as "men of professional skill, whose services are absolutely indispensable for the manufacture of medicines . . . and alcoholic stimulants."[84] Often the directors of these larger plants (especially those located in port cities) had dual duties of manufacture and inspection of imports arriving on the blockade-runners. Charles T. Mohr (1824-1901) (Figure 9.5), one of the South's most industrious and talented druggists, reported from Mobile that he had plenty of apparatus, a grinding mill to process crude drug product, and "a contrivance for the production

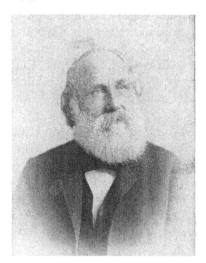

FIGURE 9.5. Charles T. Mohr ran an important Confederate laboratory in Mobile. One of the South's most accomplished pharmaceutical chemists, Mohr not only manufactured drugs but also evaluated imports smuggled past the Union blockade. Photo courtesy of the Alabama Department of Archives and History.

of high grade alcohol from corn whisky."[85] The only thing he lacked were "glass vessels." Besides his production facilities, Mohr added that he had the task of examining the quality of drugs smuggled into the Mobile port, mainly opium, morphine, and quinine.[86]

Much of what we know of these laboratories is sketchy. Records of day-to-day operations have been lost to time; but what is known of the large depot lab at Lincolnton, North Carolina, yields some interesting details.[87] A Southern sympathizer from the North, surgeon A. S. Piggott, operated this lab. He, along with a Mr. Wizzel who served as his assistant, processed tinctures and extracts of the indigenous crude drugs forwarded to them. The plant itself consisted of an oblong brick building constructed on the right bank of the Catawba River and running parallel with it.[88] The work was performed by local workers (either young boys or men too old to serve in the Confederate army) with grinding mills and other machinery powered by the river.[89] With local towns and surrounding villages serving as collection points, residents recalled large wagonloads of medicines coming into and out of the Lincolnton lab; they also recalled a large poppy and sorghum field proximate to the facility.[90] As the Union blockade tightened, efforts to complete a second building were initiated, but the war concluded before the roofing and woodwork of the building were completed.

A second method used by the Confederacy to manufacture its own drugs was the creation of a network of smaller labs supportive of those located by the larger depots. Surgeon R. M. Johnson ran such a plant at Tyler, Texas; surgeon Prioleau first operated one first in Savannah and later in Macon, Georgia; surgeon James King Hall headed a lab in Demopolis, Alabama; and there were others in Arkadelphia, Arkansas; Knoxville, Tennessee; and elsewhere.[91] These smaller labs were added rather frantically toward the end of the war as needs for medicines grew increasingly urgent. The state of Louisiana acquired the Mount Lebanon Female College for $64,000, and Governor Henry W. Allen hastily directed surgeon Bartholomew Egan to

> purchase and put up such machinery as you may think proper, in order to meet the wants of the suffering. I have this matter very much at heart, and wish you to enter at once on the duties of your office. I suggest you make your headquarters at Minden and immediately advertise for indigenous barks, roots, herbs.[92]

Egen employed a distiller, potter, two coopers, a chemist to manufacture castor oil, and a supervisor of turpentine production; he also impressed twenty-nine blacks into service.[93]

Not all of the products issuing from the Confederate labs were botanical or "galenical" preparations. The surgeon general, for example, announced in July 1863 that J. Julian Chisolm had commenced the manufacture of blue mass, mercurial ointment, and sweet spirit of nitre at his laboratory in Columbia, South Carolina, and ordered purveyor Blackie to make no more purchases of these articles but rather to requisition them directly from Chisolm.[94]

Most of the larger laboratories produced a mix of chemical and botanical products. But the smooth operations of both were often problematic. In order to manufacture the former, the requisite materials had to be on hand; to make botanical tinctures and extracts, the necessary processing equipment and personnel had to be in place in order to keep pace with processing the raw materials. William H. Anderson told Blackie that he could manufacture spirits of nitre but needed nitric acid and that he could make aque ammonium but lacked the muriate of ammonium from which it was derived.[95] But, for Anderson, botanical supplies were plentiful. His list to purveyor Blackie of available articles included only one nonherbal product and shows both the interrelatedness of various substances in the manufacturing process as well as the degree of commitment and pride the purveyors could have for their products:

I can send you—

Fluid Ext. Sarsaparilla	Tinct. Muriat of Iron
Fluid Ext. Blackberry	Tinct. of Dogwood, Willow & Poplar
Solid Ext. Podophyllum	Syrup of Squills
Solid Ext. Dogwood	Syrup of Wild Cherry

All these I am manufacturing in considerable quantity. I am now making Æther Sulph. in order to make *Tannin*—and Chloride of Lime for making Chloroform—both of which I will manufacture this month.

The Fluid Ext. Blackberry I can recommend as a capital astringent in Dysentery and Diarrhea. The Ext. Dogwood is a good substitute for Quinine. The Tinct. of Dogwood, poplar,

and willow is used in the hospitals here in large quantities. All
these preparations are made with care.[96]

Whereas Anderson urged Blackie to use the products of his lab, J.
Julian Chisolm had to put the brakes on Blackie's well-intentioned
efforts in forwarding indigenous barks to his Columbia lab: "I have
63,000 pounds of barks to reduce which will occupy sometime. You
will therefore be kind enough to keep your stock until I have made
some room for it."[97] Indeed, Chisolm recommended that those plants
not requiring further preparation be forwarded directly where needed
and not to him at all. In particular he suggested that boneset and
snakeroot could be issued as is and made into teas and that wild
cherry needed only to be steeped in water for twenty-four hours, a
task any hospital steward could readily perform.[98]

As the purveyors tried desperately to keep up with demand under
trying circumstances, the issue of product quality was certainly perti-
nent. The record here is a mixed one. Porcher found the opium he had
examined from a South Carolina lab "of very excellent quality, having all the smell and taste of opium (which I have administered to the
sick)."[99] The isinglass plaster (a medical adhesive) manufactured by
J. H. Zeilier and presented to E. W. Johns, medical purveyor in Richmond, was found to be "superior to any specimen shown him by other
parties as being of Southern origin."[100] Hunter Holmes McGuire,
praising Chisolm's sulfuric ether operation in South Carolina, insisted that the Southern chloroform he was familiar with had been administered on more than 40,000 occasions without a single death.[101]
But perhaps assistant surgeon William Taylor's assessment was more
accurate. He praised the diligence of the Confederate laboratories in
their efforts, but he admitted that in their haste and labors under
"great disadvantages" that the end product often was "not surpass-
ingly excellent."[102]

FIGHTING MORE WITH LESS: AN APPRAISAL

Despite laboring against insurmountable odds, the Confederacy's
resourcefulness in the acquisition of medicines was remarkable. The
medical corps showed no little ingenuity and courage in their efforts
to obtain pharmaceuticals deemed contraband by a much larger and
better-equipped foe. A total appraisal of the most quantitatively pro-

ductive means of acquiring pharmaceuticals would indicate (in order of importance) that the labs came first, then imports from the blockade-runners, and finally overland smuggling and enemy capture. Of the three methods the best qualitative drugs, however, were obtained either from foreign imports or enemy capture. The laboratories provided a good supply of indigenous botanical remedies, but their chemical productions were irregular at best and often of substandard quality. Still, the efforts of Surgeon General Moore, Porcher, and the many purveyors to provide a dependable supply of drugs for a large and widely dispersed army were truly commendable. However, the lack of material resources and poor transportation prohibited them from attaining *and* maintaining the all-important standards of quality and quantity necessary to fulfill the needs of their military.

Chapter 10

The Materia Medica

As important as the acquisition and regular supply of medicines were, the real story of the materia medica resided in both camp and hospital. There all the efforts of the blockade-runners, smugglers, raiders, manufacturers, and purveyors were applied and put to the test. For all of the issues of supply, the one most important facet of the materia medica came into sharp focus in the nature of the actual pharmaceutical care delivered to the men in the field.

PRESCRIBING AND DISPENSING
IN CAMP, HOSPITAL, AND HOME

Although the South clearly had to contend with serious and sustained shortages and labored under conditions of extreme difficulty that were unknown to its Northern adversary, it is important to bear in mind that through much of the war (especially before 1863), supplies were normally obtainable. In fact, twenty-four-year-old John Samuel Apperson remarked of his 1st Virginia Brigade, "I am sure I do no violence to the truth when I say that I have never seen anything so abused in my life as medicine is here. Men take it entirely too much."[1] But sickness *was* real and efforts—however crude—to alleviate it were attempted. Apperson's prescriptions of blue mass, opium, morphine, tannin, "G. pill" (probably gamboge pills), castor oil, "plumbs. Acct." (acetate of lead), and others, seem pretty routine for the period.[2] Yet Apperson's diary record covering the entire period of the Civil War gives the historian a unique opportunity to view the conflict from the perspective of a Confederate hospital steward, and thus witness firsthand pharmaceutical conditions as they existed at least for the Army of Northern Virginia. The first thing that becomes obvious is

that sickness was present throughout the war for Apperson. Sometimes disease could run rampant through a camp. As early as July 11,
1861, the beleaguered hospital steward wrote, "A great many were on
hand to be prescribed for this morning. I had to go to town to-day to
see about receiving the quarterly supply of medicine for our regiment."[3] By July 28 he had 105 men "to be examined, prescribed for,
and administered to,"[4] and the next day the number rose to 130.[5] Six
days later Apperson was exhausted and concerned:

> The weather is very oppressive now. I feel very much debilitated
> from the effect of the heat and exercise. Many of our boys are
> giving way also. I fear fever will commence its ravage in the
> army. . . . Our water here is good [it probably tasted and looked
> fine but was infested with microbes and amoeba] but a long way
> off. I hope our men will soon now be relieved of diarrhea.[6]

In September, Apperson reported that the sick lists were finally sub-
siding.

Times were not always so trying. When the regiment was healthy
the hospital steward had plenty of time on his hands. Apperson read,
studied medicine with his mentor Dr. Harvey Black, attended reli-
gious services, and speculated on everything from politics to philoso-
phy. The steward's job was made easier by having plenty of medicines
on hand. Even late in 1862, Apperson's inventory of his dispensary
found the medical stores better than expected,[7] and he reported, "We
have a good supply of stimulants, sedatives, and antiseptics."[8]

Again, as elsewhere, 1863 was a turning point for the hospital
steward's fortunes. In March 1863 a rather brief but interesting comment is entered into Apperson's diary. He describes a doctor who
takes a village woman's advice to use lily leaves instead of the usual
mustard for a plaster.[9] Although he makes no specific mention of medicinal shortages, the physician's quick acceptance of the laywoman's
suggestion implies that he probably had no mustard available. If the
dispensary was becoming bare, it was soon relieved when the Union
army consisting of General Robert Huston Milroy's cavalry left all
their artillery and a large number of supply wagons near Winchester.
Dr. Black eagerly collected a "large amount [of] . . . medicines and
confectionaries."[10] They would be needed; Gettysburg was approaching.

The Battle of Gettysburg, sometimes referred to as the "high-water mark" of the Confederacy, raged from July 1 through July 3, 1863. The month opened with the South's prospects good and its officers' spirits high. In an ironic twist, Independence Day would dawn with the Confederacy's hope for the same permanently dashed. A defeated Lee headed for the Potomac with some 20,000 casualties. Much has been written about the military disposition of troops at Gettysburg, but little of their respective medical corps. In the North, Jonathan Letterman's medical department was outside Gettysburg with medical trains assembled between Union Mills and Westminster.[11] The Confederate medical corps was shadowing their regiments. Surgeon S. G. Welch of the 20th South Carolina Volunteers noted that most of the casualties of his brigade occurred on the first day of fighting.[12] Although the fighting on the second day did not begin until around noon, surgeon Welch observed that it "raged with great fury" until night.[13] Apperson noted on this day:

> I have never seen so many wounded at any place as I saw wounded Yankees here. Our Ambulance train was put to hauling the wounded of the enemy from the field. . . . We move [sic] our Hosp't near the Cashtown road. We had to remove the wounded from Early's Division [of the 2nd Corps] and consequently took but very few from any other part of the [Ewell's] Corps. We had no medical force anyway.[14]

Apperson follows the retreat along the Emmitsburg Pike trying to reach the safety of his Old Dominion. A wet and dreary Sunday morning greeted the hospital steward, who was now separated from the rest of the medical corps and left with four ambulance-loads of men to treat and only "some two or three nurses" to help him.[15] The diary breaks off at this point, the result no doubt of pressing duties and demoralization. One is left to imagine the ensuing cases of pyemia, erysipelas, and gangrene that the hospital steward had to treat with limited medical stores and little prospect of replenishment.

Apperson's account from a pharmaceutical standpoint is interesting. What he does say about the medicines he worked with seems to indicate that they were usually not from the regular supply table. Apperson mentions compounding; making pills and poultices; and dispensing laudanum, chloroform liniment, castor oil, mercury in various forms, and quinine. No mention is made of indigenous remedies, nor does he give any hint of a foraging expedition for such articles. Presumably he worked with what was supplied to him. Following Hippocrates' admonition to "do no harm," he was fearful of trying unproven remedies when certain medicines were unavailable. Thus, although a broad sense of the hospital steward's life in camp can be gleaned from Apperson, other sources are needed to give more therapeutic details to clarify specific aspects of pharmacy care to the sick and wounded.

That can be found in the letters of B. W. Allen. Not much is known of Allen. That he was a surgeon tending patients in a Confederate hospital in or near Charlottesville, Virginia, is clear enough from his two-volume casebooks covering part of 1862 through early 1864.[16] Allen bitterly recalled his hospital experience years later:

> No one could imagine fully the labor required, unless they had gone through with it. The constant, unremitting drudgery, the "wear and tear" of both mental and physical energies, both by day and by night; the tainted atmosphere in spite of ventilation and disinfectants; the want of proper medicines; the lack of necessaries and comforts upon the sick and wounded; the moans of the dying—all were calculated to break down the strongest Surgeons and arouse the sympathies of the most callous. . . . I have often wondered how with comparatively nothing, *we* the Surgeons, who went through with it all and always saw the darkest side ever got along as well as we did.[17]

Thus were the general conditions under which surgeon Allen labored. As for his therapeutics, he gave whisky and quinine in relatively low doses (typically one or two grains three times a day), although a serious case of pneumonia was treated with eight grains of quinine.[18] Other prescriptions included Dover's powder for rheumatic symptoms, catechu (*Acacia catechu*, a powerful astringent native to India and Ceylon but naturalized in Jamaica) and opium for diarrhea, and the ever-popular whisky and quinine for fever.[19] For constipation he gave fifteen grains of rhubarb and one grain of podophyllum (mayapple).[20] Some of Allen's treatments suggest that he adjusted his medicines according to availability. When J. S. Hale presented "troublesome diarrhea" he gave three drops of laudanum (a tincture of opium) instead of the previous catechu/opium combination.[21] For Private L. T. Goodwin's foot wound he performed an amputation and directed the following postoperative care: "Wound to be washed with a weak sol. of chloride soda (Labarraque's) and the sulph. of iron to be applied at each dressing. The patient to take whisky and 2 grs. quinine [three times a day]."[22] But just three days later Allen reported that his patient "is sinking rapidly,"[23] and forty-eight hours after that Goodwin was found "barely alive this morning. He is still conscious and takes his medicine. Pulse very feeble and fluttering. Breathing very difficult."[24] Entries on Goodwin cease at this point.

Captain T. L. Haynes, suffering from general debility and "profuse night sweating," fared better. Allen prescribed his favorite fifteen-drop dose of elixir of vitriol.[25] Three days later Allen noted that the patient "looks pretty bright this morning."[26] But the healing process was often a seesaw battle calling for much encouragement on the part of the physician. Allen reported on one day of his patient's convalescence that Haynes was refusing all food and medication, insisting, "[I]t will do no good."[27] But Allen ended on a bright note, concluding the next day that he "[l]ooks much better. His case much more promising than before."[28]

So-called hospital gangrene was an especially difficult problem, as seen in the last few days in the life of Corporal W. T. Anderson, age twenty-four, member of Company C, Cutt's Georgia Artillery. Admitted December 3, 1863, with an amputated right arm, suffering from gangrene, Allen ordered a "disinfecting powder" of coal tar and gypsum and whisky ℥ j and quinine one grain every four hours.[29] The next day the gangrene was seen "extending very slowly."[30] Allen continued treatment. By December 8 the situation looked better, "The gangrene has stopped and a line of demarcation is established." Allen added, "The stump may yet be a good one without further interference of the knife."[31] In medicine, however, fortunes can change quickly. Rapidly succumbing to septicemia, the next day "the patient is quite feeble" with the "end of the bone . . . now protruding and . . . necrosed." The surgeon continued the quinine and whisky.[32] On December 10, Anderson "was taken suddenly during yesterday evening with an oppressive feeling in the chest & *stentorious breathing* although awake and conscious of everything around. The wound was looking much better. This morning he is in a dying condition."[33] Allen's final entry for Anderson, on the following day, reads: "W. T. Anderson—Died yesterday morning."[34]

As with all Civil War surgeons, the recovery rate of Allen's most severely ill patients was extremely low. But in the surgeon's defense it appears he was often working with what was available rather than what was preferred. For example, in December 1863, Allen suddenly began prescribing a lot of compound cathartic pills.[35] The regimen then vanished from his casebook as suddenly as it had appeared, suggesting that the flurry of such prescriptions was the result of a single windfall capture. There are clear indications of shortages. When Allen could not get his elixir of vitriol he ordered tincture of chloride of iron as a substitute.[36] The Charlottesville Hospital was low on quinine in February 1864, as indeed was the rest of the South. On February 3, 1864, Private H. Turner of Co. D, 55th North Carolina Regiment was admitted to the hospital with symptoms of typhoid fever. Allen writes:

> He was treated for three or four days with Tinct. Veratrium [made from the seeds of *Asagraea officinalis*] which loosened the cough but had no good effect upon the pulse. The Veratrium was then discontinued and whisky ʒ j—Quinine ½ gr. were exhibited every two hours alternating with beef tea a half teacupful at the intermediate hour was pursued until no more quinine could be gotten since which time he has been taking the whiskey and beef tea alone.[37]

On February 23, Turner "bears the marks of incipient phthisis [consumption or tuberculosis]," and surgeon Allen prescribes "Iodide Potass. (96 grs.), Sulph. Iron (128 grs.) in Simple Syrup [a sugar water mixture] fʒ IV" in teaspoonful doses three times a day.[38] Allen is apparently relieved when quinine becomes available once again on March 7, and he promptly gives eight grain doses to a Lieutenant Fisher. Interestingly, no indications suggest that Allen availed himself of Porcher's plant substitutes, following the recommended indigenous supply table, or that he foraged for the botanical substitutes whenever shortages occurred.

Others, however, clearly did use botanical subsitutes. Through interviews with aged Confederate surgeons, Joseph Jacobs was able to present a valuable picture of drug conditions in the South during the war and how they coped with shortages.[39] One surgeon used red oak bark added to water as a disinfectant, slippery elm as an emollient, mayapple and strong teas of peach tree leaves as laxatives, and for "bilious fevers" he gave Virginia snakeroot when calomel could not be had. He gave butterfly root and bloodroot in cases of pneumonia—instead of Dover's powders—and boneset was his preferred substitute for quinine.[40] But the gathering and use of elaborate substitutes takes time and considerable effort, a luxury not always available in camp and field. Consider assistant surgeon William H. Taylor of the 19th Virginia Infantry. He described his standard process of diagnosis and treatment as follows:

> Early in the morning we had sick-call, when those who claimed to be ill or disabled came up to be passed upon. Diagnosis was rapidly made, usually by intuition, and treatment was with such drugs as we chanced to have in the knap-sack and were handiest to obtain. In serious cases we made an honest effort to bring to bear all the skill and knowledge we possessed, but our science could rarely display itself to the best advantage on account of the paucity of our resources. On the march my own practice was of necessity still further simplified, and was, in fact, reduced to the lowest terms. In one pocket of my trousers I had a ball of blue mass, in another a ball of opium. All complainants were asked the same question, "How are your bowels?" If they were open, I administered a plug of opium; if they were shut, I gave a plug of blue mass.[41]

Of course these shortages affected everyone. Subsequent to the war many reminisced about the harsh conditions and the many efforts to "make due."[42] Women played a significant role in this regard, and have already been discussed, but it affected pharmacists as well. H. B. Metcalfe of Montgomery, Alabama, gives a typical example of the effects of war on a fairly large drugstore operation:

> We were able to secure some drugs and chemicals during the war by attending the blockade sales at Charleston and Mobile. We did not have to substitute to a great extent in putting up prescriptions—those of us who were fortunate enough to be supplied at the sales. We found great difficulty in securing vials and corks, and were compelled to use second-hand vials, and corks made from tupelo trees answered very well. Prices were, of course, high. For instance, during the last year of the war all tinctures were sold at $1.00 an oz.; quinine, $25.00 per oz.; mor-

phine, $10.00 per dr.; quinine pills, $1.00 each, and other pills $5.00 a dozen. Prescriptions ranged from $5.00 to $15.00. Whiskey sold at $150.00 a bottle. You must recollect that greenbacks were worth about twenty times our money, gold 100 times. I imported a great many goods through Evans' Sons, Liverpool, and regret exceedingly I now have none of the invoices.[43]

The prices cited here were comparatively low to those of the interior, where scarcity and demand commanded prices ten times those quoted by Metcalfe (see p. 197).

If pharmaceutical conditions were poor for Southern druggists and bad for the medical corps, they were worse still for those in Southern prisons. An interesting glimpse is provided in the diary of Solon Hyde, hospital steward for the 17th Regiment Ohio Volunteer Infantry.[44] Hyde was captured at the Battle of Chickamauga, September 20, 1863, and remained a prisoner until his exchange on February 27, 1865, at Wilmington, North Carolina.[45] He was transferred to a number of prisons, but his account chiefly deals with his experiences at Libby, Pemberton, Danville, and Andersonville.

Hyde's description of pharmaceutical conditions at Andersonville are especially illuminating. Although shortages were evident, drug supplies did not appear to be appreciably worse than in some of the more deprived infantry units. Hyde admits to having only an assortment of "roots and yarbs" and a very limited quantity of quinine, opium, and mercurial preparations—"though what we had were generally good and bore the stamp of English manufacture," suggesting that these were obtained through blockade-runners.[46] Hyde also pointed out that Andersonville was the only dispensary for miles around, "and citizens sometimes came, with orders from headquarters, to draw from us for family use."[47] Hyde's daily routine suggests that pharmacists' duties were performed regularly:

The manner in which the surgeons performed their duty was to visit their wards every morning, visiting each patient and writing their prescriptions in a book which was then turned over to a ward-master. This officer made a computation of the number of doses, if of roots, barks, or herbs, and we in the dispensary issued them in bulk. It was rather a unique way, but we could do no better, as we had no paper in which we could divide the doses. Every other day we made pills of various kinds, generally about seven thousand in number. This work generally kept us busy until the middle of the afternoon.[48]

Hyde's description of the paucity of medicines accords with prisons elsewhere. Writing to surgeon E. D. Eiland, in charge of the 1st Division Confederate States Military Prison Hospital, assistant surgeon J. Crews Pelot pleaded, "We have but little more than indigenous barks and roots with which to treat the numerous forms of disease to which our attention is daily called. For the treatment of wounds, ulcers, and c.," he added, " we have literally nothing except water."[49] Pelot also mentioned the extreme privation in diet that was affecting the men and insisted that two ounces of boiled beef and a half-cup of rice was making all the work of his medical staff of no avail. Solon Hyde experienced much the same and bore the scars of scurvy the remainder of his life to prove it.

There was an ironic twist to all this. The war and the shortages caused therefrom could be a double-edged sword. The Confederacy took its revenge by restricting the flow of Southern botanicals northward. When it is recalled that 67 percent of the substances listed in the *United States Pharmacopoeia* were botanical, the impact can readily be seen. John Maisch saw it too. The head of the Philadelphia lab chided his colleagues for not taking more energetic measures to grow medicinal plants on a systematic basis. Pointing out that many of the most frequently used native American plants such as Seneca snakeroot *(Polygala senega)*, Indian-pink *(Spigelia marilandica)*, Virginia snakeroot *(Aristolochia serpentatria)*, and American ginseng *(Panax quinquefolium)*—were either extinct in the East or obtainable only in the South, Maisch concluded that "we had been compelled to look to the South for a sufficient supply, and since this source has been shut off, to the young and growing states of out great West [we must look]."[50] Maisch added:

It is within this writer's knowledge that, in certain localities in the immediate neighborhood of Philadelphia, cimicifuga [black cohosh, *Cimicifuga racemosa*], sanguinara [bloodroot, *Sanguinaria canadensis*] and veratrum viride [American hellebore, *V. viride*] have almost entirely disappeared, and it is likely to be similar in other places.[51]

Thomas Potts James (1803-1882), a struggling apothecary in Philadelphia, knew this all too well. Almost as soon as hostilities broke out, ardent Unionist James feared for his business. "I am in very great need of means and am compelled to urge my customers to assist me all in their power. My Southern resources being all cut off," pleaded James, "I call earnestly upon loyal ones to come forward and relieve the pressure."[52] James had a wide and varied clientele. One interesting customer was a Dr. Burbower of Bruceton, Virginia. This region would eventually break away from the Old Dominion to become West Virginia, and Burbower, reflecting the sentiments of many of his neighbors, was apparently as strong a Unionist as James. But politics and patriotism aside, business was business. James writes to the doctor that the remittance he sent in Virginia bank notes was discounted at 16 percent, "but as heretofore," he continues, "I have shared the cost with you. I do this willingly for a loyal Virginian engaged in the sacred cause of Liberty."[53] When cash flows were not troubling the Philadelphia druggist, supplies were. By mid-November he was complaining that "camphor is now high & will be higher," "flaxseed has advanced," "nutmeg & mace have duty of 25 cents per lb.," and "wintergreen is very scarce."[54] The remainder of the war was difficult for James and his family. After the war he gave up the drug business to move his family in with his father-in-law in Cambridge, Massachusetts.

WARTIME SHORTAGES TAKE THEIR TOLL

James was just one of many north of the Mason-Dixon line hurt by the internecine conflict, but no matter how hard the Northern druggists might be hit, the South unquestionably suffered more severely and directly. From a pharmaceutical standpoint this comes into sharpest focus through the three chief factors that plagued the South throughout the war: (1) the blockade; (2) the breakdown in transportation; and (3) the breakdown in communications.

Historians have argued the effectiveness of the blockade since the war itself. Some claim the blockade was progressively effective in slowly strangling the South of its resources to wage war;[55] others insist that attempts to seal off the Confederacy from the rest of the world amounted to a "paper" or "hapless blockade."[56] None of them paused to look at the effectiveness of the blockade from the vantage point of its effects on the drug supply. The records of the purveyor's offices in Macon, Georgia, Memphis, Tennessee, and Jackson, Mississippi, show progressively dwindling drug supplies.[57] Writing in August 1864, Lafayette Guild, medical director of the Army of Northern Virginia, felt the impact of medical store deficits and warned the surgeon general,

> There are almost daily complaints from the medical officers particularly from those of General Beauregaurd's command of the great scarcity of medical supplies, especially such as tonics and antiperiodics, much disease at present prevails among the troops in the trenches consisting principally of Intermittent & Remittent Fever and bowel affection. Yet it is believed that the strength of the army would not be naturally influenced if suitable remedies could be obtained for the treatment of cases in camp. The scarcity of Sulphate of Quinea is assuming a very serious character, all of its substitutes that can be procured, are being used yet with little permanent benefit. The necessity of sending so many patriots to General Hospital arises only from the want of medicines suitable for their treatment in camp & the field infirmaries.[58]

Although the shortages of medicine were depleting men from the field, perhaps no better view of the extent of the drug shortages in the Confederacy can be seen than in the inventory of captured medical stores found in Richmond at war's end.[59] Below is a partial list of the main items:

Lobelia 178 lb	Tr. Verat Veridi ½ lb
Acid Acetic 1 lb	Acid Nitric 1 lb
Acid Tartaric 2 lb	Ether sulph. 2 ½ lbs
Ether spiritus ½ lb	Spts. Ether Nitrici 9 lb
Ammon. Carb. 3 lb	Ammon Murias ¾ lb
Asafoetida tinct. 32 oz	Bismuth Subcarb. 12 oz
Camphor 5 lb	Podophylin ¼ lb
Strmonii 1 ½ lb	Lig. Stryrax 1 ½ lbs
Ext. Sarsaparilla 3 lb	Creasotum 1 lb
Ext. Colocynth C. 1 lb	Ext. Conii ¼ lb
Ext. Gentian 20 lb	Ext. Prunii Virgin. ½ lb
Ext. Rhii Flor 24 oz	Ext. Ginger 16 oz

Ferri pwer sulph. 16 oz
Hydrarg. iodid. ½ oz
Diaphoretic antimony 2½ lb
Lini pulvis 15 lb
Potas. acetas 1 lb
Scillae 1 lb
Soda chlor. Lip 1 oz
Potas sulph. ¼ oz
Calamini ¼ oz
Calaminis 1 oz
Ext. Logwood 100 lb
Tr. Cinchona 15 gal

Glycerine 2 oz
Ferri citras 3 oz
Hydrarg. cum creta 4 oz
Opii tinct. 17 oz
Potas. chloras 1 ½ oz
Scillae syripis 5 oz
Soda bicarb. 1 oz
R. Colchici ½ oz
Colocynthidis ½ oz
Pulv. Jalap ¾ oz
Solut. Quinine 1 lb
Poplar bark 18 lb

For a principal supply depot such as Richmond *none* of the quantities appear sufficient to supply a large army, except perhaps the supplies of lobelia and logwood. The shortage problem was mirrored elsewhere. Medical purveyor William H. Prioleau experienced steadily declining acquisitions of quinine sulfate: on June 30, 1862, he reported 1,127 ounces on hand; in September 1863 he had 1,114 ounces; and by March 1865 a mere 6 ounces.[60] Historians may continue to argue the impact and effectiveness of the blockade in other areas, but the drug shortages it caused thereby were real and their impacts demonstrable.

The paucity of many indigenous medicines—such as *Podophyllum peltatum* (mayapple), *Acorus calamus* (sweetflag), *Aralia nudicaulis* (sarsaparilla), and others—suggests an additional problem: namely, transportation. The significance of the breakdown in transportation in the collapse of the Confederacy has long been recognized. Historian William Diamond pointed out that "the Confederacy's inability to solve its railroad problem contributed to its defeat."[61] Chief commissary for Virginia, B. P. Noland, recalled

> that our condition was almost desperate, not because our supplies were exhausted . . . but because our transportation from points where supplies were accumulated had almost entirely failed us. All the railroads were in bad condition, and several of the most important ones had been so damaged by the enemy's cavalry as to be unavailing for the transportation of supplies for weeks at a time."[62]

The general problem with the Southern transportation system outlined above was experienced by the medical corps specifically. For example, George Blackie complained to Major Winnermore of lost medical supplies via the South Carolina Rail Road. Perplexed at the loss, the major could only request of Blackie the value of the loss with the promise of a "claim for payment."[63] The difficulty of obtaining adequate and reliable supply deliveries was no small source of trouble for J. Julian Chisolm, who admitted, "I find my accounts give me a great deal of trouble. . . . I report stock on hand to correspond with the account for which I am responsible whilst in some cases I am far short and in a few overrun."[64] The problem of poor transportation by road and rail caused huge discrepancies to appear in drug supplies, and prevented the Confederate Medical Department from distributing essential medicines evenly and where needed. In some areas quinine was so abundant it was used prophylactically, in others it was practically nonexistent. This situation was exacerbated as the transportation infrastructure collapsed late in the war. "Wagon as well as railroad transportation broke down almost completely," concluded H. H. Cunningham, "and needed supplies arrived tardily, if at all."[65]

Closely related to the problem of transportation was the problem of communications. The extant records of the Confederate purveyor's offices are replete with shipments of medicines that were incomplete, inaccurate, or just plain wrong. Much of this was caused by a general breakdown in communications. Orders were not received, received late, or miscarried. Just as disease proved more lethal to the Confederacy than shot or shell, so too was a failure of communications *and* a failure in supplies the South's true death knell. The real end came when Lee's 35,000 exhausted and starving men beat a hasty retreat toward much-needed rations at Amelia Court House. Arriving early the morning of April 4, 1865, the beleaguered army found Confederate boxcars loaded with munitions instead of receiving the expected 135,000 rations.[66] A communications mix-up essentially spelled the end for the Army of Northern Virginia's determined defense; five days later Lee would formally surrender to Grant at Appomattox Court House. For the medical corps as well the end was the result of a lack of supplies, bad transportation, and poor communications that brought the purveying system to the breaking point.

Nevertheless, a nagging question persists. If the indigenous supply table so urgently and persistently advocated by Surgeon General

Moore really had been implemented, might the Southern medical stores been saved? After all, if plants could have been harvested proximate to most camps, hospital stewards could easily have prepared their own tinctures, decoctions, and infusions. The only pressing need would have been a steady supply of alcohol, the universal solvent and suspension medium. Without addressing the complex issue of availability, the crux of the matter comes down to how useful these indigenous substitutes really were.

Writing years later, from a physician's perspective, Dr. C. J. Edwards of Abbeville, Alabama, claimed that to be one of the few bright sides to the war in that it called "attention to the wealth of medicinal agents and remedies in our own fields, forests and plains."[67] Confederate surgeon Edwin S. Gaillard's postwar opinion was less sanguine. He felt that the blockade proved only that most of the botanical tonics and other medicines taken by Southerners were worthless.[68] Historians have generally sided with Gaillard,[69] but perhaps a fresh approach is called for.

THE MEDICINES OF THE SOUTH: AN APPRAISAL

Norman Franke, in his 1956 dissertation on Confederate pharmacy, stated:

> The merits of these substitutes in some cases speak for themselves; and a few are actually dangerous. It was not difficult to find satisfactory astringents, diuretics, local anodynes, emetics, and laxatives in the Southern woodlands, but their indigenous plants failed to produce adequate and effective narcotics, analgetics [sic], and antimalarials. Indeed, despite this concentrated effort, no new valuable indigenous drug was discovered by the Confederate physicians."[70]

Elsewhere, his analysis of the *Confederate Recipe Book* (1863) concluded that the recommended remedies were either worthless, questionable, unnecessary, or "decidedly dangerous."[71]

Franke's indictment of the Confederate materia medica deserves some comment. First of all, Franke's distinction between anodynes and analgesics is unclear, since both terms essentially mean the same thing. Second, Franke seems to indict the Confederate indigenous supply table (see Appendix A) on the basis that it contained no *new* medicinal plants. In this sense, Franke is correct. As already mentioned, around one-third of all the substances listed on the indigenous supply table were already on the primary list of the *United States Pharmacopoeia* and were, in fact, in keeping with a long tradition of an essentially botanical materia medica that did not markedly decline until the twentieth century (see Figure 10.1). These items were considered substitutes because they were offered in exclusion of imported, often preferred remedies. Thus, an indictment of the Confederacy's indigenous supply table is in some measure an indictment of nineteenth-century therapeutics in general. The Confederate surgeon general did not offer these medicinal plants on the basis of their novelty, though some undoubtedly were. They were offered on the basis of their availability and presumed likelihood of serving as reliable therapeutic substitutes for less available minerals or imported exotic botanicals.

Although the value of these Confederate drug substitutions cannot be broadly characterized as either efficacious or safe from a modern scientific perspective, it should be pointed out that of the sixty different plants listed on the supply table, over one-third still hold some current therapeutic use.[72] *Lobelia inflata* is an interesting example. The supply table recommends its use as an expectorant and it had a well-established reputation as a useful remedy for respiratory disorders.

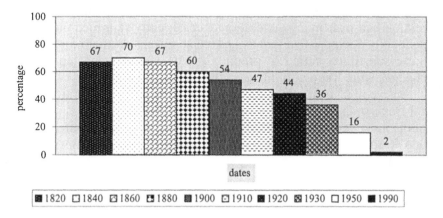

FIGURE 10.1. Botanicals in the USP (*Source:* Adapted from Wade Boyle, *Official Herbs: Botanical Substances in the United States Pharmacopoeias, 1820-1990* [East Palestine, OH: Buckeye Naturopathic Press, 1991]).

Today, *Lobelia inflata* (Indian tobacco) or its derivatives (lobeline hydrochloride and lobeline sulfate) are used for much the same purpose and are marketed throughout Europe in a number of multi-ingredient preparations.[73] Similarly, *Polygala senega* (Seneca snakeroot), listed in the supply table as an expectorant, is widely marketed throughout Europe and South Africa for respiratory-tract complaints.[74] A popularly prescribed diuretic on the supply table was *Juniperus communis* (juniper); it is still widely manufactured and dispensed for the same purpose today.[75]

The examples are numerous, but suffice it to say that some of the substances listed on the indigenous supply table are still therapeutically alive and well. Of course manufacture and sale do not necessarily equal efficacy and safety, but many of these substances have been the subjects of favorable pharmacognostic studies.[76] This is not to imply that the entire supply table remains full of viable remedies. Many of the active substances are used for very different purposes today than those recommended on the supply table. Others were and are of no value whatsoever, but it does suggest that these botanicals deserve more than the summary dismissal that they were all either worthless, dangerous, or, in the words of one recent historian, simply the product of "wishful thinking."[77] The fact that the medical corps of the Civil War did not know of pharmacology, germ theory, virology, or Koch's postulates did not also mean that they were therapeutic knaves and fools. By careful empirical observation, the medical profession had over many generations occasionally stumbled on therapeutically appropriate dose/response relationships. Furthermore, when these substitutes failed to produce the desired or expected result, changes were frequently made in the prescribed regimen.

An excellent example of this is presented in the Confederate Medical Department's struggle to find a viable substitute for quinine. One of the most common preparations for fevers among the Confederates was "tincture of indigenous barks." In its original form it consisted of the following:

> Dried dogwood bark, 30 parts; dried poplar bark, 30 parts; dried willow bark, 40 parts; whisky, 45 degrees strength; two pounds of the mixed bark to one gallon of whisky. Macerate fourteen days. Dose for tonic and anti-febrifuge [i.e., febrile] purposes, one ounce three times a day.[78]

The Confederate medical corps knew the antifebrile properties of quinine and had recommended its distribution to troops in malarial regions, just as the North had.[79] The prospects of dwindling supplies in quinine sulfate and its crude drug derivative cinchona (both of which had to be imported) sent Moore and his colleagues in search of a reliable substitute. Because of its equally bitter taste, dogwood *(Cornus florida)* became their first choice. This was by no means a new discovery. Dogwood had been conjectured to be a viable substitute for quinine from the very first edition of the U.S. *Dispensatory* of 1833.[80] This suggestion was carried to the *Dispensatory* active during the war.[81] But the four-year conflict would put this repeated assertion to the test. Though they did not know it, dogwood contains none of the constituents of cinchona or quinine and so its frequent use met with consistent and repeated failure. By early summer of 1864 the verdict on dogwood was virtually unanimous—it did *not* work— and alternatives were quickly tried. In despair, assistant surgeon W. T. Grant concluded, "Our efforts to procure a reliable substitute for quinine, has thus far proved a failure, unless the turpentine, as recently recommended in this journal, should answer; or common salt, (chloride of sodium), which has been very highly recommended to me."[82] The fact is, *nothing* worked. Quinine or cinchona simply had no substitute.

Sometimes in their efforts to modify formulae and find other equivalents, the surgeons made improvements. For example, the original tincture of indigenous barks included willow *(Salix* spp.) and popular barks *(Populus* spp.), two products that contain the basic chemical constituents of aspirin and would have helped with fevers but not specifically with those of the malarial type.[83] With dogwood increasingly recognized by surgeons as worthless, by late 1864 we find an important change. In a letter to surgeon Thomas S. Latimer, the surgeon general's office substituted logwood *(Haematoxylon campechianum)* for dogwood.[84] The designation is clear and is unmistakably not an inadvertent error (see Figure 10.2). The change was an obvious recognition of the utter failure of dogwood as a medicinal equivalent for quinine; the addition of a known astringent such as logwood was included in place of dogwood to aid in alleviating the diarrhea that so often accompanied febrile conditions. Logwood, long known for its mildly astringent properties,[85] was often given by Union surgeons in cases of dysentery and diarrhea, and its

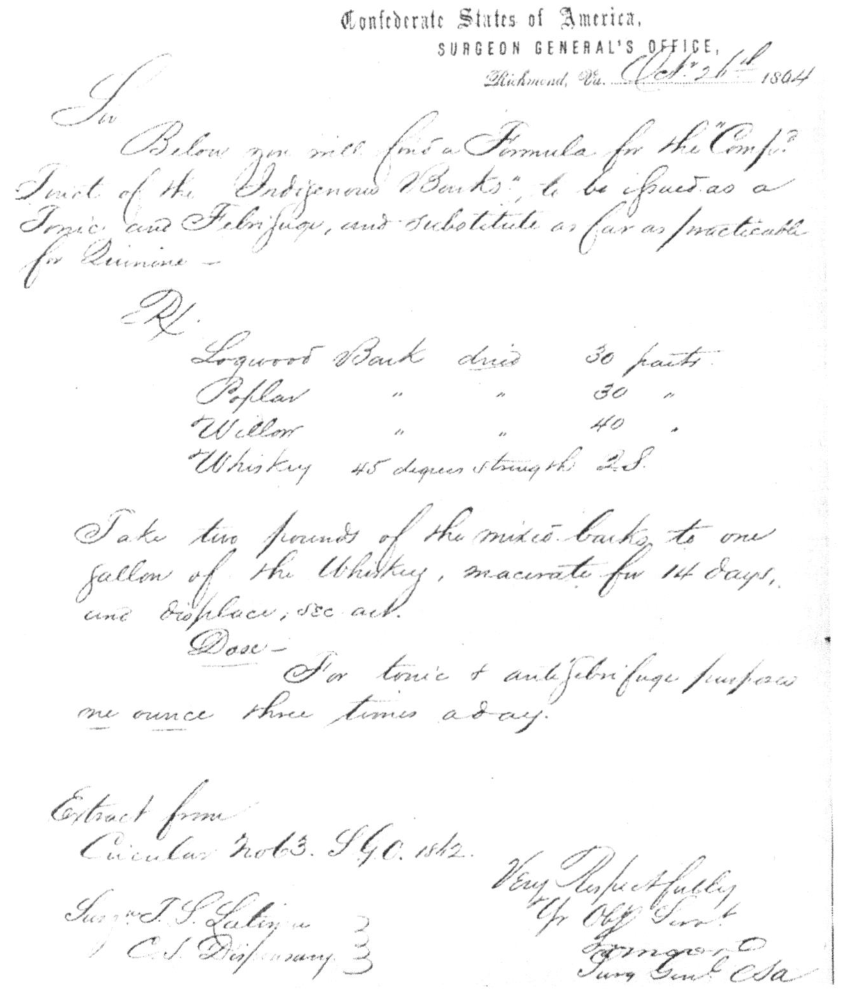

Confederate States of America,
SURGEON GENERAL'S OFFICE,
Richmond, Va. Oct 26th 1864

Sir

Below you will find a Formula for the "Comp.d Tinct of the Indigenous Barks", to be issued as a Tonic and Febrifuge, and substitute as far as practicable for Quinine –

R.

Logwood Bark	dried	30 parts
Poplar	"	"	30 "
Willow	"	"	40 "
Whiskey	45 degrees strength	q.s.

Take two pounds of the mixed bark to one gallon of the Whiskey, macerate for 14 days, and displace, &c act.

Dose –
For tonic & antifebrifuge purposes one ounce three times a day.

Extract from
Circular no. 13. S.G.O. 1862.

Very Respectfully
Yr Obt Servt
Junge,
Surg Genl CSa

Surg. T.S. Latimer
C.S. Dispensary 3

FIGURE 10.2. By 1864, dogwood had been discarded as a substitute for quinine and was being replaced by other ingredients such as logwood (shown above). Photo courtesy of the National Library of Medicine, History of Medicine Division.

use in Confederate practice was neither novel nor unexpected.[86] As we have seen from the list of captured supplies at the Richmond dispensary, logwood was in reasonably abundant supply, despite the fact that logwood is native to Central America. That it was readily obtainable is also attested to by its suggested use as reliable litmus test paper.[87] Thus, a remedy that in reality had only a general antifever action was improved into a tincture that would have helped treat the symptoms of a nonmalarial condition of fever accompanied by diarrhea.

In the end, what *can* be said with some certainty regarding the Confederate materia medica is that it was a reasonable and concerted effort to deal with the harsh realities of providing a well-stocked supply table of reliable remedies. Its effectiveness in doing so must be evaluated on an item-by-item basis, and no broad generalization can do it justice (for details, see Appendix E). The historians' harsh indictments of the indigenous drug substitutes of the Civil War are, in any case, too superficial to be taken at face value. If an evaluation must be rendered, it can be said that the indigenous supply table probably assisted the medical staff in managing symptoms if not effecting cures. Compared with the administration of antimony and assorted mercurials, the indigenous substitutes probably did less overall harm. Nevertheless, the evaluation of indigenous Southern plants had the valuable effect of serving as a proving ground for many items that had never really been put to the therapeutic test. Sometimes one of the greatest benefits an experiment can serve—and this surely was an experiment, even if it was the product of necessity—is that it tells us where *not* to look. After the Civil War no responsible physician ever seriously suggested dogwood as a substitute for quinine; the *USD* of 1884 referred to dogwood as "nearly banished" from regular practice.[88] Indeed, many of the other failed efforts at finding substitutes for narcotics and other medicinal agents allowed the medical profession to proceed advancing the healing art a bit more wisely.

Epilogue

"The Consciousness of Duty Faithfully Performed": An Appraisal of Civil War Pharmacy

On April 10, 1865, the day after his surrender to Ulysses S. Grant, General Robert E. Lee composed his last general order to the Army of Northern Virginia. The war was over he told them, but they could return to their homes with "the satisfaction that proceeds from the consciousness of duty faithfully performed."[1] The commander wanted his men to depart the battlefield without shame or remorse. Perhaps this is how we should leave the thousands of men and women, from both sides, who had provided their armies and navies with pharmaceutical care. All the surgeons, assistant surgeons, nurses, U.S. Sanitary Commission relief workers, medical purveyors, hospital and surgeon's stewards, manufacturers, and blockade-runners provided medicines to the largest collective military force ever assembled in North America. They could with some confidence return to postwar America with the satisfaction of "duty faithfully performed."

THE IMPACT OF THE WAR

But did their many sacrifices matter in the long run? Detractors could say that these men and women left the war in as sorry a therapeutic condition as they had found it: no new drug was discovered, no new treatment was adopted, and the science of pharmacy had not appreciably advanced. Perhaps, but they could take solace in the fact that they had advanced the healing art in other ways. The following are among the most important impacts of the war on American pharmacy:

1. The war provided an effective proving ground for the use of therapeutic substances, old and new. Long-established remedies such as calomel and antimony were openly questioned by Surgeon General Hammond. Although he paid a serious price for his removal of these substances from the standard supply table, the future of both were placed squarely within the forum of professional debate for the allopathic community rather than as a matter merely of sectarian contention. It would take years for physicians to change their favored use of mercurials, but the concerted challenge to the use of antimony and calomel within regular ranks may justly be said to have begun with Hammond's Circular No. 6. Other remedies, such as a wide range of botanicals and chemicals like the bromides, were also put to the test. Some actions already suspected were confirmed; others were shown to be false. The one important drug with real therapeutic value (quinine sulfate) was also put to a field test of unprecedented proportions. While quinine remained in use for a range of fevers, questions of effective dosage were, however, largely resolved and its value against malaria confirmed.

2. The government laboratories, especially the one managed by John Maisch in Philadelphia, had important implications for future pharmaceutical developments in the United States. Far from impeding growth in the private sector, the U.S. government's first effort at pharmaceutical manufacturing actually stimulated entrepreneurial activity after the war. In the words of historian George Winston Smith:

> Maisch's departments were administered by brilliant young civilian pharmacists who went on to responsible positions in the pharmaceutical manufacturing industry after the war. The laboratory was, in fact, an important in-training experience for those young men who were able to grasp the significance of pharmacy in connection with the new industrialism that the war was helping to bring into being.[2]

3. The immediate years following the war found the drug market generally healthy and returning to an especially bright peacetime normalcy. Even in cities such as Charleston that had experienced serious disruptions in both the quantity and quality of drugs, times were

markedly improving.[3] For crude drug products such as barks, the American Pharmaceutical Association's Committee on the Drug Market could report, "The market is better supplied of late, at reduced prices, for nearly every variety."[4] Roots and herbs "are in far better supply," the committee wrote, "of good quality, and generally at greatly reduced prices." Of chemicals, they announced reductions in prices and products "constantly improving in quality, and rarely adulterated."[5]

The broader impulses of industrialization and urbanization spawned by the war effort further developed the pharmaceutical industry north of the Mason-Dixon. Established firms such as Squibb, Rosengarten and Sons, Scheiffelin and Sons, Powers and Weightman, Sharp and Dohme, McKesson, Frederick Stearns, and John Wyeth were launched as major drug concerns in postwar America based on the profits accrued from wartime demands. But the valuable lessons learned in large-scale drug manufacturing during the war—and the booming economy immediately following it—spawned other companies. Mallinckrodt began its St. Louis plant in 1867 and would become a major producer of fine chemicals for years to come. S. P. Duffield's partnership with H. C. Parke in that same year would also grow into the large, Detroit-based Parke-Davis Company. Similarly, a pharmacist and Civil War veteran, Eli Lilly, would soon amass his fortune when he established his pharmaceutical manufacturing operations in Indianapolis in 1876.

The unprecedented demands for medicines caused by the war created equally unprecedented commercial activity in the North, as entrepreneurs created what Dennis Worthen has called an "eponymous industry."[6] The postwar pharmaceutical industry would no longer be clustered in Philadelphia, but would take on a truly national character based on the proliferation of a vastly enlarged arena of business opportunities. The alcohol industry also emerged from the war bigger than ever,

> with inflated capacity and an excise tax that had been advanced from 20¢ a gallon in 1862 to $2.00. Henceforth industrial alcohol was a weighty factor in the whisky business and the tax an integral part of the alcohol situation. The rate was cut sharply to 50¢ a gallon in 1868, but advanced to 70¢ in 1875, where it held for over 20 years.[7]

4. With these larger economies of scale the role of the pharmacist was forever changed. Large companies of mass-produced drugs marketed product lines resulting from sophisticated extraction processes supported and sustained by complex apparatus; a cadre of *professional* workers to manage these operations was increasingly needed after the war. This need was fulfilled through a greater sense of unity and collegial identity, along with improved educational opportunities. Indeed, the effects of these could be seen in the establishment of state pharmaceutical associations in the 1870s and 1880s, a similar expansion of state pharmacy laws, and with this a tremendous growth in formalized pharmaceutical education, as schools blossomed across America in the 1880s and 1890s.[8] Even the South was a beneficiary of this professionalization process, as state associations were established in Mississippi in 1871, Tennessee in 1873, Georgia in 1875, South Carolina in 1876, and so on. By 1887 every state of the former Confederacy had its own state association.

5. Although the pharmaceutical industry did not extend to the South, the region developed its own unique postwar environment. As with virtually every other part of the economy, the big drug manufacturers kept their operations north of the Mason-Dixon line. By 1890, census data suggests that only in Baltimore (at best a border city of the South) was there any pharmaceutical manufacturers of any size. The bulk centered in New York and Philadelphia, and so in some very real senses the contrasts witnessed in drug provision and distribution during the war remained thereafter.

This industrialization pattern meant that the South would become a chief supplier of crude vegetable drug product for the nation and the world. The challenge of alternative medicine launched prior to the Civil War by men such as Samuel Thomson, Alva Curtis, Wooster Beach, Hans Gram, and others (see pages 144-145) had the practical effects of (1) introducing botanicals into the mainstream pharmacopoeia and (2) fueling sectarian contention. This meant that the laity, disgruntled and unimpressed over the profession's own lack of therapeutic confidence, simply sought their own relief. Soldiers often brought their own homemade or store-bought medicines to camp and field, believing them to be at least as good and perhaps better than anything the surgeons could offer. These cure-all nostrums (often herbal) were boosted by wartime necessities, but after the war they became a veritable craze. Thus the dual influences of botanicism on regular medicine and the general public sustained plant-based drugs into the early decades of the next century. The patent medicine market exploded following the war, rising from 2,700 different items in 1880 to 38,000 different items by 1916.[9] Even by World War I, one-third of the U.S. standard supply table remained botanically based.[10] By the 1920s it was estimated that plant drugs from the Southern states, particularly the Blue Ridge and southern Appalachian regions, provided producers with 75 percent of the medicinal plants native to North America.[11]

These consumer-driven patent medicines had a profound and long-term effect on the retail businesses of the South. As thousands of ex-Confederate veterans returned to civilian life, many turned to store-keeping. Indeed, it became almost a fad in the postwar years. These small entrepreneurs throughout the South stimulated and provided a ready outlet to an expanding nostrum industry in the North. They sold cure-all elixirs and potions carrying names such as Dr. Kilmer's Swamp Root, Kickapoo Oil, and Mecca Compound. But all of them stocked ample supplies of distinctly Southern products such as: the Chattanooga Medicine Company's Black-Draught and Cardui; Pellagricide, manufactured by a South Carolina firm; Baughan's Pellagra Cure of Jasper, Alabama; Dr. Bell's Anti-Pain drops of Paducah, Kentucky; and the Brown Medicine Company's N and B Liniment of Morristown, Tennessee.[12] They captured the hearts, minds, and dollars of their Southern customers with ads touting the noble "Lost Cause" and printed descriptions of the curative wonders of their products on facsimiles of Confederate dollar bills. Although their Northern competitors produced product lines that dwarfed patent medicines of Southern manufacture, certain patent medicines and their promotional gimmicks remained as unique an expression of Southern distinctiveness as the diseases that plagued it.

6. Finally, the wartime demands laid the groundwork for America's role as a leader of the pharmaceutical industry worldwide. Indeed, it is quite possible that without the Civil War as a catalyst to pharmaceutical development (both in its manufacture and in its professionalization) that American pharmacy might well have languished in a comparatively primitive state for several more generations to come. The connections between pharmaceutical manufacturers and academia were largely twentieth-century phenomena, as was the active role of industry in research;[13] however, the economies of

scale necessary to develop meaningful partnerships between scientific and business enterprise were rooted in the catalytic forces of the Civil War.

The war is believed to have one very serious pharmaceutical consequence, and one for which the patent medicine trade was at least partially responsible—drug addiction. The "army disease" or "soldier's sickness" was regarded as synonymous with addiction to opiates, morphine, and other narcotics so frequently prescribed by Civil War surgeons. One historian has called the rate of addiction in the South a "hidden epidemic" and blames the problem on diseases endemic to the region, physicians quick to prescribe pain relief for illnesses with no other remedy, and an unregulated patent medicine industry.[14] This notwithstanding, Mark A. Quinones does not ascribe this scourge to service-related prescriptions.[15] Quinones points out that statistics show a higher rate of addiction among Southern women than men and that many Civil War veterans developed drug problems who had no record of addiction during their tour of duty.[16] Quinones concludes:

> From a careful review of the existing literature, there is insufficient evidence to credit the Civil War as the catalyst for the onset of drug addiction in America. On the contrary, it is clear that while the Civil War may have contributed to the problem, drugs were already on the scene and being consumed at alarming rates long before the start of the war.[17]

CONCLUSION

Taking everything into consideration, it is a fair conclusion that more had happened to American pharmacy in the four years from 1861 to 1865 than had happened to it in all the years since the nation's birth. Pharmacy came into the war with an industry concentrated almost exclusively in Philadelphia and dominated by just a few major firms; it left the war poised to develop into an industry of national proportions, one that would eventually compete as a major player in the international market. Largely spawned by wartime demands, urban expansion, unprecedented growth in transportation, a massive influx of immigrant workers, and a rising middle class, postwar socioeconomic forces combined to keep pharmacy's economies of scale large and burgeoning. Historians have continued to argue the importance of the Civil War to the economic life of the nation (progress or impediment),[18] but for pharmacy there can be no question: it was the spark that drove the industry's phenomenal expansion in the last quarter of the nineteenth and into the twentieth century.

For the individual pharmacist, a new age had also dawned. Hospital stewards had tried to gain professional recognition in the military, and failed. The road to commissioned officer rank and standing would be a long one, but the foundations of professional cooperation and identity had been laid. The march from tradesman to professional practitioner, initiated with the founding of the American Pharmaceutical Association in 1852, was advanced through wartime necessity and finally bore fruit in the rapid establishment of state societies and formal schools of pharmacy. Just as Philadelphia pharmaceutical manufacturers shared the postwar stage with major competitors in New York, Detroit, St. Louis, and Indianapolis, would-be pharmacists also had an increasing number of educational choices beyond the venerable Philadelphia College of Pharmacy.

Of course all this was not readily apparent to all those who had labored so arduously on behalf of the apothecary's art throughout the war, but the sheer exhaustion must have somehow spawned relief. So it was on April 10 that while Lee was penning his final farewell to his men, hospital steward John N. Henry of the 49th New York Infantry was writing from Burkesville, Virginia, to his wife Diana: "Our arduous labors are closed & I write with a more buoyant heart than for the last three years & eight months."[19] Indeed, for pharmacists everywhere, North and South, better days lay ahead.

Appendix A

Union and Confederate Standard Supply Tables

TABLE A.1.The U.S. Army Standard Supply Table for Field Service

Articles	In medicine wagon	In army wagon
Acaciæ	Oz. 8	
Acid sulphuricum aromat.	Oz. 8	
Acid tannic	Oz. 1	
Acid tartaricum	Oz. 8	
Æther sulphuric	Oz. 32	Oz. 32
Æther spirit: comp.	Oz. 16	Oz. 16
Æther spirit nitrici	Oz. 32	Oz. 32
Alcohol	Botts. 12	
Alumen	Oz. 8	
Ammoniæ carbonas	Oz. 8	
Ammoniæ liquor	Oz. 32	Oz. 64
Ammoniæ spirit: aromat.	Oz. 4	Oz. 16
Argenti nitras	Oz. 1	
Argenti nitras fusum	Oz. 1	
Bismuth subnitras	Oz. 16	
Camphora	Oz. 8	
Cantharides ceratum	Oz. 8	
Capsici pulvis	Oz. 8	
Cera alba	Oz. 4	
Ceratum adipis	Lbs. 3	Lbs. 4
Ceratum resinæ	Lbs. 1	
Chloroformum (in 8 oz. bottles)	Oz. 32	Oz. 192

TABLE A.1 *(continued)*

Articles	In medicine wagon	In army wagon
Cinchonæ sulphas	Oz. 24	
Collodium	Oz. 1	
Copiaba	Oz. 32	
Creosotum	Oz. 4	
Cupri sulphas	Oz. 2	
Extractum aconiti rad: fluidum	Oz. 4	
Extractum belladonnæ	Oz. 1	
Extractum cinchonæ fluidum	Oz. 16	
Extractum colchici sem: fluid.	Oz. 4	
Extractum colocynthidis comp.	Oz. 8	
Extractum ipecacuanhæ fluid	Oz. 8	
Extractum senegæ fluid	Oz. 8	
Extractum zingiberis fluid	Oz. 16	
Ferri chloridi tinctura	Oz. 8	Oz. 16
Ferri et quiniæ citras	Oz. 1	
Ferri persulphatis liquor	Oz. 4	
Ferri persulphatis pulvis	Oz. 1	Oz. 16
Glycerina	Oz. 8	
Hydrargyri pilulæ	Oz. 8	Oz. 16
Hydrargyri unguentum	Lb. 1	
Hydrargyri unguentum nitratis	Oz. 4	
Hydrargyrum c. creta	Oz. 8	
Iodinum	Oz. 2	
Ipecachuanæ et opii pulvis	Oz. 8	Oz. 48
Ipecachuanæ pulvis	Oz. 8	
Lini pulvis	Lbs. 8	
Magnesiæ sulphas	Lbs. 8	Lbs. 16
Morphiæ sulphas	Oz. ½	Lbs. 4
Oleum olivæ (in 32 oz. bottles)	Botts. 2	Botts. 4
Oleum ricini (in 32 oz. bottles)	Botts. 4	Botts. 4
Oleum terebinthinæ	Bott. 1	

Articles	In medicine wagon	In army wagon
Oleum tiglii	Oz. 1	
Opii pulvis	Oz. 8	Oz. 16
Opii tinctura	Oz. 16	
Opii tinctura camphorata	Oz. 16	Oz. 32
Pilulæ camphoræ (gr. 2) et opii (gr. 1)	Doz. 8	Doz. 8
Pilulæ cathart: comp.	Doz. 8	Doz. 24
Pilulæ opii	Doz. 8	Doz. 24
Plumbi acetas	Oz. 8	Oz. 32
Potassæ arsenitis liquor	Oz. 8	
Potassæ bicarbonas	Oz. 8	
Potassæ chloras	Oz. 8	Oz. 32
Potassæ permanganas (crystals)	Oz. 2	
Potassii iodidum	Oz. 8	Oz. 32
Quinæ sulphas	Oz. 10	Oz. 48
Quinæ sulphas (in pills, 3 grs. each)	Doz. 8	Doz. 24
Sapo	Lbs. 8	Lbs. 4
Scillæ syrupus	Lbs. 4	Lbs. 4
Sinapis nigræ pulvis	Lbs. 6	Lbs. 6
Sodæ bicarbonas	Oz. 8	Oz. 64
Sodæ chlorinat: liq. (in one pound bottles)	Lb. 1	Lbs. 6
Sodæ et potassæ tartras	Oz. 16	
Spiritus frumenti	Botts. 24	Botts. 24
Spiritus vini gallici	Botts. 6	Botts. 24
Sulphur		Oz. 32
Zinci chloridii liquor	Oz. 16	Oz. 96
Zinci sulphas	Oz. 2	

Source: "Standard Supply Table for Field Service" in Charles R. Greenleaf, *A Manual for Medical Officers of the United States Army* (Philadelphia: J. B. Lippincott, 1864), pp. 143-144.

TABLE A.2. The U.S. Army Standard Supply Table for General Hospitals (Allowance for Three Months)

Articles	100 beds	200 beds	300 beds	400 beds	500 beds	1,000 beds
Acaciæ Pulvis, in ½ lb. bottles (oz.)	32	56	80	104	128	232
Acidum Aceticum, in ½ g. s. bottles (oz.)	8	16	24	32	40	72
Acidum Citricum, in ½ lb. bottles (oz.)	16	32	48	56	64	120
Acidum Muriaticum, in ½ lb. g. s. bottles (oz.)	2	2	3	3	4	7
Acidum Nitricum, in ½ lb. g. s. bottles (oz.)	8	16	16	24	32	56
Acidum Phosphoricum Dilutum, in 2 oz. g. s. bottles (oz.)	2	2	3	3	4	7
Acidum Sulphuricum, in ½ lb. g. s. bottles (oz.)	8	8	16	16	24	40
Acidum Aromaticum, in ½ lb. g. s. bottles (oz.)	16	32	48	56	64	120
Acidum Tannicum, in 1 oz. bottles (oz.)	4	6	8	10	12	22
Acidum Tartaricum, in 8 oz. bottles (oz.)	32	56	80	104	128	232
Æther Fortoir, in ½ lb. g. s. bottles and ½ lb. tins, soldered (lbs.)	64	112	160	208	256	464
Ætheris Spiritus Compositus, in ½ lb. g. s. bottles (oz.)	16	32	48	56	64	120
Ætheris Nitrici, in ½ lb. g. s. bottles (oz.)	48	96	144	176	208	384
Alcohol Fortius, in 32 oz. bottles (bottles)	24	36	48	60	72	144
Aloes Pulvis, in 2 oz. bottles (oz.)	2	4	6	6	8	14
Alumen, in ½ lb. bottles (oz.)	16	32	40	48	56	104
Ammoniæ Carbonas, in ½ lb. bottles (oz.)	16	32	40	48	64	112
Ammoniæ Liquor, in ½ lb. g. s. (oz.)	96	164	224	288	352	640

Articles	100 beds	200 beds	300 beds	400 beds	500 beds	1,000 beds
Ammoniæ Murias, in ½ lb. bottles (oz.)	8	16	24	32	40	72
Ammoniæ Spiritus Aromaticus, in 4 oz. g. s. bottles (oz.)	4	8	12	16	20	36
Argenti Nitras, in 1 oz. g. s. bottles (oz.)	2	3	4	5	6	11
Argenti Fusum, in 1 oz. bottles (oz.)	2	3	4	5	6	11
Arsenitis Potassæ Liquor, in 4 oz. bottles (oz.)	4	8	12	16	20	36
Asafœtida, in 4 oz. bottles (oz.)	4	8	12	16	16	32
Bismuthi Subcarbonas, in 2 oz. bottles (oz.)	2	4	6	8	10	18
Camphora, in 8 oz. bottles (oz.)	8	16	24	32	40	72
Cantharidis Pulvis, in 2 oz. bottles (oz.)	2	2	2	4	4	8
Cantharidis Ceratum, in 8 oz. tins (oz.)	24	40	56	72	88	160
Capsici Pulvis, in 8 oz. bottles (oz.)	8	16	24	24	32	56
Catechu, in 8 oz. bottles (oz.)	8	16	24	24	32	56
Cera Alba in paper (oz.)	32	32	48	48	64	112
Ceratum Adipis, in 1 lb. pots (lbs.)	10	18	26	32	40	72
Ceratum Resinæ, in 1 lb. pots (lbs.)	2	4	5	6	8	14
Chlorinium (the materials for preparing) in a package (no.)	1	2	3	4	5	9
Chloroformum, in ½ lb. g. s. bottles and ½ lb. tins (oz.)	32	64	80	96	112	208
Cinchonæ Calisayæ Pulvis, in ½ lb. bottles (oz.)	16	24	32	40	48	88
Cinchonæ Sulphas, in 2 oz. bottles (oz.)	40	50	60	70	80	150
Collodium, in 1 oz. bottles (oz.)	2	3	4	5	6	11

TABLE A.2 (continued)

Articles	100 beds	200 beds	300 beds	400 beds	500 beds	1,000 beds
Copaiba, in 1 lb. bottles (oz.)	64	96	102	128	144	272
Creasotum, in 2 oz. g. s. bottles (oz.)	4	6	8	10	12	22
Creta Præparata, in ½ lb. bottles (oz.)	16	24	32	40	48	88
Cubebæ Oleo-resina (ex. Cubebæ Fl. U.S.P., 1850) in 8 oz. g. s. bottles (oz.)	8	16	24	32	40	72
Cupri Sulphas, in 2 oz. bottles (oz.)	2	4	6	8	10	18
Extractum Aconiti Radicis Fluidum, in ½ bottles (oz.)	8	16	24	32	40	72
Extractum Belladonnæ, in 1 oz. pots (oz.)	1	2	3	4	5	9
Extractum Buchu Fluidum, in ½ lb. bottles (oz.)	16	24	32	40	48	88
Extractum Cinchonæ Fluidum, (with aromatics) in ½ lb. bottles (oz.)	16	32	48	56	64	120
Extractum Colchici Seminis Fluidum, in 4 oz. bottles (oz.)	8	12	16	20	24	44
Extractum Colocynthidis Compositum, in 8 oz. pots (oz.)	8	16	24	32	32	64
Extractum Conii, in 1 oz. pots (oz.)	1	2	3	4	5	9
Extractum Ergotæ Fluidum, in 2 oz. bottles (oz.)	2	4	6	8	8	16
Extractum Gentianæ Fluidum, in ½ oz. bottles (oz.)	16	32	48	64	80	144
Extractum Glycyrrhizæ, in paper (oz.)	64	96	128	160	192	352
Extractum Hyoscyami, in 1 oz. pots (oz.)	1	2	3	4	5	9
Extractum Ipecacuanhæ Fluidum, in ½ lb. bottles (oz.)	8	16	24	32	40	72

Articles	100 beds	200 beds	300 beds	400 beds	500 beds	1,000 beds
Extractum Nucis Vomicæ, in 1 oz. pots (oz.)	1	2	3	4	5	9
Extractum Pruni Virginianæ Fluidum, in ½ lb. bottles (oz.)	8	16	24	32	40	72
Extractum Rhei Fluidum, in ½ lb. bottles (oz.)	8	16	24	32	40	72
Extractum Senegæ Fluidum, in ½ lb. bottles (oz.)	8	16	24	32	40	72
Extractum Spigeliæ Fluidum, in ½ lb. bottles (oz.)	8	16	16	24	24	48
Extractum Valerianæ Fluidum, in ½ lb. bottles (oz.)	8	16	24	32	40	72
Extractum Veratri Viridis Fluidum, in 2 oz. bottles (oz.)	2	4	6	6	8	14
Extractum Zingiberis Fluidum, in ½ lb. bottles (oz.)	16	24	32	40	48	88
Ferri Chloridi Tinctura, in ½ g. s. bottles (oz.)	16	32	48	56	64	120
Ferri Iodidi Syrupus, in ½ lb. g. s. bottles (oz.)	16	24	24	32	32	64
Ferri Et Quiniæ Citras, in 1 oz. bottles (oz.)	4	6	8	10	12	22
Ferri Persulphatis Liquor, in 4 oz. g. s. bottles (oz.)	4	8	12	16	20	36
Ferri Pulvis, in 1 oz. g. s. bottles (oz.)	1	2	8	4	5	9
Ferri Sulphas, in 4 oz. bottles (oz.)	4	4	8	8	12	20
Ferri Oxidum Hydratum (the material for) in package (no.)	1	1	1	1	1	2
Glycyrrhizæ Pulivs, in ½ oz. bottles (oz.)	8	16	24	32	32	64
Glycerina (pure and inodorous), in ½ lb. g. s. bottles (oz.)	16	24	32	40	40	80
Hydrargyri Chloridum Corrosivum, in 1 oz. g. s. bottles (oz.)	1	2	2	3	3	6
Hydrargyri Iodidum Flavum, in 1 oz. bottles (oz.)	1	1	2	2	2	4
Hydrargyri Oxidum Rubrum, in 1 oz. bottles (oz.)	1	1	2	2	3	4

TABLE A.2 *(continued)*

Articles	100 beds	200 beds	300 beds	400 beds	500 beds	1,000 beds
Hydrargyri Pilulæ, in 8 oz. pots (oz.)	8	16	24	32	40	72
Hydrargyri Unguentum, in 1 lb. pots (lbs.)	1	2	3	4	4	8
Hydrargyri Nitratis, in 4 oz. pots (oz.)	4	8	8	12	16	28
Iodinium, in 1 oz. g. s. bottles (oz.)	4	6	6	8	8	16
Ipecacuanhæ Pulvis, in ½ oz. bottles (oz.)	8	16	16	24	24	48
Ipecacuanhæ Pulvis et Opii Pulvis, in ¼ lb. bottles (oz.)	8	16	24	32	40	72
Linum, in tins (lbs.)	6	12	18	24	30	54
Lini Pulvis, in tins (lbs.)	16	32	48	48	56	104
Magnesia, in 4 oz. bottles (oz.)	8	16	16	20	24	44
Magnesiæ Sulphas, in ½ oz. papers and 8 lb. tins (lbs.)	16	24	32	40	48	88
Morphæ Sulphas in ¼ oz. bottles (oz.)	½	½	¾	1	1¼	2¼
Olei Menthæ Piperitæ Tinctura, in ½ lb. bottles (oz.)	16	24	32	40	48	88
Oleum Cinnamomi, in 1 oz. g. s. bottles (oz.)	1	1	2	2	3	5
Oleum Morrhuæ, in 32 oz. bottles (bottles)	10	15	20	25	30	55
Oleum Olivæ, in 32 oz. bottles (bottles)	4	8	12	16	20	36
Oleum Ricini, in 32 oz. bottles (bottles)	8	12	16	20	24	44
Oleum Terebinthinæ, in 32 oz. bottles (bottles)	2	4	6	8	10	18
Oleum Tiglii, in 1 oz. g. s. bottles (oz.)	1	1	2	2	3	5
Opii Pulvis, in ½ lb. bottles (oz.)	8	16	16	24	24	48

Articles	100 beds	200 beds	300 beds	400 beds	500 beds	1,000 beds
Opii Tinctura, in ½ lb. bottles (oz.)	16	32	48	56	64	120
Opii Camphorata, in ½ lb. bottles (oz.)	16	32	48	56	64	120
Pilulæ Catharticæ Comp., in g. s. bottles (doz.)	6	16	24	32	40	72
Plumbi Acetas, in ½ lb. bottles (oz.)	6	16	24	32	40	72
Podophyll Resini, in 1 oz. bottles (oz.)	1	1	2	2	3	5
Potassæ Acetas, in ½ lb. bottles (oz.)	8	16	24	32	40	72
Potassæ Bicarbonas, in ½ lb. bottles (oz.)	8	16	24	32	40	72
Potassæ Bitartras, in ½ lb. bottles (oz.)	16	32	32	48	48	96
Potassæ Chloras, in ½ lb. bottles (oz.)	16	32	32	48	48	96
Potassæ Nitras, in ½ lb. bottles (oz.)	8	8	16	16	24	40
Potassii Iodidum, in ½ lb. bottles (oz.)	24	48	64	80	96	176
Quinæ Sulphas, compressed in 5 oz. tins (oz.)	20	30	40	50	60	110
Rhei Pulvis, in 4 oz. bottles (oz.)	4	8	12	16	16	32
Rheum (oz.)	4	4	4	8	16	4
Sapo, in paper (lbs.)	8	12	16	20	24	44
Scillæ Pulvis, in 1 oz. bottles (oz.)	4	4	6	6	8	14
Scillæ Syrupus, in 1 lb. bottles (oz.)	8	14	20	26	42	58
Sinapis Nigræ Pulivs, in 6 lb. tins (lbs.)	6	12	18	18	24	42
Sodæ Clorinatæ Liquor, in 1 lb. g. s. bottles (lbs.)	6	9	12	15	15	30
Sodæ Bicarbonas, in ½ lb. bottles (oz.)	16	32	40	48	56	104

TABLE A.2 (continued)

Articles	100 beds	200 beds	300 beds	400 beds	500 beds	1,000 beds
Sodæ Boras, in ½ lb. bottles (oz.)	8	16	16	24	24	48
Sodæ et Potassæ Tartras, in ½ lb. bottles (oz.)	32	64	64	80	96	176
Spiritus Lavandulæ Comp., in ½ lb. bottles (oz.)	16	24	32	40	48	88
Spiritus Frumenti, in 32 oz. bottles (bottles)	72	120	168	216	264	480
Spiritus Vini Gallici, in 32 oz. bottles (bottles)	12	24	24	36	36	72
Strychnia, in ⅛ oz. bottles (oz.)	⅛	⅛	¼	¼	¼	½
Sulphur, in ½ lb. bottles (oz.)	16	24	32	40	48	88
Vinum Acetas, in 1 oz. bottles (bottles)	24	36	48	60	72	132
Zinci Acetas, in 1 oz. bottles (oz.)	2	4	5	6	7	13
Zinci Carbonas, in 1 oz. bottles (oz.)	1	2	3	4	5	9
Zinci Chloridi Liquor, in 1 lb. g. s. bottles (oz.)	48	80	96	112	128	240
Zinci Sulphas, in 1 oz. bottles (oz.)	2	4	5	6	7	13

Source: "Standard Supply Table." In William Grace, The Army Surgeon's Manual (New York: Bailliere Brothers, 1864), pp. 128-130.

TABLE A.3. C.S.A. Standard Supply Table of the Indigenous Remedies for Field Service and the Sick in General Hospitals

SURGEON GENERAL'S OFFICE, *Richmond, Va.*, March 1, 1863.

The articles of this Supply Table are intended as adjuncts to, or substitutes for those of the original Supply Tables of the Regulations for the Medical Department.

When the articles of the original Supply Tables cannot be procured from the Purveyors, or when they are deficient in quantity, Medical Officers are instructed to make requisition for such indigenous preparations from the following table as will supply the deficiencies.

The interests of the government which they serve, and the importance of relying upon the internal resources of their own country, should prompt the adoption, as far as practicable, of these remedies as substitutes for articles which now can be obtained only by importation.

As much care has been taken in the collection and preparation of these remedies, in order that they might be recommended in form as well as quality, it is hoped that Medical Officers will lay aside all prejudice which may exist in their minds against their use, and will give them a fair opportunity for the exhibition of those remedial virtues which they certainly possess.

Much reliable information on this subject may be obtained from the work on Medical Botany, entitled "Resources of the Southern Fields and Forests," prepared by Surgeon F. P. Porcher, P. A. C. S., under instructions from this office.

S. P. MOORE, Surgeon General C. S. A.

TABLE A.3 (continued)

Articles/Quantities for One Year, for Commands of 500 Men in the Field, or 100 Sick in General Hospital

Botanical Names	Common Names	Medical Properties	Dose	Form for Issue	Quantities
Acorus calamus,	Calamus,	Aromatic, stimulant and stomachic,	10 to 20 grs.	Pulv.	1 [lb.] 0 [oz.]
Acorus calamus,	Calamus,	Aromatic, stimulant and stomachic,	1 fl. drachm,	Fl. ext.	1[lb.] 0[oz.]
Aristolochia serpentaria,	Virginia snake root,	Stimulant, tonic and diaphoretic; in infusion,	1 or 2 ozs.	Rad.	2[lb.] 8[oz.]
Arum tryphillum,	Wake robin, or indian turnip,	Expectorant; stim. to gland, system, lungs and skin; in emulsion,	10 grs.	Pulv.	1[lb.] 0[oz.]
Asarum canadense,	Wild ginger,	Aromatic stimulant, tonic and diaphoretic,	20 to 30 grs.	Rad.	1[lb.] 0[oz.]
Asarum canadense,	Wild ginger,	Aromatic stimulant, tonic and diaphoretic,	½ to 1 fl. drachm,	Fl. ext.	1[lb.] 8[oz.]
Asclepias tuberosa,	Pleurisy root, or butterfly weed,	Diaphoretic; in decoction,	1 teacupful,	Rad.	1[lb.] 8[oz.]
Asclepias tuberosa,	Do. Do.	Expectorant,	20 to 60 grs.	Pulv.	1[lb.] 8[oz.]
Capsicum,	Pepper,	External irritant,	—	Pod,	4[lb.] 0[oz.]
Capsicum,	Pepper,	Stim. stomachic; in gargles,	½ to 2 drachms,	Tinct.	2[lb.] 0[oz.]

Botanical Names	Common Names	Medical Properties	Dose	Form for Issue	Quantities
Cassia marilandica,	American senna,	Cathartic; in infusion,	1 to 3 ounces,	Fol.	1[lb.] 8[oz.]
Cassia marilandica,	American senna,	Cathartic; in infusion,	1 to 4 drachms,	Fl. ext.	4[lb.] 0[oz.]
Chenopodium anthelminticum,	Worm seed,	Anthelmintic, in emulsion with ol. ricini,	–	Sem.	1[lb.] 0[oz.]
Chimaphila umbellata,	Pipsisseway,	Diuretic; in decoction,	1 pint during 24 hours,	–	2[lb.] 0[oz.]
Conium maculatum	Hemlock,	Narcotic and sedative,	2 to 3 grs.	Solid ext.	0[lb.] 4[oz.]
Cornus florida,	Dogwood,	Tonic, astringent,	20 to 60 grs.	Pulv.	–
Cornus florida,	Dogwood,	Tonic, astringent, in decoction,	2 fl. ounces,	Cort.	40[lb.] 0[oz.]
Cornus florida,	Dogwood,	Tonic, astringent,	10 to 30 grs.	Solid ext.	0[lb.] 4[oz.]
Cornus florida,	Dogwood,	Tonic, astringent,	1 fl. drachm,	Co. fl. ext.	3[lb.] 0[oz.]
Cucurbita citrullus,	Watermelon,	Diuretic; in infusion,	Ad libitum,	Sem.	8[lb.] 0[oz.]
Cucurbita pepo,	Pumpkin,	Anthelmintic; in emulsion,	2 ounces,	Sem.	1[lb.] 0[oz.]
Cytisus scoparius,	Scotch broom,	Diuretic; in decoction,	½ to 1 pt. during 24 hours,	–	4[lb.] 0[oz.]
Datura stramonium,	Jamestown weed,	Narcotic; anti-spasmodic and anodyne; tinct. and infusion as local application,	–	Fol.	4[lb.] 0[oz.]
Datura stramonium,	Jamestown weed,	Internally (local applic. also for ung. stramorium),	¼ to ½ grain,	Solid ext.	0[lb.] 2[oz.]
Diospyros virginiana,	Persimmon,	Tonic; in comp. infusions, and gargles,	–	Cort.	8[lb.] 0[oz.]

TABLE A.3 *(continued)*

Botanical Names	Common Names	Medical Properties	Dose	Form for Issue	Quantities
Diospyros virginiana,	Persimmon,	Astringent,	½ to 1 drachm,	Tinct.	—
Diospyros virginiana,	Persimmon,	Astringent,	10 to 30 grs.	Pulv.	2[lb.] 0[oz.]
Erigeron philadelphicum,	Fleabane,	Diuretic; in infusion,	1 pint during 24 hours,	—	—
Erigeron philadelphicum canadense,	Fleabane,	Diuretic; in infusion, and astringent; in infusion,	2 to 4 fl. ozs.	Plant,	4[lb.] 0[oz.]
Erigeron philadelphicum canadense,	Fleabane,	Styptic,	—	Oil,	0[lb.] 2[oz.]
Eupatorium perfoliatum,	Boneset,	Tonic, diaphoretic; in infusion,	2 to 4 fl. ozs.	Herb,	15[lb.] 0[oz.]
Euphorbia ipecacuanha,	Ipecacuanha spurge,	Emetic,	15 grs.	—	—
Euphorbia ipecacuanha corollata,	Large flowery spurge	Diaphoretic,	5 grs.	Rad.	2[lb.] 8[oz.]
Frasera walteri,	American columbo,	Tonic; in infusion,	1 to 2 fl. ozs.	Rad.	7[lb.] 8[oz.]
Gaultheria procumbeus,	Partridge berry, or spicy wintergreen,	Stim. aromatic,	—	Oil,	—
Gentian catesbei,	American gentian,	Tonic; in comp. infusion,	1 to 3 fl. ozs.	Rad.	5[lb.] 0[oz.]

Botanical Names	Common Names	Medical Properties	Dose	Form for Issue	Quantities
Gentian catesbei,	American gentian,	Tonic; in comp. infusion,	10 to 30 grs.	Solid ext.	4[lb.] 0[oz.]
Geranium maculatum,	Cranesbill,	Astringent; in decoction,	1 to 2 fl. ozs.	Rad.	10[lb.] 0[oz.]
Geranium maculatum,	Cranesbill,	Astringent; in decoction,	10 to 15 grs.	Solid ext.	2[lb.] 0[oz.]
Gillenia trifoliata; or gillenia stipulacea,	Indian physic,	Emetic,	20 to 30 grs.	Pulv.	2[lb.] 0[oz]
Humulus lupulus,	Hop,	Tonic, hypnotic; in infusion,	2 fl ozs.	–	10[lb.] 0[oz.]
Humulus lupulus,	Hop,	Tonic, hypnotic; in infusion,	1 to 3 drachms,	Tinct.	1[lb.] 0[oz.]
Hyosciamus niger,	Henbane,	Anodyne, soporific,	1 to 3 grs.	Solid ext.	0[lb.] 8[oz.]
Hyosciamus niger,	Henbane,	Anodyne, soporific,	1 fl. drachm,	Tinct.	2[lb.] 0[oz.]
Juglans cinerea,	Butternut,	Aperient, cathartic,	20 to 30 grs.	Solid ext.	1[lb.] 0[oz.]
Juniper communis,	Juniper,	Stim. diuretic; in infusion,	1 pint during 24 hours,	Berry,	0[lb.] 8[oz.]
Laurus sassafras,	Sassafras,	Stim. aromatic; adjunct to infusions,	–	Cort.	3[lb.] 0[oz.]
Laurus sassafras,	Sassafras,	Demulcent,	–	Pith,	0[lb.] 8[oz.]
Laurus sassafras,	Sassafras,	Stim. carminative,	2 to 10 drops,	Oil,	0[lb.] 2[oz.]
Lavandula,	Lavender,	Stim. aromatic,	30 to 60 drops,	Comp. spts.	2[lb.] 8[oz.]
Leontodon taraxacum,	Dandelion,	Alterative,	1 fl. drachm,	Fl ext.	4[lb.] 0[oz.]
Liriodendron tulipifera,	Tulip tree,	Stim. tonic, diaphoretic,	½ to 2 drachms,	Pulv.	10[lb.] 0[oz.]
Liriodendron tulipifera,	Tulip tree,	Stim. tonic, diaphoretic,	1 to 3 fl. drachms,	Co. fl. ext.	2[lb.] 0[oz.]

TABLE A.3 *(continued)*

Botanical Names	Common Names	Medical Properties	Dose	Form for Issue	Quantities
Lobelia inflata,	Lobelia,	Expectorant,	1 to 2 fl. drachms,	Tinct.	0[lb.] 8[oz.]
Mentha piperita,	Peppermint,	Aromatic, stimulant, and antispasmodic.	1 to 3 drops,	Oil,	8[lb.] 0[oz.]
Mentha viridis,	Mint,	Aromatic, stimulant, and antispasmodic; in infusion,	Ad libitum,	Herb,	2[lb.] 0[oz.]
Monarda punctata,	Horsemint,	Stim. carminative; also adjunct to liniments; internally,	2 to 3 drops,	Oil,	0[lb.] 4[oz.]
Panax quinquefolium,	Ginseng,	Demulcent,	–	Pulv.	2[lb.] 0[oz.]
Papaver,	Poppy,	Anodyne; local application,	–	Heads,	2[lb.] 0[oz.]
Phytolacca decandra,	Poke root,	Alterative; for other uses, see Dispensatory,	1 to 5 grs.	Pulv.	2[lb.] 0[oz.]
Pinckneya pubens,	Georgia bark,	Tonic and antiperiodic; in infusion,	2 to 3 fl. ozs.	Cort.	10[lb.] 0[oz.]
Pinckneya pubens,	Georgia bark,	Tonic and antiperiodic; in infusion,	1 drachm,	Pulv.	2[lb.] 0[oz.]
Podophyllum peltatum,	Mayapple,	Cathartic,	5 to 15 grs.	Solid ext.	1[lb.] 0[oz.]
Polygala senega,	Seneka snake root,	Stim. and expectorant; in decoction,	2 fl. ozs.	Rad.	2[lb.] 6[oz.]
Polygala senega,	Seneka snake root,	Stim. and expectorant; in decoction,	1 fl. drachm,	Syrup,	4[lb.] 0[oz.]
Prunus virginiana,	Wild cherry,	Tonic and sedative; in infusion,	1 to 3 fl. ozs.	Cort.	12[lb.] 0[oz.]

Botanical Names	Common Names	Medical Properties	Dose	Form for Issue	Quantities
Prunus virginiana,	Wild cherry,	Tonic and sedative; in infusion,	½ fl. oz.	Syrup,	4[lb.] 0[oz.]
Quercus alba,	White oak,	Tonic; local application, fomenta-tion, gargle, &c.	–	–	–
Quercus alba,	White oak,	Astringent; in decoction,	–	Cort.	8[lb.] 0[oz.]
Quercus alba,	White oak,	Astringent; in decoction,	½ to 1 drachm,	Pulv.	4[lb.] 0[oz.]
Rhus glabra,	Sumach,	Astringent; infusion a cooling refrigerant drink in fevers; for gargles.	–	Berries,	8[lb.] 0[oz.]
Rubus villosus, or rubus trivialis,	Blackberry, or dewberry,	Tonic, astringent; in decoction,	½ to 2 fl. ozs.	Rad.	4[lb.] 0[oz.]
Do. do.	Do.	Tonic, astringent; in decoction,	1 fl. drachm,	Comp. syr.	4[lb.] 0[oz.]
Sabbatia angularis,	American centaury,	Tonic, in infusion,	2 fl. ozs.	Herb.	6[lb.] 0[oz.]
Salix abra,	White willow,	Tonic, astringent; in decoction,	2 fl. ozs.	Cort.	7[lb.] 8[oz.]
Salvia,	Sage,	Tonic, for gargles, &c.	–	Fol.	5[lb.] 0[oz.]
Sanguinaria canadensis,	Puccoon or blood root,	Stim. expectorant, alterative,	1 fl. drachm,	Tinct.	2[lb.] 0[oz.]
Sarsaparilla, [Aralia spp.?]	Sarsaparilla,	Alterative,	1 fl. drachm,	Fl. ext.	6[lb.] 0[oz.]
Sesamum indicum,	Bene plant,	Demulcent; in infusion,	Ad libitum,	Fol.	4[lb.] 0[oz.]
Solanum dulcamara,	Bitter sweet or woody night-shade,	Narcotic, alterative; in decoction,	2 fl. ozs.	Herb.	1[lb.] 0[oz.]

Botanical Names	Common Names	Medical Properties	Dose	Form for Issue	Quantities
Solanum dulcamara,	Do. do.	Narcotic, alterative; in decoction,	5 to 10 grs.	Solid ext.	0[lb.] 8[oz.]
Spigelia marilandica,	Pink root,	Anthelmintic,	½ fl. oz.	Co. fl. ext.	0[lb.] 8[oz.]
Spiræa tomentosa,	Hardhack,	Tonic, astringent,	5 to 15 grs.	Solid ext.	0[lb.] 4[oz.]
Statice caroliniana,	Marsh rose-mary,	Astringent; in cold infusion,	–	Rad.	2[lb.] 0[oz.]
Stillingia sylvatica,	Queen's root,	Alterative; in decoction,	½ to 2 fl. ozs.	Rad.	2[lb.] 0[oz.]
Stillingia sylvatica,	Queen's root,	Alterative; in decoction,	1 fl. drachm,	Tinct.	1[lb.] 0[oz.]
Symplocarpus foetidus,	Skunk cab-bage,	Antispasmodic, narcotic, expectorant,	10 to 20 grs.	Pulv.	1[lb.] 0[oz.]
Triosteum perfoliatum,	Fever root,	Cathartic,	10 to 20 grs.	Solid ext.	0[lb.] 4[oz.]
Ulmus,	Elm,	Demulcent; in infusion,	Ad libitum,	Cort.	6[lb.] 0[oz.]
Ulmus,	Elm,	Demulcent; in infusion,	Ad libitum,	Pulv.	2[lb.] 0[oz.]
Uva ursi,	Bear berry,	Astringent, tonic, with direction to urinary organs; in decoction,	1 to 2 fl. ozs.	Fol.	1[lb.] 0[oz.]
Veratrum viride,	American Hellebore,	Sedative, expectorant; to be used with caution,	4 to 8 drops,	Norwood's tinct.	1[lb.] 0[oz.]

Source: Samuel P. Moore, "Standard Supply Table of the Indigenous Remedies for Field Service and the Sick in General Hospitals" (Richmond?: Surgeon General's Office?, 1863).

Appendix B

Circular No. 6

Surgeon General's Office
Washington, D.C., May 4, 1863

I. From the reports of Medical Inspectors and the Sanitary reports to this office, it appears that the administration of calomel has so frequently been pushed to excess by military surgeons as to call for prompt steps by this office to correct this abuse; an abuse the melancholy effects of which, as officially reported, have exhibited themselves not only in innumerable cases of profuse salivation, but in the not infrequent occurrence of mercurial gangrene.

It seeming impossible in any other manner to properly restrict the use of this powerful agent, it is directed that it be struck from the Supply Table, and that no further requisitions for this medicine be approved by Medical Directors. This is done with the more confidence as modern pathology has proved the impropriety of the use of mercury in very many of those diseases in which it was formerly unfailingly administered.

II. The records of this office having conclusively proved that diseases prevalent in the Army may be treated as efficiently without tartar emetic as therewith, and the fact of its remaining upon the Supply Table being a tacit invitation to its use, tartar emetic is also struck from the Supply Table of the Army.

No doubt can exist that more harm has resulted from the misuse of both these agents, in the treatment of disease, than benefit from their proper administration.

W. A. Hammond
Surgeon-General

Appendix C

How to Read and Fill a Civil War Prescription

All prescriptions of the Civil War period were written in Latin. Yet Edward Parrish admitted that the Latin employed in most everyday prescriptions, even those of the best classically educated physicians, was grammatically incorrect and riddled with errors. Nevertheless, because physicians and army surgeons used just a few Latin phrases repeatedly, a thorough knowledge of the language was not essential. Still, a working knowledge of Latin is very helpful in reading nineteenth-century prescriptions and some Latin terms and phrases commonly found in prescriptions of the period are listed in the following section.* A key to understanding prescriptions during the war period is a familiarity with the symbols and conventions for indicating quantities used by the medical staff. Much of this is covered in *The Hospital Steward's Manual* (1862), which follows the list of Latin phrases and approximate measures. Taken together, these should give modern readers a basic primer useful for reading and following prescriptions of the 1860s.

A GLOSSARY OF LATIN PHRASES AND APPROXIMATE MEASURES

A, aa, ana (Greek), of each; it signified equally by weight or by measure.
Abs. febr., absente febre, fever being absent.
Ad. 2 vic., ad secundam vicem, to the second time; or *ad duas vices,* two times.
Ad. def. animi, ad defectionem animi or *Ad. del. an,* to fainting.
Ad. gr. acid., ad gratam aciditatem, to an agreeable acidity.
Ad. libit., ad libitum, at pleasure.
Add., adde, or *addantur,* add, or let them be added; *addendus,* to be added.

---

*From Francis Mohr and Theophilus Redwood, *Practical Pharmacy: The Arrangements, Apparatus, and Manipulations of the Pharmaceutical Shop and Laboratory*, edited by William Procter (Philadelphia: Lea and Blanchard, 1849), pp. 478-484.

Adjac., adjacens, adjacent.

Admov., admove, admoveatur, apply, let it be added, let them be added.

Ads. febre, adstante febre, while the fever is present.

Alter. hor., alternis horis, every other hour.

Alvo adstr., alvo adstricta, when the bowels are confined (restricted).

Aq. astr., aqua astrica, frozen water.

Aq. bull., aqua bulliens, boiling water.

Aq. com., aqua communis, common water.

Aq. ferv., aqua fervens, hot water.

Aq. fluv., aqua fluviatilis, river water.

Aq. font., aqua fontana, spring water.

Aq. mar., aqua marina, sea water.

Aq. niv., aqua nivalis, snow water.

Aq. pluv., aqua pluviatilis, rain water.

Bib., bibe, drink.

Bis ind., bis indies, twice a day.

B.M., balneum mariœ, or *balneum maris,* a warm-water bath.

But., butyrum, butter.

B.V., balneum vapris, a vapor bath.

Cœrul., cœruleus, blue.

Calom., calomelas, calomel.

Cap., capiat, let him/her take.

C. C., cucurbitula cruenta, a cupping glass with scarificator.

C.m.s., cras mane sumendus, to be taken tomorrow morning.

C.n., cras nocte, tomorrow night.

Coch. ampl., cochleare amplum, a tablespoonful (f℥iv = 15 cc.).

Coch. infant., cochleare infantis, a child's spoonful.

Coch. med. or *mod., cohleare medium* or *modicum,* dessert spoonful (f℥ii = 8 cc.)

Coch. parv., cochleare parvum, a teaspoonful.

Cochleta., cochleatim, by spoonful.

Col., cola, strain.

Colent., colentur, let them be strained.

Colet., coletur, colat., colatur, let it be strained; *colaturœ,* to the strained liquid.

Color., coloretur, let it be colored.

Comp., compositus, compounded.

Cong., congius, a gallon.

Cont. rem. or *med., continuentur remedia* or *medicamenta,* continue the remedy or medicine.

Coq., coque, boil; *coquantur,* let it be boiled.

Coq. ad. med. consumpt., coqatur ad mediatatis consumptionem, let it be boiled to the consumption of one-half.

Coq. in S.A., coque in sufficiente quantitate aquæ, boil in a sufficient quantity of water.

Cort., cortex, bark.

Crast., crastinus, for tomorrow.

Cuj., cujus, of which.

Cujusl., cujuslibet, of any.

C.v., cras vespere, tomorrow evening.

Cyath., cyathus vel or *C. vinar,* in a wineglass (f ℥ ii = 60 cc.)

Cyath. theæ, cyatho theæ, in a teacup of tea (f ℥ iv = 120 cc.) sometimes referred to as a gill.

D., dosis, a dose.

D. in 2 plo., deter in duplo, let it be given in double doses.

D. in p. æq., dividatur in partes æquales, let it be divided in equal parts.

De d. in d., de die in diem, from day to day.

Deb. spiss., debita spissitudo, due consistence.

Dec., decanta, pour off.

Decub. hor., decubitus hora, at bedtime.

Deglut., deglutiatur, let it be swallowed.

Dej. alv., dejectiones alvi, stools.

Det., detur, let it be given.

Dieb. alt., diebus alternis, every other day.

Dieb. tert., diebus tertiis, every third day.

Dil. or dilue., dilutus, dilute or thin.

Diluc., diluculo, at break of day.

Dim., dimidius, one-half.

Donec. alv. bis. dej., donec alvus bis dejecerit, until the bowels have been twice opened.

Donec. dol. neph. exulv., donec dolor nephriticus exulavert, until the nephritic pain has been removed.

Ejusd., ejusdem, of the same.

Elect., electuarium, electuary.

Enem., enema, enema or clyster.

Exhib., exhibeatur, let it be administered.

F., fiat, to make.

F. H., fiat haustus, let a draught be made.

F. M., fiat mistura, let a mixture be made.

F. pil., fiat pilulæ, make pills.

F. venæs., fiat venæsectio, perform a venesection.

Feb. dur., febre durante, during the fever.

Fem. intern., femoribus internis, to the inside of the thighs.

Fil., filtrum, a filter.

Fist. arm., fistula armata, a clyster pipe and bladder fitted for use.

Fl., fluidus, fluid.

G. G. G., gummi guttæ gambæ, gamboge.

Gel. quav., gelatina quavis, in any jelly.

Gr., granum, a grain.

Gr. vi. pond., grana sex pondere, six grains by weight.

Gtt., gutta, a drop.

Gtt. quibusd., guttis quibusdam, with some drops.

Guttat., guttatim, by drops.

H. D., hora decubitus, at bedtime.

H. P., haustus purgans, purging draught.

H. S., hora somni, at the hour of going to sleep.

Har. pil. sum. iij, harum pilularum sumantur tres, of these pills let three
be taken.

Hor. 11 *ma. mat., hora undecima matutina,* at 11 o'clock in the morning.

Hor. un. spatio, horæ unius spatio, at the expiration of one hour.

In pulm., in pulmento, in gruel.

Ind., indies, daily.

Inf., infunde, infuse.

Jul., julepus, julep.

Lat. dol., lateri dolente, to the affected side.

M., misce, mix, or *mensura,* measure, or *manipulus,* a handful, or
minimum, a minim.

M. P., massa pilularum, a pill mass.

M. R., mistura, a mixture.

Man., manipulus, a handful.

Mana pr., mane primo, early in the morning.

Min., minimum, a minim or a sixtieth of a drachm.

Mitt., mitte, send.

Mitt. sang. ad ℥ xij., mitt. sanguinum ad ℥ xij, take blood to 12 ounces.

Mod. præscr., modo præscripto, in the manner prescribed.

Mor. dict., more dicto, in the way ordered.

Mor. sol., more solito, in the usual way.

No., numero, number.

O., octarius, a pint.

O. M. or omn. man., omni mani, every morning.

O. N. or omni noct., every night.

Omn. bid., omni biduo, every two days.

Omn. bih., omni bihorio, every two hours.

Omn. hor., omni hora, every hour.

Omn. quadr. hor., omni quadrante horæ, every quarter of an hour.

Oz., an avoirdupois ounce (common weight) as opposed to a troy ounce
(apothecary weight).

P., pondere, by weight.

P. æ. part., parte æquales, equal parts.

P. r. n., pro re nata, occasionally or as needed.

P. rat. ætat., pro ratione ætatis, according to the age.

Part. vic., partitis vicibus, in divided doses.

Past., pastillus, a pastil or ball of paste.

Per. op. emet., peractu operatione emetici, the operation of the emetic being over.

Pocill., pocillum, a small cup.

Pocul., poculum, a cup.

Pocul. ampl., poculum amplum, a large cup or tumblerful (f℥ viii = 240 cc.)

Post sing. sed. liq., post singulas sedes liquidas, after every loose stool.

Ppt., præparata, prepared.

Pulv., pulvis, a powder.

Q. l., q. p., or *q. s., quantum libet, placet, sufficiat,* as much as you please.

Q. v., quantum vis, as much as you will.

Quor., quorum, of which.

Red. in pulv., redactus in pulverem, reduced to powder.

Redig. in pulv., redigatur in pulverem, let it be reduced to powder.

Repet., repetatur, to repeat.

S. A., secundum artem, according to the art.

S. S. S., stratum super stratum, layer upon layer.

S. v., spiritus viniv, spirits of wine.

S. V. T., spiritus vini tenius, proof spirit.

Scat., scatula, a box.

Semidr., semidrachma, half a drachm.

Semih., semihora, half an hour.

Sesquih., sesquihora, an hour and a half.

Sesunc., sesuncia, half an ounce.

Si n. val., si non valeat, if it does not answer.

Si op. sit., si opus sit, if it be necessary.

Signat., signatura, a label.

Sing., singulorum, of each.

Ss., semis, a half.

St., stet, let it stand or *stent,* let them stand.

Sub fin. coct. or *sub finem coctionis,* toward the end of boiling, when the boiling is nearly finished.

Sum., sume, sumat, sumatur, sumantur, take, let him/her take, let it be taken.

Sum. tal., sumat talem, let the patient take one like this.

Tabel., tabella, a lozenge.

T. O., tinctura opi, tincture of opium.

T. O. C., tinctura opii camphorata, camphorated tincture of opium.

Ult. præscr., ultimo præscriptus, last prescribed.

V. O. S., vitello ovi solutes, dissolved in the yolk of an egg.

Vom. urg., vomitione urgente, the vomiting being troublesome.

EXCERPT FROM THE HOSPITAL STEWARD'S MANUAL,* 1862

Part IV
The Dispensary
Chapter 2
Hints on Pharmacy for Hospital Stewards

Section I.—Remarks on Prescriptions

Upon the steward in charge of the drugstore devolves the responsibility of compounding the prescriptions of the medical officers. The following brief remarks on this subject may perhaps, therefore, be found useful.

The prescription is headed with the name of the patient for whom it is intended. Then follows the list of ingredients and quantities, preceded by the character ℞, which is an abbreviation of the Latin word *recipe*, "take." The officinal names of the several ingredients are employed. The steward will, however, generally notice a difference between the termination of the officinal name and that of the name employed in the prescription. This is owing to the names being written in Latin genitive case, the verb *recipe* governing the genitive.

Thus, the surgeon writes, ℞ Chloroformi ℥ j, instead of "Chloroformum," which is the nominative, *chloroformi* being in the genitive case, and meaning "of chloroform."

This, also, ℞ Zinci sulphatis grs. xx: Zinci sulphas being nominative.

A still greater difficulty in the way of the steward occurs from the fact that surgeons very frequently abbreviate the officinal names for convenience, in writing their prescriptions, writing, for example, Hyd. Chl. Mit. for Hydrargyri chloridum mite; Potas. Iod. for Potassæ iodidum, & c. and c. As these abbreviations are, unfortunately, not always made in the same manner by different surgeons, a very long list of abbreviations might here be given, without exhausting the subject; and as it is directed in army regulations that no person shall be enlisted a hospital steward unless he is *sufficiently skilled in pharmacy* for the proper performance of his duties, it is presumed that such a list would be unnecessary here. Most of the abbreviations, moreover, at once explain themselves to anyone familiar with the officinal names of the articles, and the steward should certainly be with those on the army supply table. The general rule may, however, be laid down, that the steward should under no circumstances allow himself to put up a prescription containing any abbreviation of the meaning of which he entertains the slightest doubt. In all such cases he should go at once to the surgeon for an explanation. By so doing, he not only avoids, at the time, mis-

---

*From Joseph Janvier Woodward, *The Hospital Steward's Manual* (Philadelphia: J. B. Lippincott, 1862), pp. 278-294.

takes which might be fatal, but gradually becomes thoroughly acquainted with all the abbreviations employed by the surgeon under whom he serves.

The quantities of the several ingredients employed are indicated by the usual symbols with Roman numerals affixed. Thus:

Weights	**Measures**
gr. a grain	*gtt.* a drop
℈, a scruple	ℳ, a minim
ʒ, a drachm	fʒ, a fluidrachm
℥, an ounce	f℥, a fluidounce
℔, a pound	O, a pint
	Cong., a gallon

The Roman numerals follow these signs, thus: ℥vj, i.e., six drachms; f℥xj, i.e., eleven fluidrachms.

The following tables may be given for reference:

Apothecaries Weight

Pounds		Ounces		Drachms		Scruples		Grains
℔ 1	=	12	=	96	=	288	=	5,760
		℥ 1	=	8	=	24	=	480
				ʒ 1	=	3	=	60
						℈ 1	=	20

Avoirdupois Weight

Pound		Ounces		Drachms		Grains (Apothecaries)
℔ 1	=	16	=	256	=	7,000
		oz. 1	=	16	=	437.5
				dr. 1	=	27.34375

Weighing for prescriptions is always done in accordance with apothecaries' weight. Medical purveyors in the U.S. Army, however, are in the habit of employing, in the issue of medical stores, a pound which corresponds neither with the apothecaries' pound nor with that of the avoirdupois weight. It is composed of 16 ounces apothecaries' weight, and contains, therefore, 7,680 grains,—being 1,920 grains heavier than the apothecaries' pound, and 680 grains heavier than the avoirdupois pound.

Apothecaries' Measures

Gallons	Pints	Fluidounces	Fluidrachms	Minims
Cong. 1 =	8 =	128	=	1,024	=	61,440
	0.1 =	16	=	128	=	7,680
		f℥ 1	=	8	=	480
				f℈ 1	=	♏ 60

The following remarks may be added with regard to certain domestic measures frequently alluded to in the administration of remedies.

A *teacup* is estimated to contain about four fluidounces or one gill. A *wineglass,* two fluidounces. A *tablespoon,* half a fluidounce. A *teaspoon,* a fluidrachm.

The steward may here be cautioned against the frequent mistake of identifying the drop with the minim. The minim is a fixed and unchangeable measure, which varies neither with the nature of the liquid nor the manner in which it is poured out. The drop, on the other hand, is exceedingly variable, differing in size considerably for different liquids, and even for the same liquid, in accordance with the shape of the bottle from which it is poured, and many other circumstances.

As an illustration of the variation caused by the nature of the liquid, it may be stated that in the experiments of Mr. E. Durand, of Philadelphia, on this subject, it was found that while 150 drops of sulphuric ether were necessary to make a fluidrachm, it required 132 of the tincture of chloride of iron, 120 of aromatic sulphuric acid, 120 of laudanum, 78 of black drop, 57 of Fowler's solution, and but 45 of distilled water, for the same purpose.

The list of the articles and their quantities is followed in the prescription by short directions as to compounding it. These are generally written in Latin, and are frequently abbreviated. The following are the abbreviations most commonly employed:

> *M.*—Misce.—Mix.
> *Ft. pulv.*—Fiat pulvis.—Make a powder.
> *Ft. pulv. Xij.*—Fiat pulveres xij.—Make twelve powders.
> *Ft. pulv. et divid. in chart. xij.*—Fiat pulvis et divde in chartulas xij—Make twelve powders.
> *Ft. pulv. in ch. xij. div.*—Fiat pulvis in chartulas xij. Dividenda—Make twelve powders.
> *Ft. ch. xij.*—Fiat chartulæ xij.—Make twelve powders.
> *Ft. solut.*—Fiat solutio.—Make a solution.
> *Ft. inject.*—Fiat injectio.—Make an injection (for urethra).
> *Ft. collyr.*—Fiat collyrium.—Make an eye-wash.
> *Ft. enema.*—Fiat enema.—Make an injection (for rectum).

Ft. mas.—Fiat massa.—Make a mass.

Ft. mas. in pil. xij. Dive.—Fiat massa in pilulas xij. Dividenda— Make twelve pills.

Ft. mas. etdiv. in pil. xij.—Fiat massa et divide in pilulas xij.—Make twelve pills.

Ft. infus.—Fiat infusum.—Make an infusion.

Ft. haust.—Fiat haustus.—Make a draught.

Ft. troch. xxiv.—Fiat trochisci xxiv.—Make twenty-four lozenges.

After the directions as to compounding, follow those as to administration. These are always written in English, the direction being prefixed by the abbreviation *S.*—Signatura.

The directions are followed by the date and the signature of the medical officer.

The prescription, therefore, consists properly of three parts:

1. The list of ingredients and quantities prefixed by the sign ℞.
2. The directions as to compounding, generally a Latin abbreviation.
3. The directions for administration. These are preceded by the name of the patient, and followed by the date and the signature of the medical officer.

Section II.—Compounding and Distribution of Prescriptions.

Having read the prescription, the steward proceeds to compound it, varying his process according as it is a solution, a mixture, powders, or pills, & c., that he is to prepare.

Where the prescription consists of *liquids only,* they are measured seriatim in the graduated measure and poured into the phial which is to receive them, when the process is completed by corking and gently agitating the mixture.

In performing this duty, but one bottle should be taken down from the shelves at a time. The measure should be held by the thumb and finger of the left hand, and the stopper should be seized by the little finger of the same hand. The bottle is held in pouring with the right hand. The measure is held up well up before the eye, so as to observe the quantity with accuracy; and, when it is obtained, the stopper is replaced, and the bottle put back in its place upon the shelf before proceeding to the next ingredient.

Where the ingredients of the prescription are partly solids and partly liquids, the quantities of the solids are to be determined by weight.

If the solids are saline or other solid substances, and a solution is to be made, it is generally best to bruise them in a mortar with the liquids until their solution is effected, after which the product is transferred to a phial.

Where insoluble solid matters are to be suspended in the form of a mixture or emulsion, the mortar becomes still more important. The ingredients are to be rubbed steadily together until a smooth and uniform liquid is obtained, and the label of the phial into which the mixture is introduced should contain directions to shake well before administration.

When the prescription directs the preparation of a given number of *powders,* the ingredients in powder are carefully weighed out and thoroughly mixed together on a pill-tile with a spatula, or, preferably, in a mortar. The mixture having been completed, the product is to be divided into the number of equal parts called for by the prescription, the division being effected by the scales or the eye, according to the nature of the ingredients and the importance of accuracy. Each portion is then transferred to the paper in which it is to be folded. The papers for each set of powders should be neatly cut and of equal size. The folding is effected in the following manner. A crease is made by folding over the edge along the long side of the paper, at about one-third of an inch from the margin. The opposite edge is then laid in this crease, and the paper folded over longitudinally, so as to give the proper width. The ends are then folded over a spatula, to make the flaps of a proper width.

Uniformity in the size of the powders is exceedingly desirable. It may readily be attained by cutting out a small wooden gauge of the desired size, by which both the length and width of the powder may accurately be determined.

In the preparation of *pills,* the materials for the whole number of pills, as directed by the prescription, are first to be weighed separately, then worked into a mass of the proper consistence, and afterwards divided into the number of pills called for.

To make a pill-mass where the ingredients are all dry powders, without increasing unnecessarily the size of the pills, requires often considerable ingenuity.

In the case of certain vegetable powders, such as aloes, rhubarb, and opium, a mass suitable for rolling into pills may readily be formed by the aid merely of a small quantity of water, the powder being beat into a mass in a mortar during the gradual addition of the fluid.

Where, however, the powder is of an unadhesive character, as is the case, for example, with many vegetable powders and metallic salts, some adhesive ingredient must be added to them to enable a mass of pillular consistence to be formed.

Molasses answers an excellent purpose in very many cases. It must be added carefully, as an excess will make the pill-mass too fluid for manipulation. Gum Arabic in small quantities may be added where the molasses does not give the mass sufficient cohesion. It is frequently used alone for this purpose, either in the form of powder or of thick mucilage, but is objectionable, as the pills produced by its use are apt to become excessively hard on drying.

For many vegetable powders castile soap answers very well, a small quantity readily imparting the necessary consistence. Resinous powders are particularly adapted to its use.

Where the prescription presents among its constituents one or more semi-solid extracts, it will frequently be found that these impart sufficient tenacity, and that by simply beating the ingredients together a suitable mass is obtained. But it sometimes happens, on the one hand, that the quantity of the soft extract is too small for the purpose, and then the addition of some such articles as those above enumerated becomes necessary; and, on the other hand, the extract may be of such quality and consistence as to make the mass entirely too soft to be rolled into pills. In the latter case addition of some dry powder, which shall not interfere with the medicinal value of the prescription, becomes necessary. Powdered liquorice-root or wheat flour are well adapted for this purpose.

Where the materials to be made into pills are wholly semi-solid or liquid, the addition of some dry powder becomes yet more necessary. Wheat flour is very generally available, and is on the whole preferable to the crumb of bread, which is recommended by many pharmaceutists. Powdered liquorice-root, arrow-root, starch, and gum Arabic are also used for the same purpose.

Other articles may be necessary in special cases, as, for example, magnesia in making pills out of balsam of copaiva.

Many other articles are used by pharmaceutists in giving elegance and consistence to pills. It is not, however, considered desirable to enumerate them in this place, because in most general hospitals treatises on pharmacy are accessible, and because those above mentioned comprise the chief that will be found accessible to the hospital steward in the field and at remote posts.

The pill-mass, having been properly formed, is next to be divided into the number of pills directed. This may be done either by a spatula upon a pill-tile, or with a pill-machine.

In the first case the pill mass is rolled out upon the tile into a cylinder corresponding in length to the number of pills to be made, which is ascertained by measuring it upon a scale which is marked upon the surface of the tile. The rolling may be commenced with the hand and finished with the spatula. The cylinder is then cut by the spatula into equal pieces, one for each pill, in accordance with the same scale, which is generally ruled up to 18 or 24 pills. The pills are then finished by rolling them separately between the fingers or on the palm of the hand.

In general hospitals the steward is furnished with a pill-machine, by which pills may be made neatly with considerable rapidity. It consists of a smooth base-piece, in one part of which a number of parallel grooves (18 to 24) are made, and of a roller with a handle on each end, the back of which is smooth and the under surface grooved to correspond with the grooves in the base-piece. The pill-mass having been rolled on the smooth surface of the base-piece with the back of the roller until it is long enough to cover as many grooves as it is to make pills, the cutting surface of the grooves is adjusted, and by the motion of the roller the cylinder is at once divided into the requisite number of pills, which, if the operation has been properly conducted, will be so round as to require no further rolling.

The pills, having been completed either by hand or the machine, are, if very moist, to be spread out upon a sheet of paper with the edges turned up, or upon the bottom of a shallow box, to dry somewhat: they are finally introduced into a pill-box, if for dispensing, or into a bottle if made to keep on hand. In either case, some dry powder, such as starch, liquorice-root, or pulverized sugar, should be introduced to keep them from sticking together.

Where *ointments* and *cerates* are prescribed containing several ingredients, they may very often be compounded upon the pill-tile by means of the spatula. Occasionally, however, the employment of heat is necessary to make the ingredients combine.

Cerate of Spanish flies may be spread for blisters by means of a spatula slightly warmed. Perhaps the best substance to spread it upon is ordinary adhesive plaster, spreading the cerate so that a margin of half an inch is left uncovered. This will serve to keep the blister in its place.

Plasters proper usually require heat to spread them upon the prepared sheep-skin which is furnished for that purpose. The heat is best obtained by means of a hot iron of the proper shape (plaster-iron). Care must be taken not to heat the iron too hot, or the sheep-skin is shriveled and the adhesiveness of the plaster diminished.

The prescription, having been put up, must not, whatever its nature, be allowed to leave the dispensary without a label. The labels usually employed in civil practice are not adapted to military hospitals, where the label should at once indicate whom the prescription is for, and give information to the nurse as to its administration, and to the surgeon as to its composition. The label must therefore be, in fact, a copy of the prescription, and should be made out in the following form:

FOR PRIVATE JAMES SIMPSON

WARD 2, BED 14.

R—Pulveris opii, grs. vj.
Cupri sulphatis, grs. ix.
Ft. mas. in pil. xxiv div.
S. One pill to be taken every three hours.

2, 16, 1862

_____ *Surgeon, U.S.A.*

This label should be written upon a neat slip of white paper, about two inches wide by five or six long. It may be pasted upon bottles if considered desirable; but, as the same bottles in a military hospital are to be used again and again, it will save labor in cleaning the bottles to tie the labels upon them. The corners of the label may be folded obliquely at one end, so as to form a point, and this may be tied to the neck of the phial by a thread. The label for pill-boxes may be secured in the same way to the bottom part of the box, leaving the lid free. For packages of powders or other packages, the label should be pasted upon the proper wrapper.

In putting up prescriptions, those for each ward should be put up together, attending to the wards *seriatim* in the order in which their prescription-books come to the dispensary in the morning. So soon as the prescriptions for any ward are complete, the chief nurse of the ward is to be notified, and will send an attendant to bring the medicines to the ward, where they will be distributed to the beds to which they belong, and administered strictly in accordance with directions.

Appendix D

Circular No. 3

Confederate States of America, Medical Purveyor's Office
Richmond, Va., April 12, 1862

The instructions contained in this circular are issued for the guidance of the Medical Purveyors and will be duly observed.

I. For the convenience of collecting supplies and for the purposes of the Purveying Department, Medical Purveyors are classified as Department Purveyors and field Purveyors, and districts are assigned to them in which to collect supplies, as follows, and for the present:

Depot Purveyors

	District	**Depot**	**Purveyor**
No. 1	Virginia	Richmond	[Edward W. Johns]
No. 2	N. Carolina	Charlotte	
No. 3	S. Carolina S. Georgia	Charleston	Surg. J. J. Chisolm
No. 4	Georgia Cen. R. R. & East Florida N. Georgia	Savannah	Surg. W. H. Prioleau
No. 5	Georgia Cen. R. R. & East Tennessee	Atlanta	Surg. G. S. Blackie
No. 6	Alabama & Middle Tennessee	Montgomery	Surg. Richard Potts
No. 7	Mississippi & West Tennessee	Jackson	Surg. Richard Potts
No. 8	Louisiana	New Orleans	Surg. Howard Smith
No. 9	Texas	San Antonio	Surg. Howard Smith

Field Purveyors

Names	**Army**	**Station**
Surg. J. T. Johnson	Army Potomac	Gordonsville, North Carolina

Surg. E. Warren	North Carolina	Goldsboro, North Carolina
Surg. W. H. Wilson	Norfolk	Norfolk, Virginia
Surg. F. Morrow	East Tennessee	Knoxville, Tennessee
Ast. E. R. Duval		Fortsmith, Arkansas
Ast. Wm. H. Geddings		Fredericksburg, Virginia
Ast. D. P. Ramsier		Williamsburg, Virginia
Ast. Wm. H. Anderson		Mobile, Alabama
Ast. W. B. Robertson		Wytherville, Virginia

II. Depot Purveyors at Marine ports of entry, when they have opportunities to import supplies will immediately avail themselves of such occasion, should there be a probability of losing the chance of procuring supplies by waiting to report at this office.

When there is time, however, they will not fail to report to this office for instructions in relation to such opportunities in order that some control of the market may be had if possible by combined action.

Depot Purveyors will also send weekly price currents of the general market in the principal cities, and always keep the undersigned well advised of the prices they are paying. They will make monthly and bi-monthly reports to this office of their supplies on hand, the monthly report will be a simple report of the number of men for which they have supplies on hand according to the Supply Table.

The bi-monthly reports will include the monthly report, due for the second month of the bi-monthly period, and will also state in an enumerated list of the articles, the amount of all supplies on hand at the end of the bi-monthly period. The bi-monthly periods are to be considered as commencing with the year.

Depot Purveyors are expected to keep themselves well advised as to, and to avail themselves, without loss of time, of all sources of supplies within their districts; and each Purveyor will use every endeavor to have, if possible always in hand, a reserve of supplies for 50,000 men for one month, over their issues.

The Purveyors stationed at Marine Ports of entry will assist, when they are able to do so, those stationed inland, by issuing necessary supplies. In such cases the request for the transfer of such supplies will be sent to this office for approval.

III. Field Purveyors will provide by timely requisition on the depot Purveyors nearest them, for such supplies only as are necessary for one month, for the Army Corps with which they may be serving. When there is a reasonable probability that their commands may be distant from a Purveyor's depot, and transportation difficult from such depot to them, they should provide supplies for two months, reporting the necessity to this office. They will require for, and issue only, such supplies as are necessary to meet special requisitions from regiments, or to furnish regiments that may not have been able to obtain supplies upon regular requisitions.

Field Purveyors will always so dispose their supplies on hand that they may be moved to the rear, or some other place of safety, when there is a danger of losing them, and will give preference always to the preservation of surgical instruments, quinine, morphine & the other leading articles. They will endeavor to obtain if possible & keep under their control special transportation to move their supplies, and to this end they should urgently represent to commanding Generals the great scarcity of medical supplies in the Confederacy & the pressing necessity that what we have should be saved.

Regimental medicine chests & Hospital Knapsacks (which latter are being manufactured for issue) will probably be sufficient for all the medicines a regiment in the field can carry.

IV. Purveyors to whom the pamphlets prepared in the Surgeon General's Office are sent are instructed to distribute them to the best advantage through their districts to such persons as would be likely to carry out the collection & to such Apothecaries as would not use them for speculation; each Depot Purveyor to employ from one to three trustworthy agents to go through the country in their districts, to collect and encourage the country people to cultivate, collect, and prepare the indigenous plants needed. A special list of such indigenous plants as may have been collected will be forwarded monthly to this office in order that when necessary the plants may be sent to the Laboratory, that preparations may be made from them.

V. The undersigned expecting and not doubting that the Purveyors will use all means in their power to meet pressing exigencies of the service to which they are assigned, will be at all times, glad to receive from them suggestions that are brief and to the point.

Appendix E

A Materia Medica for the South:
A Selected List of Medicinal Substances
from Porcher's *Resources*
of the Southern Fields and Forests

Common Name	Botanical Name	Therapeutic Action	Symptomatic Activity
birch leaves	*Betulacea* spp.	heamaturia, dyspepsia, and bowel complaints	likely[a]
boneset	*Eupatorium perfoliatum*	fever	no
dittany	*Cunila Mariana*	diaphoretic, fever, colds	no
dogwood		fever	no
evening primrose	*Oenthera* spp.	skin conditions	possibly[b]
fleabane	*Erigeron anadensis*	diuretic, astringent	possibly[c]
fringe tree	*Chionanthus virginica*	intermittent fever	no
gentian	*Gentiana lutea*	dyspepsia	possibly[d]
Georgia bark	*Pinckneya pubens*	tonic and anti-periodic	no
geranium (cranesbill)	*Geranium maculatum*	astringent (useful in diarrhea/dysentery)	likely[e]
goldenseal	*Hydrastis Canadensis*	tonic	possibly[f]
Indian tobacco	*Lobelia inflata*	diaphoretic, expectorant, use in bronchial asthma	likely[g]

Jamestown weed	*Datura stramonium*	anti-spasmodic, anodyne, narcotic	likely[h]
pink root	*Spigelia marilandica*	anthelmintic	likely[i]
pleurisy root	*Asclepias tuberosa*	expectorant and diaphoretic	possibly[j]
raspberry/black-berry	*Rubus* spp.	astringent for treating diarrhea	likely[k]
sassafras	*Sassafras officinalis*	tonic	no
scullcap	*Scutellaria lateriflora*	rabies	no
tansy	*Tanacetum vulgare*	tonic, anthelmintic (i.e., verminfuge)	likely[l]
valerian	*Valeriana* spp.	sedative	likely[m]
watermellon	*Curcubita citrullus*	diuretic	no
yellow dock	*Rumex crispus*	laxative	likely[n]

Notes: [a]The plant contains a number of flavinoids thought to have an effect on the urinary tract and has been endorsed by German Commission E for this purpose. See Varro E. Tyler, *Tyler's Herbs of Choice: The Therapeutic Uses of Phytomedicines* (Binghamton, NY: Pharmaceutical Products Press, 1994), pp. 77-78.

[b]Evening primrose contains 14 percent fixed oil, nine of which is an unusual one referred to as GLA (*cis*-linolenic acid). Some studies suggest it may improve atopic eczema. See Varro E. Tyler, *The Honest Herbal,* Third Edition (Binghamton, NY: Pharmaceutical Products Press, 1993), pp. 123-125.

[c]Contains some tannins, volatile oils, and gallic acid. See *The Merck Index,* Twelfth Edition (Whitehouse Station, NJ: Merck, 1996), p. 623. The plant may also be antiphlogistic; see the *PDR for Herbal Medicines* (Montvale, NJ: Medical Economics, 1998), p. 831.

[d]Some studies suggest that gentian works on the membranes of the stomach and mouth as a digestive stimulant. See Daniel B. Mowrey, *The Scientific Validation of Herbal Medicine* (New Caanan, CT: Keating Publishing, 1986), p. 250; and *PDR for Herbal Medicines,* pp. 866-867.

[e]*Geranium maculatum's* 10-18 percent tannin content would make it a useful astringent. See *The Merck Index,* p. 4412.

[f]This plant contains the alkaloids hydrastine and berberine, both of which have antiseptic amoebicidal properties. See Tyler, *Tyler's Herbs of Choice,* p. 162; and *PDR for Herbal Medicines,* pp. 903-904.

[g]Lobelia contains an alkaloid lobeline. Several studies suggest that lobeline is a bronchial dilator in humans. See Melvyne R. Werbach and Michael T. Murray, *Botanical Influences on Illness: A Sourcebook of Clinical Research,* Second Edition (Tarzana, CA: Third Line Press, 2000), pp. 137-138.

[h]Contains more than thirty different tropane alkaloids, but would have to be used with caution as overdose could be lethal. See Andrew Pengelly, *The Constituents of Medicinal Plants,* Second Edition (Muswellbrook, NSW: Sunflower Herbals, 1997), p. 87. See also *PDR for Herbal Medicines,* p. 802.

[i]Contains spigeline, resins, tannin, and volatile oils. Still listed as an anthelmintics in *The Merck Index,* p. 8900; and *PDR for Herbal Medicines,* p. 1155.

[j]Several studies support its use in this regard. See Mowrey, *Validation of Herbal Medicine,* p. 240; and *PDR for Herbal Medicines,* pp. 672-673.

[k]*Rubus* spp. all contain polyphenols called tannins that are known to be effective against diarrhea. According to Tyler, "They effect this by binding to the surface protein layer of the inflamed mucous membranes, causing it to thicken, thereby hindering resorption of toxic materials and restricting secretions." See Tyler, *Tyler's Herbs of Choice,* pp. 51-52.

[l]Tansy contains a volatile oil known as thujone, which is responsible for the anthelmintic properties of the plant. Thujone level can be highly variable between plants, and therefore proper dosage can be very difficult. Overdoses can be quite dangerous. See Tyler, *The Honest Herbal,* pp. 305-306.

[m]Although *Valeriana officinalis* is the official pharmacopoeial form, others contain the active sedative principles and thus the several species suggested by Porcher undoubtedly had the same effect. See Tyler, *The Honest Herbal,* pp. 315-316.

[n]The plant's laxative properties are due to anthraquinone derivatives. See Tyler, *The Honest Herbal,* pp. 325-326.

Appendix F

Some Common Prescriptions of the Civil War Period Including the Basic Syrups with Monographs on the Principal Substances: Alcohol, Cinchona, Hydrargyrum (Mercury), Opium, and Quinine

(With Ingredients Translated and/or Identified from the Latin)

COMMON PRESCRIPTIONS

For Diarrhea and Dysentery

R Olei Ricini [castor oil] f℥ iss
Tincturæ Opii [Tincture of opium] ℳ xxx
Pulv. Acaciæ [powdered acacia],
Sacchari, āā ℥ ii
Aquæ Menthæ Viridus f ℥ iv.

Acacia and sugar with a little water of spearmint; finally, pour in oil and repeatedly triturate; at last, pour in water to the rest little by little and mix it all together.

S. A tablespoonful to be taken every hour or two hours till it operates, the mixture being each time well shaken. (Used as a gentle laxative in dysentery and diarrhea. It is usually known by the name *oleaginous mixture*.)*

---

*Source: Prescriptions for diarrhea and dysentery; diarrhea and upset stomach, upset stomach, constipation, and gas; "biliousness" and as a laxative; and a fever remedy of quinine in solution from *USD*, Eleventh edition (Philadelphia: J. B. Lippincott, 1858), pp. 1514, 1515, 1515, 1513, and 1515, respectively.

For Diarrhea and Upset Stomach

℞ Pulveris Kino [powdered *Pterocarpus marsupium*] ℨ ii
Aquæ bullientis [boiling water] f℥ vi
Make an infusion and strain; finally, mix accordingly,
Cretæ Præparatæ [prepared chalk] f℥ iii.
Tincturæ Opii fℨ ss.
Spiritus Lavandulæ Compositii [compound spirit of lavender] f℥ ss.
Pulveris Acacia [powdered acacia],
Sacchari, āā ℨ ii.

S. A tablespoonful to be taken for a dose, the mixture being well shaken. (Astringent and antacid, useful in diarrhea.)

For Upset Stomach, Constipation, and Gas

℞ Columbæ contusæ [bruised columbo],
Zingiberis contusi [ginger, bruised], āā ℥ ss.
Sennæ [senna] ℨ ii.
Aquæ bullientis [boiling water] Oi.

Macerate for an hour in a vessel closed to like (darkened glass) and strain.
S. A wineglassful to be taken morning, noon, and evening, or less frequently if it operates too much. (An excellent remedy for dyspepsia with constipation and flatulence.)

For "Biliousness" and As a Laxative (Blue Mass Pills)

℞ Massæ Pilularum Hydrargyri [blue mass or mercury],
Pulveris Aloes [powdered aloe],
Pulveris Rhei [powdered rhubarb], āā Э i.

Mix and with water make a pilular mass and divide into twenty pieces of equal parts.
S. Three to be taken at bedtime. (An alterative and laxative, useful in constipation with deranged or deficient hepatic secretion.)

A Fever Remedy of Quinine in Solution

℞ Quiniæ Sulphatis [quinine sulfate] ℥ gr. xii.
Acidi Sulphurici Aromatici [sulfuric acid, aromatic] gtt. xxiv.
Syrupi f℥ ss.

Aquæ Menthæ Piperitæ [peppermint water] f℥ i.
Misce. [mix]

S. A teaspoonful to be taken every hour or two hours. (A good mode of administering sulphate of quinia in solution.)

For Congestion Due to the Common Cold, Etc. (Catarrh)

℞ Polygalæ Senegæ Pulv. [powdered Seneca snakeroot], ℨij.
Ipecacuanhæ Pulv. [powdered Ipecac], ℨj.
Mel. Opt. [best honey], ℥ ij.
Aquæ fervent [hot water], ℥ vj.

Make a mixture of which a small spoonful should be taken at the beginning signs of congestion.*

For Worms and Intestinal Parasites

℞ Spigeliæ Mariland [pinkroot], ℥ ss.
Aquæ ferventis, Oj.

Macerate an hour, of which take a large spoonful every three or four hours.

If a moderate dose of Calomel be given in the evening, sufficient to produce a mild cathartic effect, and its operation followed the next day by the administration of Pinkroot, in doses of from half a fluid ounce to a fluid ounce, once in three or four hours, we have found this plan altogether more efficient than when the Spigelia is given without Calomel.

For Pneumonia

According to Dr. Norwood, this prescription is "as much a specific as Quinine is for intermittent fever."

℞ Tict. Veratri Viride [tincture of American hellebore]
Syrupi Scillæ [syrup of squills—see below for recipe]

Mix together intimately.

Source: Prescriptions for congestion due to the common cold; worms and intestional parasites; and pneumonia, from Horace Green, *Selections from Favorite Prescriptions of Living American Practitioners* (New York: J. Wiley, 1860), pp. 123, 161, 94, respectively.

Of this mixture to an adult male, Dr. Norwood advises to begin with from four to six drops, increasing the amount from one to two drops at each subsequent dose, until the pulse is reduced, or nausea and vomiting are occasioned, when the medicine is to be diminished one-half, and continued as long as necessary to prevent a return of symptoms.

For Intermittents (Intermittent Fevers)

> R Cinchonæ flavæ [yellow cinchona bark] p. ℥ j.
> Antim. Potass.-tart. [tartar emetic] gr. ij.
> Opii pulv. [powdered opium] gr. j.

Mix, and divide into four powders. One to be given every second hour.*

In Obstinate Intermittents

> R Cinchonæ pulv. [powdered cinchona] ℥ ss.
> Syrupi Auranti [syrup of orange], q. s. [as much as sufficient]

Make an electuary: a teaspoonful to be taken every hour, drinking after it a spoonful of wine. (Many other combinations of bark might be given, containing from ℈ss to ℈j of bark, with 1-12 of camphor, 1-6 or 1-8 of ginger or of cinnamon, 1-2 valerian, & c.)

Antiperiodics [for Fever] or Tonic

> R Quinæ Disulph. [quinine dissulfate or basic sulfate of quinia] gr. ij.
> Pulv. Cinnam. [powdered cinnamon] ℥ ss.
> Extr. Cinchonæ, q. s. [as much as sufficient] to make thirty pills.

Four, every fourth, third, or second hour.

BASIC SYRUPS

Syrup of Blackberry Root

> Take of blackberry root, in moderately fine powder, eight
>   troyounces.
> Syrup a pint and a half.
> Diluted alcohol a sufficient quantity.

---

*Source: Prescriptions for intermittents, obstinate intermittents, and antiperiodics (for fever) or tonic from Henry Beasley, *The Book of Prescriptions* (Philadelphia: Lindsay and Blackiston, 1865), p. 197.

Introduce the powder, previously moistened with four fluidounces of diluted alcohol, into a glass percolator, and pour diluted alcohol upon it until a pint and a half of tincture have passed. Evaporate this by means of a water bath, at a temperature not exceeding 160°, to half a pint; then mix it while hot with the syrups previously heated, and strain.*

Compound Syrup of Sarsaparilla

> Take of sarsaparilla, in moderately coarse powder (1 lb. 10 ozs.
>   comb.), twenty-four troyounces.
> Guiacum wood, in moderately coarse powder, three troyounces.
> Pale rose, in moderately coarse powder,
> Senna, in moderately coarse powder,
> Liquorice root, in moderately coarse powder, each, two troyounces.
> Oil of sassafras,
> Oil of anise, each, five minims.
> Oil of gaultheria three minims.
> Sugar, in coarse powder (6 lbs. 9 ozs. com.), ninety-six troyounces.
> Diluted alcohol in sufficient quantity.

Mix the solid ingredients, except the sugar, with three pints of diluted alcohol, and allow the mixture to stand for twenty-four hours; then transfer it to a cylindrical percolator, and gradually pour diluted alcohol upon it until ten pints of tincture have passed. Evaporate this by means of a water bath, to four pints, filter, and, having added the sugar, dissolve it with the aid of heat, and strain the solution while hot. Lastly, rub the oils with a small portion of the solution, and mix them thoroughly with the remainder.

Syrup of Squills

> Take of vinegar of squill a pint.
> Sugar, in coarse powder (1 lb. 10 oz. com.), twenty-four troyounces.

Dissolve the sugar in the vinegar of squill, with the aid of a gentle heat, and stain the solution while hot.

Compound Syrup of Squills

> Take of squill, in moderately coarse powder,
> Seneka [Seneca snakeroot], in moderately fine powder, each, four
>   troyounces.

---

*All taken from Edward Parrish, *A Treatise on Pharmacy*, Third Edition (Philadelphia: Blanchard and Lea, 1864), pp. 249-251.

Tartrate of antimony and potassa forty-eight grains.
Sugar, in coarse powder (2 lbs. 14 ozs. com.), forty-two troyounces.
Diluted alcohol,
Water, each, a sufficient quantity.

Mix the squill and seneka, and, having moistened the mixture with half a pint of diluted alcohol, allow it to stand for an hour. Then transfer it to a conical percolator, and pour diluted alcohol upon it until three pints of tincture have passed. Boil this for a few minutes, evaporate it by means of a water bath to a pint, add six fluidounces of boiling water, and filter. Dissolve the sugar in the filtered liquid, and, having heated the solution to the boiling point, strain it while hot. Then dissolve the tartrate of antimony and potassa in the solution while still hot, and add sufficient boiling water, through the strainer, to make it measure three pints. Lastly, mix the whole thoroughly together.

Syrup of Seneka

Take of Seneka [Seneca snakeroot], in moderately fine powder, four
troyounces.
Diluted alcohol two pints.

Moisten the seneka with two fluidounces of the diluted alcohol; then transfer it to a conical percolator, and gradually pour on it the remainder of the diluted alcohol. When the tincture has ceased to pass, evaporate it, by means of a water bath, at a temperature not exceeding 160°, to half a pint; then filter, and, having added the sugar, dissolve it with the aid of a gentle heat, and strain the solution while hot.

Syrup of Tolu

Take of tincture of tolu two fluidounces.
Carbonate of magnesia one hundred and twenty grains.
Sugar, in coarse powder (1lb. 12½ oz. com.), twenty-six troyounces.
Water, a pint.

Rub the tincture of tolu first with the carbonate of magnesia and two troyounces of the sugar, then with the water, gradually added, and filter. To the filtered liquid add the remainder of the sugar, and, having dissolved it with the aid of a gentle heat, strain the solution while hot.

Syrup of Ginger

Take of tincture of ginger six fluidounces.
Carbonate of magnesia half a troyounce.

Sugar, in coarse powder, one hundred and eight troyounces (7 lbs. 6½ oz. com.).
Water, four pints.

Evaporate the tincture to three fluidounces with a gentle heat; then rub it first with the carbonate of magnesia and two troyounces of the sugar, and afterwards with the water, gradually added, and filter. To the filtered liquid add the remainder of the sugar, and, having dissolved it with the aid of a gentle heat, strain the solution while hot.

ALCOHOL

In the form of Rectified Spirit and Proof Spirit, alcohol is used in many pharmaceutical preparations, which are noticed under the several drugs.* Largely diluted spirit is used in evaporating and other lotions, in gargles, collyria [eye wash], & c. Ardent Spirits (brandy, rum, gin, whisky, & c.) may be regarded as diluted alcohol. Of their dietetic use it is not necessary to speak here; but we many notice Dr. Paris's opinion that the habitual use of them induces "more than half of all our chronical diseases." Medicinally, they are sometimes prescribed, particularly brandy, to rouse the system in some cases of extreme debility, the sinking stage of typhus fever, & c. *Mistura Spiritus Vini Galli* [mixture of spirit of French wine] is given in the dose of half an ounce to an ounce, frequently repeated.

HYDRARGYRUM (MERCURY)

The compounds of mercury are alterative, deobstruent, cathartic, antiphlogistic, anthelmintic, and antisyphilitic. They are all of them (with the exception, perhaps, of the sulphurets) capable of inducing a state of mercurialism, of which salivation is the most prominent symptom. Their action requires to be carefully watched. Some of the preparations of mercury are corrosive poisons; and most of them are capable of doing serious injury when incautiously used.

Mercurials are supposed directly to promote the secretion of bile, or its flow into the intestines. They increase the effect of diuretics and diaphoretics. The following are the principal preparations and their doses:

Source: Prescriptions for alcohol, hydragyrum (mercury), cinchona, opium, and quinine and its salts from Henry Beasley, *The Book of Prescriptions* (Philadelphia: Lindsay and Blackiston, 1865), pp. 62-63, 282-284, 195-196, 371-372, 422-423, respectively.

Pilula Hydrargyri [blue mass]: as an alterative, three to five grains; as a cathartic, eight to fifteen grains, but usually conjoined with purgatives, or followed by them; as a sialogogue [salivating agent], five grains three times a day, till the gums are affected, adding a little opium, if necessary, to prevent the pills from acting on the bowels.

Hydrargyrum cum Creta [mercury with chalk] and *Hydr. Cum Magnesia* [mercury with magnesia]: these are mild preparations, yet capable of producing salivation by their continued use. Dose, five to thirty grains; or two to five grains for children. They are much employed in diseases of children attended with deficient biliary secretion . . .

Hydrargyri Chloridum (Calomel). It is impossible to specify here the cases in which this remedy is given, or the intentions it is designed to effect. Dose, as an alterative, half a grain to a grain, every or every other night; as an antiphlogistic, three to five grains; as a cholagogue cathartic, three to six grains; but as its operation is uncertain, it is usual to combine it with vegetable purgatives, or to follow it with a draught of salts and senna. In some cases, as in cholera, yellow fever, & c., calomel has been given in scruple doses. *Pilula Hydrargyri Chloridi* [subchloride?] *composita* [compound calomel pills], five to ten grains; *Pilulæ Calomelanos et Opii* [pills of calomel and opium], one or two pills repeatedly.

Hydrargyri Bichloridum. Corrosive sublimate. A few grains are sufficient to cause death. It is given as an alterative, in lepra and other chronic cutaneous diseases, old ulcers, chronic rheumatism, visceral diseases, and in syphilis. Dose, from one-twentieth or one-sixteenth of a grain to one-eight, two or three times a day. *Liquor Hydrargyri Bichloridi,* half a fluid-drachm to two drachms.

Hydrargyri Amminio-chloridum (white precipitate). This is for outward use only.

Hydrargyri Bromidum (Sub-bromidum). A grain twice a day.

Hydrargyri Perbromidum; from one-twentieth to one-fourth of a grain.

Hydrargyri Bicycanidum; one-sixteenth to one-eighth of a grain.

Hydrargyri Iodidum (flavum, aut *viride)* [yellow and green iodide of mercury]; one to three grains.

Hydraryri Biniodidum (rubrum) [red iodide of mercury]; from one-sixteenth to one-eighth of a grain.

Hydrargyri Acetas; from one-sixth of a grain to one grain.

Hydrargyri Pro-nitras; one-tenth of a grain.

Hydrargyri Phosphas; one-sixth to half a grain.

Hydrargyri Sulphas flavus [yellow sulfate of mercury]; quarter to half a grain as an alterative; as a rough emetic, two or four grains; one grain with five of starch as an errhine [an agent to induce sneezing].

Hydrargyri et Quinæ Chloridum [mercury and quinine]; half a grain three times a day as a sialogogue.

Potassii Hydrargyro-Iodidum (Dr. Channing, U.S.) [iodide of mercury in potassium] is employed as the iodide. It is soluble in water, and given in doses of one-twelfth to one-twentieth of a grain.

CINCHONA

Peruvian Bark is taken from several species of Cinchona. The kinds principally used are the yellow, the pale, and the red. The first is the most powerful; the pale is used where a lighter tonic is required; the red is now seldom employed. All of them are tonic and antiperiodic; and are used in intermittent fevers (after due evacuations, and during the intermissions), and in diseases of debility unattended with local inflammation, especially of the stomach or bowels; in acute rheumatism, after depletions; in the advanced stage of malignant fevers and exanthemata [rashes like those attending the "eruptive" fevers, i.e., measles]; in scrofula [a morbid condition usually affecting the lymph nodes]; in amenhorrhœa [suppressed menstruation]; and in painful neuralgic affections recurring at stated intervals.

The dose of *Pulvis Cinchonæ* is from five grains to two drachms, according to the purpose intended, and the ability of the patient's stomach to bear it. As a general tonic, it is usual to begin with a few grains, and increase the dose, as may be practicable or necessary, to fifteen, twenty, or thirty grains. In intermittents the medium dose is a drachm, more or less frequently during the intermission. In acute rheumatism, Dr. D. Davis has successfully given, after bleeding, & c., from twenty to thirty grains, three or four times a day.

The two principal alkaloids on which the virtues of Peruvian Bark depend, Quinia and Cinchonia, are used as substitutes for the bark itself. Quinia and its salts will be noticed elsewhere. See Quinia [next monograph]. The following are the officinal preparations of Bark, with their doses:

> *Decoctum Cinchonæ* [decoction of cinchona], one to three ounces.
> *Extractum Cinchonæ* [extract of cinchona], five to twenty grains.
> *Extractum Calisayicum* [extract of calisaya bark (yellow cinchona)], one to four grains.
> *Infusum Cinchonæ* [infusion of cinchona] one to three ounces.
> *Calce, et Magnesiæ* [light magnesia and cinchona] one to three ounces.
> *Infusum Cinch. Spissatum* [infusion of freshly expressed cinchona], ten to twenty minims.
> *Syrupus Cinchonæ concent.* [concentrated cinchona concentrate] one-half ounce.

Syrupus Cinchonæ vinosus [syrup of cinchona wine], one ounce.
Tinctura Cinchonæ [tincture of cinchona], one to three drachms.
Tinctura Cinchonæ Am. [ammoniated tincture of cinchona?]
  one-half drachm to one drachm.
Tinctura Cinchonæ comp. [compound tincture of cinchona]
  one to three drachms.
Vinum Cinchonæ [wine of cinchona], one ounce.
Vinum Cinchonæ et Valerianæ [wine of cinchona and valerianic
  acid], one oz. every eight hours.
Cinchonaæ Disulphas, c. [cinchona sulfate], three to five grains.
Cinchonaæ Disulphas, Syrupus [cinchona syrup], a spoonful.
Cinchonaæ Disulphas, Tinctura [tincture of cinchona sulfate],
  a drachm.
Cinchonaæ Disulphas, Vinum [wine of cinchona sulfate],
  a wineglassful.

OPIUM

Opium is perhaps the most important drug in the whole Materia Medica. It is the half-dried juice obtained by cutting the unripe capsule of the White or Eastern Poppy, *Papaver somniferum* (Nat. Ord. *Papaveraceæ*). There are many kinds of opium on commerce. The Turkey or Smyrna Opium, which occurs in small irregular masses, covered outside with the capsules of a species of dock, is of excellent quality, and generally preferred. The various kinds of Opium produced in India are also very good.

Opium, applied externally, acts as a sedative, lulling pain. Given internally in moderate doses, it first produces some excitement, quickening of the pulse, and heat of skin. This effect is quickly followed by a tendency to sleep, and a diminution of sensibility. It abates or banishes pain, if present. It diminishes irritation, and relaxes the muscular system. It diminishes the secretion of the bowels, but increases that of the skin, acting as a sudorific [an agent producing sweating]. Taken continually in small doses, it causes a kind of intoxication, as in opium-eaters. Taken in an over-large dose, it is a dangerous narcotic poison, causing deep sleep, with contraction of the pupil of the eye, succeeded by coma and death.

When not contraindicated, it is the best anodyne and soporific with which we are acquainted. A state of high fever or inflammation forbids its use, as its primary operation is that of a stimulant. It is seldom given when there is a parched tongue and dry skin. In most cases of great pain or irritation, in moderate fever with a moist skin and no cerebral disorder, in delirium tremens, in cancer, in bronchitis (combined with camphor or ipecacuanha, as in Paregoric and Dover's powder), opium may be prescribed. It is given to check the discharge in dysentery and diarrhea, as a diaphoretic in many cases, and as an antispasmotic in convulsive disorders. It may be combined with calomel [see entry on *Hydrargyri Chloridum*] in severe inflammations, as pleurisy; and Dr. Graves gave it in fevers with tartar emetic.

In cases of poisoning by opium, the stomach pump should first be used, or an emetic of sulphate of zinc given; the patient must be kept awake by continual walking between attendants; after the vomiting, cold water may be poured on the face and chest, and an infusion of gall-nuts given, followed by brandy and coffee. Artificial respiration may succeed when all other means have failed.

Opium contains many peculiar chemical principles, but its narcotic properties are chiefly owing to one of these, the alkaloid *Morphia*. Of this, good opium contains about twelve percent, in combination with Meconic acid. This morphia may be extracted from opium, and used separately, either in the pure form or in combination with various acids, with which it forms salts soluble in water and spirit. Morphia resembles opium in its action, but is rather less stimulating. It may be used in the same cases.

The usual dose of opium for the adult is about one grain, but as much as three grains may be given in urgent cases. It acts powerfully on children, and should be given to them either in very small doses, or not at all.

QUININE AND ITS SALTS

Quina and cinchonia are the two bitter alkaloids to which the medicinal properties of the Cinchona barks are owing. The yellow barks (as the Calisaya) contain most Quina; the red barks most Cinchonia. They exist naturally in combination with Kinic acid. Quina is extracted from the bark by a chemical process, and being subsequently combined with sulphuric acid, forms the crystalline Disulphate of Quina, or common Quinine [the same as quinine sulfate]. In this form it is perhaps more used than any other medicine, except Opium. Though itself rather insoluble in water, it becomes very soluble on the addition of a drop of dilute sulphuric acid for each grain of Quinine in the mixture.

As a tonic in simple debility, and loss of appetite from atonic dyspepsia, Quinine is unrivaled. It is rarely given where there is much irritation of the stomach, or in high inflammatory fever. It has lately been highly recommended in typhoid fever, though its employment in this case was deprecated by the late Dr. Graves. It is the best antiperiodics with which we are acquainted. It may be given between the paroxysms of ague, in moderate or in large doses. It is useful in neuralgia and other affections, when marked by periodicity.

The Valerianate of Quina [quinine combined with valerianic acid] has been recommended as an antiperiodic. The Arsenite combines the antiperiodic action of Arsenious acid with that of Quinine. The Citrate of Quinine and Iron may be given in debility when attended with anemia, or in facial neuralgia.

The ordinary dose of *Dispulphate of Quinia* is two grains three times a day. As much as ten grains or more may be given in particular cases. (Quinidia is an alkaloid found in some kinds of bark, which much resembles Quina. What has been called *Amorphous Quinine* is impure Quinidia. It may be prescribed and used like Quinine.)

> *Tinctura Quinæ composita* (L.) [compound tincture of quinine]: dose, one to three drachms.
>
> *Quinæ Arsenis* [arsenite (white arsenic) of quinine: dose, one-fifth of a grain.
>
> *Quinæ Citras* [citrate of quinine], one to five grains.
>
> *Syrupus Quinæ Citratis* (Majendie) [syrup of quinine citrate], one to two drachms.
>
> *Ferri et Quinæ Citras* [iron, quinine, and citric acid], five grains.
>
> *Quinæ Ferrocyanas* (Paris Codex) [Ferrocyanate of quinine, ferrocyanic acid $H_4 Fe(CN)_6$], one to five grains.
>
> *Quinæ Iodidum (Hydriodized)* [iodized hydriodate of quinine*], two to three grains.
>
> *Quinæ et Ferri Iodidum* [quinine and iodide of iron], two to three grains.
>
> *Quinæ Murias* (D.) [muriate of quinine], one to two grains.
>
> *Quinæ et Hydrargyri Chloridum* [quinine and mercurous chloride (calomel)], half to one grain.
>
> *Quinæ Kinas* [quinine and kino or kinoic acid?], three to five grains.
>
> *Quinæ Lactas* [lactate of quinine†], three to nine grains in the day.
>
> *Quinæ Nitras* [nitrate of quinine] (Paris).
>
> *Quinæ Phosphas* [phosphate of quinine‡].
>
> *Quinæ Sulphas (neutra)*. These three are prescribed as the disulphate.
>
> *Quinæ Tannas* [tannate of quinine], one to five grains.

---

*Hydriodate of quinine consists of sulfate of quinine, 95 parts; iodide of potassium, 40 parts. The product corresponds to 100 parts of hydriodate of quinine. Iodized hydriodate of quinine consists of 70 parts; iodide of potassium, 50 parts; iodine, 20 parts. To be triturated together with a little alcohol. Corresponds to 100 parts of the above quinine salt. See *USD,* Fifteenth Edition, 1884, p. 1216.

†Lactate of quinine consists of pure quinine, 70 parts; lactic acid, 35 parts. To be triturated together, if necessary, with a few drops of alcohol. See Ibid., p. 1217.

‡Phosphate of quinine consists of sulfate of quinine, 94 parts; phosphate of sodium, 80 parts. See Ibid., p. 1217.

Quinæ Tartras [tartrated quinine] (Paris Codex), one to five grains.
Quinæ Valerianas (D.) [valerianate of quinine], half to one grain.
Cinchonæ Dispulphas and *Quinidiæ* (vel *Chinoidinæ*) *Dispulphas*
    are prescribed in the same manner as common quinine.

Notes

List of Abbreviations

Am. J. Pharm. = *American Journal of Pharmacy*

Med. Surg. Hist. = *The Medical and Surgical History of the War of the Rebellion* (1861-1865) (2 volumes in 6 parts: volume 1, *Med. Hist.*; volume 2, *Surg. Hist.*)

NA = National Archives (organized by Record Group, designated RG)

NLM = National Library of Medicine

Pharm. Hist. = *Pharmacy in History*

Proc. APhA = *Proceedings of the American Pharmaceutical Association*

SHSP = *Southern Historical Society Papers*

USD = *Dispensatory of the United States of America*

USP = *Pharmacopoeia of the United States of America*

War Reb. = *The War of the Rebellion: A Compilation of the Official Records of the Union and Confederate Armies* (in 4 series)

Chapter 1

1. George Worthington Adams, *Doctors in Blue: The Medical History of the Union Army in the Civil War* (1952; reprint, Louisiana State University Press, 1996); H. H. Cunningham, *Doctors in Gray: The Confederate Medical Service,* Second Edition (1960; reprint, Louisiana State University Press, 1993); C. Keith Wilbur, *Civil War Medicine, 1861-1865* (Philadelphia: Chelsea House Publishers, 1995); Mark J. Schaadt, *Civil War Medicine: An Illustrated History* (Quincy, IL: Cedarwood Publishing, 1998); Alfred J. Bollett, *Civil War Medicine: Challenges and Triumphs* (Tucson, AZ: Galen Press, 2002). These do not include more specialized studies relating to field hospitals, ambulance corps, nursing, surgery, nor the many personal memoirs and diary accounts of medical service during the war. For an excellent annotated bibliography on all aspects of Civil War health care, see Frank R. Freemon, *Microbes and Minie Balls: An Annotated Bibliography of Civil War Medicine* (Rutherford, NJ: Fairleigh Dickinson University Press, 1993). For details see the bibliographical essay.

2. Allan Nevins, *The Organized War, 1863-1864,* volume 3 of *The War for the Union* (1971; reprint, New York: Konecky and Konecky, 2000), p. 313.

3. Bollett, *Civil War Medicine,* pp. 231-255.

4. Norman Franke, "Medico-Pharmaceutical Conditions and Drug Supply in the Confederate States of America 1861-1865." Unpublished PhD dissertation (Madison: University of Wisconsin, 1956).

5. George Winston Smith, *Medicines for the Union Army: The United States Army Laboratories During the Civil War* (1962; reprint, Binghamton, NY: Pharmaceutical Products Press, 2001).

6. Bruce A. Evans, *A Primer of Civil War Medicine: Non Surgical Medical Practice During the Civil War Years,* Revised Enlarged Edition (Knoxville, TN: Bohemian Brigade Bookshop, 1998), p. ix.

7. Guy Hasegawa, "Pharmacy in the American Civil War," *American Journal of Health-System Pharmacy* 57 (2000): 475-489.

8. Charles A. Beard and Mary R. Beard, *The Rise of American Civilization,* One-Volume Edition (New York: Macmillan, 1930), pp. 52-121; Louis M. Hacker, *The Triumph of American Capitalism* (New York: Columbia University Press, 1940); and James M. McPherson, *Battle Cry of Freedom: The Civil War Era* (New York: Oxford University Press, 1988), pp. 452-453.

9. Beard and Beard, *American Civilization,* p. 54.

10. Richard B. Morris, ed., *Encyclopedia of American History,* Bicentennial Edition (New York: Harper and Row, 1976), p. 648.

11. Inter-University Consortium for Political and Social Research (ICPSR). United States Historical Census Data. Available at <http://fisher.lib.virginia.edu/census>.

12. Ibid.

13. Ibid.

14. Emerson David Fite, *Social and Industrial Conditions in the North During the Civil War* (New York: Macmillan, 1910), p. 99.

15. Ibid., p. 97.

16. Williams Haynes, *American Chemical Industry,* 6 Volumes (New York: Van Nostrand, 1954), *Background and Beginnings,* 1: 401.

17. Ibid.

18. Ibid., p. 320.

19. Frederick Allen, *Secret Formula* (New York, HarperCollins, 1994), pp. 18-39.

20. See obituary notice, "James Vernor," *Journal of the American Pharmaceutical Association* 16 (1927): 1124-1125.

21. See, for example, John S. Haller Jr., *American Medicine in Transition, 1840-1910* (Urbana: University of Illinois Press, 1981); and Lester S. King, *American Medicine Comes of Age, 1840-1920* (n.p.: American Medical Association, 1984).

22. Haller, *American Medicine,* p. vii.

23. An excellent overview of the changes in medical thinking through the nineteenth century is provided in Lester S. King's *Transformations in American Medicine: From Benjamin Rush to William Osler* (Baltimore: Johns Hopkins University Press, 1991).

24. These groups have been subjected to extensive analysis. See Martin Kaufman, *Homeopathy in America: The Rise and Fall of a Medical Heresy* (Baltimore: Johns Hopkins University Press, 1971); John S. Haller Jr., *Medical Protestants: The Eclectics in America, 1825-1939* (Carbondale: Southern Illinois University, 1994); Haller, *Kindly Medicine: Physio-Medicalism in America, 1836-1911* (Kent, OH: Kent State University Press, 1997); Haller, *The People's Doctors: Samuel Thomson and the American Botanical Movement, 1790-1860* (Carbondale: Southern Illinois University Press, 2000); and Alex Berman and Michael A. Flannery, *America's Botanico-Medical Movements: Vox Populi* (Binghamton, NY: Pharmaceutical Products Press, 2001), pp. 17-31.

25. A complete discussion is offered in Michael A. Flannery, "Another House Divided: Union Medical Service and Sectarians During the Civil War," *Journal of the History of Medicine and Allied Sciences* 54 (1999): 478-510.

26. On Wood's role in the *USP* and *USD,* see Lee Anderson and Gregory J. Higby, *The Spirit of Voluntarism: A Legacy of Commitment and Contribution: The United States Pharmacopeia, 1820-1995* (Rockville, MD: The United States Pharmacopeial Convention, 1995), pp. 43-84 passim.

27. See biographical sketch in Joseph W. England, ed., *The First Century of the Philadelphia College of Pharmacy, 1821-1921* (Philadelphia: The College, 1922), pp. 397-398.

28. George B. Wood, *A Treatise on the Practice of Medicine,* Fifth Edition, 2 Volumes (Philadelphia: J. B. Lippincott, 1858), 1: 17-142.

29. Ibid., 1: 26.

30. Ibid., 1: 30.

31. Ibid., 1: 85.

32. Ibid. 1: 144.

33. Ibid., 1: 144-145.

34. Ibid., 1: 154-163.

35. Ibid., 1: 165.

36. Ibid., 1: 168.

37. Ibid., 1: 171.

38. Ibid.

39. Pierre C. A. Louis, *Researches on the Effects of Bloodletting in Some Inflammatory Diseases and on the Influence of Tartarized Antimony and Vesication in Pneumonitis,* trans. by C. G. Putnam (Boston: Hilliard, Gray and Company, 1836).

40. For a complete discussion of Farr's zymotic theory, see John M. Eyler, *Victorian Social Medicine: The Ideas and Methods of William Farr* (Baltimore: Johns Hopkins University Press, 1979), pp. 97-122.

41. Wood, *Treatise,* 1: 172.

42. *Med. Surg. Hist.,* Part. 2, Volume 1, *Med. Hist.* (Washington, DC: GPO, 1879).

43. In explaining the link between "zymotic" and its Greek origin, meaning ferment, Farr and his disciples proposed that disease proceeded from an altered state of the blood (induced by a minute quantity of this so-called "zymotic agent"), and "not from the direct agency of the foreign matter admitted into circulation" (Wood, *Treatise,* 1: 172). With the advent of our knowledge of microbes, the above statement is challenged: Microbes carry the capacity to multiply through genetic material (either DNA or RNA) and the action on their host is much more direct than Farr or Wood anticipated. One example of such direct action is the secretion of bacterial toxins, which can interfere with important physiological processes of the body and/or overwhelm our immune system. The interesting thought is that, in contrast to the direct action of microbes such as bacteria, viruses, and parasites, the suggested mechanism of a "zymotic agent" may resemble the mechanistic insights we know thus far of "mad cow" disease. Mad cow disease, or bovine spongiform encephalopathy (BSE), is part of a new class of diseases termed transmissible spongiform encephalopathies or TSE. The causative agent of TSE appears to be a "prion" protein. Prion proteins are normal host-encoded proteins; however the disease-causing prion protein appears to have taken on an altered conformational state. A prion-related disease, called scrapie, was first discovered in sheep, and the trouble actually may have begun when remains of scrapie-affected sheep were entered into cattle feed. This is believed to have caused the mad cow disease outbreak in cattle, and, after sub-

sequent consumption of BSE-tainted meat, cases of another prion-related phenomena, Creutzfeldt Jakob disease, in humans. Researchers have tried hard to find any genetic material associated with an invading prion protein because our own scientific paradigms dictate that an infectious agent without DNA or RNA cannot cause disease on its own; to suggest otherwise flies in the face of all conventional wisdom. Stanley Prusiner, whose discovery of the prion concept won him a Nobel prize in 1997, lends credibility to a potentially revolutionary concept that received wide skepticism from many scientists. Here is the interesting link between past and present: Because there is no genetic material associated with this invading prion protein, it cannot multiply and cause disease according to the traditional microbial model. Instead, after consuming it, it somehow manages (by acting as a "ferment" or "zymotic agent" according to Wood or Farr's description?) to induce our own healthy prion proteins to also take on this altered conformation, thereby converting them into a disease-causing state. Could this prion concept see Farr vindicated after more than 160 years? Letter to the author, August 13, 2001, from Tom Oomens, PhD, Department of Microbiology, University of Alabama at Birmingham. The author is grateful to Dr. Oomens for this observation.

44. *Dictionary of Scientific Biography,* Eight-Volume Edition, s.v. "Pasteur, Louis."

45. Ibid., s.v. "Koch, Robert."

46. Richard Harrison Shryock, *The Development of Modern Medicine: An Interpretation of the Social and Scientific Factors Involved* (1947; reprint, Madison: University of Wisconsin Press, 1979), p. 249.

47. Oliver Wendell Holmes, "Currents and Counter-Currents in Medical Science," in *Medical Essays, 1842-1882* (Boston: Houghton Mifflin, 1883), p. 203.

48. *Med. Surg. Hist.,* part 3, volume 2, *Surg. Hist.,* 899.

49. *The Photographic History of the Civil War,* 10 volumes in 5 (1911; reprint, Secaucus, NJ: The Blue and Grey Press, 1987), 4: 220.

50. Marcy C. Gillett, *The Army Medical Department, 1818-1865* (Washington, DC: GPO, 1986), p. 154.

51. John H. Brinton, *Personal Memoirs of John H. Brinton: Civil War Surgeon, 1861-1865* (1914; reprint, Carbondale: Southern Illinois University Press, 1996), pp. 29-36.

52. Adams, *Doctors in Blue,* p. 5.

53. Ibid., p. 9.

54. Ibid., pp. 10-11.

55. Charles J. Stillé, *History of the United States Sanitary Commission* (Philadelphia: J. B. Lippincott, 1866), pp. 57-60.

56. See the proclamation issued April 15, 1861, in James D. Richardson, ed., *A Compilation of the Messages and Papers of the Presidents, 1789-1902,* 10 volumes ([Washington, DC]: Bureau of National Literature and Art, 1905) 6: 13-14.

57. Facsimile reprinted in *A Newspaper History of the Civil War from Nat Turner to 1863,* volume 1 of *Civil War Extra* (Edison, NJ: Castle Books, 1999), p. 65.

58. Gillett, *The Army Medical Department,* p. 177.

59. James Evelyn Pilcher, *The Surgeon Generals of the Army* (Carlisle, PA: The Association of Military Surgeons, 1905), pp. 47-57.

60. Details on Letterman's reorganization of the U.S. Army field hospital and medical supply systems are provided in Gordon W. Jones, "The Medical History of

the Fredericksburg Campaign: Course and Significance," *The Journal of the History of Medicine and Allied Sciences* 18 (1963): 241-256.

61. *War Reb.,* series 3, volume 5 (Washington, DC: GPO, 1900), p. 150.

62. Gillett, *The Army Medical Department,* p. 156.

63. Ibid.

64. The precise number of hospital stewards is difficult to determine. The complete number does not appear in the surgeon general's reports nor is it published in any of the official records. While the numbers undoubtedly fluctuated throughout the war, it is known that at their greatest number, general hospitals numbered 205 (see *Med. Surg. Hist.,* part 3, volume 2, *Surg. Hist.,* 902) and that three to four stewards were employed in each facility (see *Med. Surg. Hist.,* part 3, volume 1, *Med. Hist.,* 957).

65. The act establishing medical storekeepers was issued as General Order, no. 55, May 24, 1862, see *War Reb.,* series 3, volume 2, p. 67; and Hasegawa, "Pharmacy in the Civil War," p. 482.

66. E. Robert Wiese, "Life and Times of Samuel Preston Moore, Surgeon-General of the Confederate States of America," *Southern Medical Journal* 23 (1930): 916-922.

67. Harris D. Riley, "Moore, Samuel P." In *Encyclopedia of Southern Culture,* ed. Charles Reagan Wilson and William Ferris (Chapel Hill: University of North Carolina Press, 1989), pp. 1374-1375.

68. Cunningham, *Doctors in Gray,* p. 75. Like their Northern counterparts, storekeepers held a rank of first lieutenant but were not to exceed six in number. The number of stewards, however, was "as many . . . as the service may require." See *War Reb.,* series 4, volume 1, pp. 326-327.

69. Joseph Jones, "The Medical History of the Confederate States Army and Navy," in *SHSP* 20 (Richmond, VA: The Society, 1892), p. 119.

70. America's involvement in World War I (1917-1918) was the first war in which the Medical Department was able to take full advantage of the many innovations in medical microbiology, immunology, and the rise of numerous specialties. For details, see James H. Cassedy, *Medicine in America: A Short History* (Baltimore: Johns Hopkins University Press, 1991), p. 120.

71. Jones, "Medical History of the Confederate States," p. 115.

72. Paul Steiner, *Disease in the Civil War: Natural Biological Warfare in 1861-1865* (Springfield, IL: Charles C Thomas, 1968), p. 8.

73. Ibid., pp. 16-25; Adams, *Doctors in Blue,* pp. 222-228, 240-241.

74. Steiner, *Disease,* p. 9.

75. William F. Fox, *Regimental Losses in the American Civil War, 1861-1865* (1898; reprinted, Dayton, OH: Morningside Bookshop, 1985), p. 129.

76. Ibid.

77. Ibid., p. 149.

78. Ibid., p. 347.

79. Ibid., p. 554.

80. Adams, *Doctors in Blue,* p. 240.

81. Andrew K. Black, "In the Service of the United States: Comparative Mortality Among African-American and White Troops in the Union Army," *Journal of Negro History* 79 (1994): 331.

82. Interesting as much for its misunderstandings as for its discussion is Joseph Janvier Woodward's *Outlines of the Chief Camp Diseases of the United States Army* (Philadelphia: J. B. Lippincott, 1863).

83. Black, "In the Service of the United States," p. 325.

Chapter 2

1. Glenn Sonnedecker, *Kremers and Urdang's History of Pharmacy,* Fourth Edition (1976; reprinted, Madison: AIHP, 1986), p. 193.

2. Editorial Dept., *Am. J. Pharm.* 33 (1861): 476.

3. William C. Bakes, December 10, 1861, Philadelphia College of Pharmacy, Minute Book, p. 24.

4. Quoted in Michael A. Flannery and Dennis B. Worthen, *Pharmaceutical Education in the Queen City: 150 Years of Service, 1850-2000* (Binghamton, NY: Pharmaceutical Products Press, 2001), p. 13.

5. Editorial Dept., *Am. J. Pharm.* 35 (1863): 92.

6. David L. Cowen and William H. Helfand, *Pharmacy: An Illustrated History* (New York: Harry N. Abrams, 1990), p. 149.

7. Gregory J. Higby, "A Brief Look at American Pharmaceutical Education Before 1900." In Robert A. Buerki, *In Search of Excellence: The First Century of the American Association of Colleges of Pharmacy* (Research Triangle Park, NC: AACP, 1999), p. 7. Issued as the Fall Supplement to the *American Journal of Pharmaceutical Education* 63 (1999).

8. Sonnedecker, *History of Pharmacy,* p. 244.

9. Ibid., p. 230.

10. Gregory J. Higby, "A Brief Look at American Pharmacy Education Before 1900," p. 6.

11. Sonnedecker, *History of Pharmacy,* p. 230.

12. Joseph W. England, ed., *The First Century of the Philadelphia College of Pharmacy, 1821-1921* (Philadelphia: The College, 1922), p. 143.

13. Robert G. Mrtek, "Pharmaceutical Education in These United States—An Interpretive Historical Essay of the Twentieth Century," *American Journal of Pharmaceutical Education* 40 (1976): 340.

14. Cowen and Helfand, *Pharmacy,* pp. 161-162.

15. Evan Tyson Ellis, "The Story of a Very Old Philadelphia Drug Store," *American Journal of Pharmacy* 75 (1903): 65. As an interesting aside, the Charles Ellis Company served as the business that gave Joseph P. Remington (1847-1918), one of America's important leaders of pharmacy, his four-year apprenticeship.

16. Ibid., p. 66. An excellent historical review of the patent medicines mentioned by Ellis is found in George B. Griffenhagen and James Harvey Young, "Old English Patent Medicines in America," *Pharm. Hist.* 34 (1992): 199-228.

17. Ellis, "Old Philadelphia Drug Store," pp. 67-68.

18. Philip D. Jordan, "Purveyors to the Profession: Cincinnati Drug Houses, 1850-1860," *Ohio Archæological and Historical Quarterly* 54 (1945): 371-380.

19. Ibid., p. 377.

20. Ibid., p. 378.

21. A synopsis of the company's history is available in Williams Haynes, *American Chemical Industry,* 6 volumes (New York: D. Van Nostrand, 1947), *The Chemical Companies,* 6: 423-424.

22. [William Procter], "New Lebanon; Its Physic Garden and Their Products," *Am. J. Pharm.* new series, 17 (1851): 387-388.

23. Tilden and Company, *Formulæ for Making Tinctures, Infusions, Syrups, Wines, Mixtures, Pills, & c., Simple and Compound, from the Fluid & Solid Extracts Prepared at the Laboratory of Tilden & Co.* (New York: Tilden, 1861).

24. Procter, "New Lebanon," 388.

25. Ibid.

26. Haynes, *American Chemical Industry,* 6 volumes, *The Chemical Companies,* 6: 397.

27. Ibid., 275.

28. Sonnedecker, *History of Pharmacy,* p. 295.

29. Wade Boyle, *Official Herbs: Botanical Substances in the United State Pharmacopoeias, 1820-1990* (East Palestine, OH: Buckeye Naturopathic Press, 1991), p. 57.

30. See George B. Wood and Franklin Bache, *USD,* Eleventh Edition (Philadelphia: J. B. Lippincott, 1858), pp. 226-273, 1233-1243.

31. Ibid., pp. 549-571. Details on Sertürner's discovery of morphine are available in Rudolf Schmitz, "Friedrich Wilhelm Sertürner and the Discovery of Morphine," *Pharm. Hist.* 27 (1985): 61-74.

32. Wood and Bache, *USD,* pp. 605-607.

33. Ibid., pp. 763-765.

34. Ibid., pp. 381-382.

35. Ibid., pp. 442-446.

36. Edward Parrish, *An Introduction to Practical Pharmacy,* Second Edition (Philadelphia: Blanchard and Lea, 1859), p. 587.

37. Robert A. Buerki and Gregory J. Higby, "History of Dosage Forms and Basic Preparations." In *Encyclopedia of Pharmaceutical Technology,* edited by James Swarbrick and James C. Boylin, volume 7 (New York: Marcel Dekker, 1993), p. 333.

38. Buerki and Higby, "History of Dosage Forms," p. 325; and Parrish, *Practical Pharmacy,* p. 587.

39. Parrish, *Practical Pharmacy,* p. 91.

40. Alfred Stillé, *Therapeutics and Materia Medica,* Second Edition, 2 volumes (Philadelphia: Blanchard and Lea, 1864), 2: 501.

41. Ibid.

42. Parrish, *Practical Pharmacy,* p. 628.

43. Ibid., pp. 244-246.

44. Buerki and Higby, "History of Dosage Forms," p. 309.

45. Stillé asserts the conventional wisdom regarding counter-irritation by saying, "apart from all theoretical or analogical illustrations of the subject, the fact is patent that spontaneous inflammations aggravate, while artificial inflammations, duly regulated, palliate or cure those which arise primarily or idiopathically." (See his *Therapeutics and Materia Medica,* 1: 223).

46. *The Merck Index: An Encyclopedia of Chemicals, Drugs, and Biologicals,* Twelfth Edition (Whitehouse Station, NJ: Merck and Co., 1996), p. 285.

47. Stillé, *Therapeutics and Materia Medica,* 1: 350-374.

48. Ibid., 1: 356.

49. Parrish, *Practical Pharmacy,* p. 130.

50. Ibid., p. 195.

51. Buerki and Higby, "History of Dosage Forms," p. 313.

52. Details on the rise and impact of elixirs can be found in Gregory J. Higby, "Publication of the National Formulary: A Turning Point for American Pharmacy," in *One Hundred Years of the National Formulary: A Symposium,* edited by Gregory J. Higby (Madison, WI: AIHP, 1989), pp. 6-9.

53. Stillé, *Therapeutics and Materia Medica,* 1: 93.

54. Ibid., 1: 144.

55. Ibid., 1: 376.

56. Ibid., 1: 529.

57. Ibid., 1: 644.

58. Ibid., 2: 143.

59. Ibid., 2: 159.

60. Ibid., 2: 221.

61. Ibid., 2: 251.

62. Ibid., 2: 317.

63. Ibid., 2: 629.

64. H. C. Wood and Franklin Bache, *USD,* Fifteenth Edition, edited by H. C. Wood, Joseph P. Remington, and Samuel P. Sadtler (Philadelphia: J. B. Lippincott, 1884), p. 741.

65. For a more detailed discussion on the use of leeches and its prevalence in the professional literature, see Margareta Modig, "The Strange Lore of Leeches," *Pharm. Hist.* 28 (1986): 99-102; and Glenn Sonnedecker, "The Beginning of American Pharmaceutical Journalism," *Pharm. Hist.* 33 (1991): 67.

66. Stillé, *Therapeutics and Materia Medica,* 1: 646.

67. For details, see Frederick William Headland, *The Action of Medicines in the System,* Third Edition (Philadelphia: Lindsay and Blakiston, 1859), pp. 422, 431-433.

68. A useful classification of medicines and treatments cross-referenced to the U.S. Army Supply Table is provided in Bruce A. Evans, *A Primer of Civil War Medicine: Non Surgical Medical Practices During the Civil War Years,* Revised Enlarged Edition (Knoxville, TN: Bohemian Brigade Bookshop, 1998), pp. 21-43.

69. See, for example, Norman Franke, "A Confederate Recipe Book," in *Three Essays on Formulaires* (Madison, WI: AIHP, 1961), p. 13; and Franke, "Medico-Pharmaceutical Conditions and Drug Supply in the Confederate States of America, 1861-1865" (Unpublished PhD dissertation, University of Wisconsin, 1956), p. 124.

70. David Madden, *Beyond the Battlefield: The Ordinary Life and Extraordinary Times of the Civil War Soldier* (New York: Simon and Schuster, 2000), p. 252.

71. Eleanor M. Tilton, *Amiable Autocrat: A Biography of Dr. Oliver Wendell Holmes* (New York: Henry Schuman, 1947), p. 255.

72. A. E. Magoffin, "Recollections of an Old-Time Druggist," *Druggists Circular* 51 (January 1907): 192-193.

73. Michael C. C. Adams, *Our Masters the Rebels: A Speculation on Union Military Failure in the East, 1861-1865* (Cambridge, MA: Harvard University Press, 1978), p. 47.

74. For a complete discussion, see John Duffy, "A Note on Ante-Bellum Southern Nationalism and Medical Practice," *The Journal of Southern History* 34 (1968): 266-276.

75. Details on antebellum justifications for racial differences are insightfully covered in John S. Haller, *Outcasts from Evolution: Scientific Attitudes of Racial Inferiority, 1859-1900,* new edition (Carbondale: Southern Illinois University Press, 1995), esp. pp. 74-84; and Stephen Jay Gould, *The Mismeasure of Man,* revised and expanded edition (New York: W. W. Norton, 1996), esp. 71-74, 101-103.

76. This concept is summarized in John Duffy, "States' Rights Medicine," in *Encyclopedia of Southern Culture,* edited by Charles Reagan Wilson and William Ferris (Chapel Hill: University of North Carolina Press, 1989), pp. 1335-1336. On this topic, see also James H. Cassedy, "Medical Men and the Ecology of the Old South," in *Science and Medicine in the Old South,* edited by Ronald L. Numbers and Todd L. Savitt (Baton Rouge: Louisiana State University Press, 1989), pp. 166-178; and John Harley Warner, "The Idea of Southern Distinctiveness: Medical Knowledge and Practice in the Old South," in *Science and Medicine in the Old South,* pp. 179-205.

77. James H. Cassedy, *Medicine in America: A Short History* (Baltimore: Johns Hopkins University Press, 1991), p. 64.

78. Quoted in Warner, "The Idea of Southern Distinctiveness," *Science and Medicine in the Old South,* p. 184.

79. David L. Cowen, "The History of Pharmacy and the History of the South," *Report of Rho Chi* 33 (November 1967): 18-24.

80. David L. Cowen, "The Trustees' Garden at Savannah," *Georgia Pharmacist Quarterly* 60 (Spring 1983): 5.

81. Ibid, p. 3.

82. Cowen, "The History of Pharmacy and the History of the South," p. 20.

83. David L. Cowen, "The British North American Colonies As a Source of Drugs," *Die Vorträge der Hauptversammlung,* Bd. 28 (Stuttgart: Wissenschaftliche Verlagsgesellschaft MBH, 1966), p. 50.

84. Ibid., p. 54.

85. Henry C. Fuller, *The Story of Drugs* (New York: The Century Co., 1922), pp. 148-149.

86. Cowen, "The History of Pharmacy and the History of the South," p. 23.

87. Ibid.

88. Ibid.

89. Ibid., p. 24.

90. Clement Eaton, *A History of the Old South: The Emergence of a Reluctant Nation,* Third Edition (New York: Macmillan, 1975), p. 11.

91. Sonnedecker, *History of Pharmacy,* pp. 71-73.

92. Eaton, *History of the Old South,* p. 181.

93. On the life of Porcher, see Jonathan M. Townsend, "Francis Peyre Porcher, M.D.," *Annals of Medical History* 1 (1939): 177-188.

94. Inter-University Consortium for Political and Social Research (ICPSR). The U.S. Census from 1860. United States Historical Census Data. Available at <http://fisher.lib.virginia.edu/census>.

95. Kenneth M. Stampp, *The Irrepressible Conflict: Essays on the Background of the Civil War* (New York: Oxford University Press, 1980), p. 243.

96. Quoted in Ibid.

97. Marion B. Lucas, *From Slavery to Segregation, 1760-1891,* volume 1 of *A History of Blacks in Kentucky* (Frankfort: The Kentucky Historical Society, 1992), p. 58.

98. Cowen, "The History of Pharmacy and of the South," p. 21.

99. Ibid.

100. Quoted in Ibid., p. 22.

101. Ibid., p. 21.

Chapter 3

1. Quoted in Jack Larkin, *The Reshaping of Everyday Life, 1790-1840* (New York: Harper and Row, 1988), p. 149.

2. Mrs. West, *Letters to a Young Lady, in Which the Duties and Character of Women Are Considered* (Troy, NY: Penniman, 1806), pp. 23-24.

3. Women were finally accorded full military rank and status with the establishment of the Army and Navy Nurse Corps in 1901 and 1908 and the entry of 13,000 women into the Corps during World War I. See Barbara A. Wilson, "Women's Military History," available at <www.undelete.org/military/timeline1.html>.

4. This estimate came from Samuel Ramsey, chief clerk for the U.S. Army Medical Department. For details see George Worthington Adams, *Doctors in Blue: The Medical History of the Union Army in the Civil War* (1952; reprint, Baton Rouge: Louisiana State University Press), p. 178; and Mary Elizabeth Massey, *Bonnet Brigades: American Women and the Civil War* (New York: Alfred A. Knopf, 1966), p. 52.

5. Susan Lyons Hughes, "The Daughter of the Regiment: A Brief History of *Vivandiers* and *Cantinieres* in the American Civil War," Ehistory.com: U.S. Civil War: "A Nation Divided," May 2000 issue, available at <www.ehistory.com/uscw/features/articles/0005/vivandieres.efm> .

6. Ibid.

7. Allen Nevins' preface to William Quentin Maxwell, *Lincoln's Fifth Wheel: The Political History of the United States Sanitary Commission* (New York: Longmans, Green, 1956), p. viii.

8. Alexis de Tocqueville, *Democracy in America,* 2 volumes in 1 (New York: Everyman's Library, 1994), 2: 106.

9. Ibid., p. 175.

10. For details on the formation of the Sanitary Commission, see Charles J. Stillé, *History of the United States Sanitary Commission* (Philadelphia: J. B. Lippincott, 1866), pp. 39-45; and Maxwell, *Lincoln's Fifth Wheel,* pp. 1-8.

11. For details on the association's formation and history, see Julia B. Curtis, "Woman's Central Association of Relief." In L. P. Brockett and Mary C. Vaughan's *Women's Work in the Civil War: A Record of Heroism, Patriotism, and Patience* (Philadelphia: Zeigler, McCurdy and Co., 1867), pp. 527-539.

12. Maxwell, *Lincoln's Fifth Wheel,* p. 2.

13. The complete notice as it appeared in the New York City newspapers is available at the U.S. Sanitary Commission Web site <www.netwalk.com/~jpr/>.

14. Ibid.

15. Quoted in Maxwell, *Lincoln's Fifth Wheel,* p. 8.

16. Ibid.

17. Stillé, *History of the Sanitary Commission,* p. 547.

18. There are three excellent overviews of the women of the Sanitary Commission: giving due allowance for a penchant toward Victorian hagiography is Brockett and Vaughan's *Women's Work* (see note 11); good biographical material on many Sanitary Commission women by a contemporary historian is available in Rebecca D. Larson, *White Roses: Stories of Civil War Nurses* (Gettysburg, PA: Thomas Publications, 1997); and a very thorough scholarly account is given in Marilyn Mayer Culpepper, *Trials and Triumphs: Women of the American Civil War* (East Lansing: Michigan State University Press, 1991).

19. Mary A. Livermore, *My Story of the War: A Woman's Narrative of Four Years Personal Experience* (Hartford, CT: A. D. Worthington, 1888), p. 129.

20. Larson, *White Roses,* p. 39.

21. The problems of the U.S. Army Medical Department are thoroughly covered in Mary C. Gillett, *The Army Medical Department, 1818-1865* (Washington, DC: GPO, 1987), chapter 8, esp. pp. 153-162.

22. Katharine Prescott Wormeley, *The Cruel Side of War with the Army of the Potomac* (Boston: Roberts Brothers, 1898), pp. 8-9.

23. Livermore, *My Story of the War,* p. 133.

24. See the following for details, Livermore, *My Story of the War,* p. 134; A. H. Hoge, *The Boys in Blue; or, Heroes of the "Rank and File"* (New York: E. B. Treat, 1867), pp. 266-267; and Emma E. Edmonds, *Nurse and Spy in the Union Army* (Hartford, CT: W. S. Williams, 1865), p. 363.

25. Maxwell, *Lincoln's Fifth Wheel,* pp. 86-87.

26. Wormeley, *The Cruel Side of War,* p. 39.

27. Ibid., p. 115.

28. For example see Wormeley, *The Cruel Side of War,* p. 91; Anon., *Notes of Hospital Life from November, 1861, to August, 1863* (Philadelphia: J. B. Lippincott, 1864), pp. 48-49.

29. See Elvira Powers, *Hospital Pencillings: Being a Diary While in Jefferson General Hospital, Jeffersonville, Ind., and Others at Nashville Tennessee* (Boston: Edward L. Mitchell, 1866), p. 64. On the opposition of physicians to women in the camp and general hospitals, see Culpepper, *Trials and Triumphs,* p. 322.

30. Quoted in Gillett, *The Army Medical Department,* p. 156.

31. John H. Brinton, *Personal Memoirs of John H. Brinton, Civil War Surgeon, 1861-1865* (1914; reprinted, Carbondale: Southern Illinois University Press, 1996), pp. 43-44.

32. Ibid., pp. 44-45.

33. Anon., *Notes of Hospital Life,* pp. 48-50.

34. *A Manual of Directions Prepared for the Use of the Nurses in the Army Hospitals* (1861; reprinted, New Market Battlefield Military Museum, 1994).

35. Ibid., pp. 15-16. Labarraque's fluid was a chlorinated soda solution made from carbonate of soda, chlorinated lime, and water.

36. Ibid., p. 17.

37. Ibid., p. 19.

38. Ibid., p. 20.

39. *Hints for the Control and Prevention of Infectious Diseases in Camps, Transports, and Hospitals,* Sanitary Commission, S (New York: Wm. C. Bryant, 1863), p. 29.

40. See, for example, *Report of a Committee of the Associate Medical Members of the Sanitary Commission on the Subject of Continued Fevers,* Sanitary Commission, K (Boston: J. E. Farwell, 1862), pp. 21-23; and *Report of a Committee of the Associate Members of the Sanitary Commission on Dysentery,* Sanitary Commission, M (Philadelphia: Collins, 1862), pp. 25-39.

41. *Quinine As a Prophylactic Against Malarious Diseases,* Sanitary Commission Report, no. 31 (New York: Wm. C. Bryant, 1861).

42. *A Report to the Secretary of War of the Operations of the Sanitary Commission,* Sanitary Commission Report, no. 40 (Washington, DC: McGill and Withrow, 1861), p. 50.

43. *A Collection of the Papers of the Sanitary Commission,* Sanitary Commission, no. 25 (n.p.: [The Commission?], 1861), p. 56.

44. *Report of the Condition of the Troops and the Operations of the Sanitary Commission in the Valley of the Mississippi,* Sanitary Commission, no. 36 (Cleveland: Fairbanks, Benedict and Co., 1861), pp. 11-12.

45. Ibid.

46. Livermore, *My Story of the War,* p. 125.

47. *U.S. Sanitary Commission* [Report] no. 22 (n.p.: [The Commission], 1861), p. 3.

48. *Two Reports Concerning the Aid and Comfort Given by the Sanitary Commission to Sick Soldiers Passing Through Washington,* Sanitary Commission, no. 35 (n. p.: [The Commission?], 1861), p. 3.

49. *Sanitary Commission* [Report] no. 48 ([n.p.: [The Commission?], 1862), pp. 1-2.

50. *Report of the Soldiers' Aid Society of Cleveland, Ohio, (and Its Auxiliaries) to the U.S. Sanitary Commission at Washington* (Cleveland: Fairbanks, Benedict and Co., 1861), p. 28.

51. Maxwell, *Lincoln's Fifth Wheel,* p. 310.

52. J. S. Newberry, *The U.S. Sanitary Commission in the Valley of the Mississippi During the War of the Rebellion* (Cleveland: Fairbanks, Benedict and Co., 1871), pp. 210-216.

53. Calculated as follows: The total value of supplies collected was $15,000,000 (see Maxwell, *Lincoln's Fifth Wheel,* p. 297). The value of medicinal supplies acquired by the Western Department of the Sanitary Commission was $95,055 of its grand total of more than $5,000,000. This would imply the commission's Eastern District acquired double the amount of supplies, thus approximately $190,000 in medicinal articles. Thus, a grand total of roughly $285,000 is a reasonable value on all medicinal stocks.

54. See John M. Maisch, "Statistics of the U. S. Army Laboratory at Philadelphia," *Proc. APhA* 14 (1866): 272-278.

55. H. H. Cunningham, *Doctors in Gray: The Confederate Medical Service* (1958; reprint, Louisiana State University Press, 1993), pp. 144-145. The Association for the Relief of Maimed Soldiers did provide Confederate-wide assistance of crutches and prosthetic devices for soldiers with injured and amputated limbs, but it did not include broad-ranging services such as those provided by the Sanitary Commission, including drug provision and pharmaceutical care. In his section on the

Confederate medical service in *The Photographic History of the Civil War*, edited by Holland Thompson, two volumes in one, volume 4, *Prisons and Hospitals* (1911; reprinted, Secaucus, NJ: Blue and Grey Press, 1987), p. 247, Deering J. Roberts claims that Mrs. Porter "collected a vast fund" for soldier relief, but absence of its mention in official and unofficial primary materials makes this doubtful.

56. Mrs. Thomas Taylor, Mrs. August Kohn, Miss Popenheim, and Miss Martha B. Washington, eds., *South Carolina Women in the Confederacy* (Columbia, SC: The State Company, 1903), pp. 45-52.

57. Biographical information on each is available in Larson, *White Roses*, s.v.

58. Letter from Ellen P. Bryce to Dr. Owen, Tuscaloosa, Alabama, February 15, 1911, Alabama Department of Archives and History, SG11144, folder #1.

59. Kate Cumming, *In the Confederate Army of Tennessee from the Battle of Shiloh to the End of the War* (Louisville: John P. Morton, 1866).

60. Alfred Stillé, *Therapeutics and Materia Medica,* Second Edition, 2 volumes (Philadelphia: Blanchard and Lea, 1864), 1: 112-113.

61. Cumming, *In the Confederate Army,* p. 21.

62. In the North, "Mother Newcomb" nursed her men back to health with her own "syrup." See Adams, *Doctors in Blue,* p. 182. Her memoirs are available in *Four Years of Personal Reminiscences of the War* (Chicago: H. S. Mills, 1893).

63. Norman Franke, "The Medico-Pharmaceutical Conditions and Drug Supply in the Confederate States of America 1861-1865" (Unpublished PhD dissertation, University of Wisconsin, 1956), p. 52.

64. Larson, *White Roses,* p. 57.

65. Franke, "Medico-Pharmaceutical Conditions and Drug Supply," p. 52.

66. *War Reb.,* serial 4, volume 2 (Washington: GPO, 1900), p. 442.

67. See, National Archives, RG 109, chapt. VI, volume 750.

68. NA, RG 109, chapt. VI, volume 6, Circular, April 12, 1862, Richmond, Virginia.

69. C. Kendrick, "Indigenous Plants Used by Southern People As Medicines During the War," *The Southern Practitioner* 31 (1909): 534-535.

70. Ibid.

71. Joseph Jacobs, "Some Drug Conditions During the War Between the States, 1861-1865," *SHSP* 33 (Richmond, VA: The Society, 1905), pp. 161-187. Originally read before the American Pharmaceutical Association at its Baltimore meeting in 1898 and published in the *Proc. APhA* 46 (1898): 192-213.

72. Ibid., p. 176.

73. Brockett and Vaughan, *Women's Work in the Civil War,* p. 91.

74. Ibid.

75. Cumming, *In the Confederate Army,* p. 136.

76. The concept of the South as an extended frontier was delineated and discussed at length by W. J. Cash, *The Mind of the South* (New York: Vintage Books, 1941).

77. Robert L. Dabney, *A Defense of Virginia and Through Her of the South in Recent and Pending Contests Against the Sectional Party* (1867; reprint, Harrisonburg, VA: Sprinkle Publications, 1991), p. 285.

78. These "Southern belles" looked a bit less pristine and refined when, on April 2, 1863, they angrily marched to Governor John Letcher's office in Richmond to demand satisfaction against high wartime prices. The ensuing riots saw hundreds of

women smash merchant windows and bash down doors looting and pillaging to the plaintive cry, "bread! bread!" For a complete account see William C. Davis, *Look Away!: A History of the Confederate States of America* (New York: The Free Press, 2002), pp. 212-215.

79. Dabney, *A Defense of Virginia,* p. 285.

80. A thorough discussion on the social effects of slavery upon white women in the South is offered in Catherine Clinton, "Women in the Land of Cotton," in *Myth and Southern History,* edited by Patrick Gerster and Nicholas Cords, Second Edition, volume 2, *The Old South* (Urbana: University of Illinois Press, 1989), pp. 107-119.

81. On this thesis, see Richard E. Beringer, Herman Hattaway, Archer Jones, and William N. Still Jr., *Why the South Lost the Civil War* (Athens: University of Georgia Press, 1986), pp. 37-102 passim.

82. Liah Greenfield, *Nationalism: Five Roads to Modernity* (Cambridge: Harvard University Press, 1992), p. 479.

83. See, Nancy Woloch, "Seneca Falls Convention," in *The Reader's Companion to American History,* edited by Eric Foner and John A. Garraty (Boston: Houghton Mifflin, 1991) pp. 981-982.

84. George C. Rable, *Civil Wars: Women and the Crisis of Southern Nationalism* (Urbana: University of Illinois Press, 1989), p. 285.

85. Adams, *Doctors in Blue,* p. 178.

86. "Proceedings of the First Confederate Congress: Second Session in Part," *SHSP* 46 (Richmond, VA: The Society, 1928), pp. 236-237.

87. Quoted in Culpepper, *Trials and Triumphs,* p. 351.

88. Quoted in Ibid., p. 352. See also Dyson-Bell Papers, 1850-1880, folder #12, Western Historical Manuscript Collection, University of Missouri, St. Louis.

89. Brockett and Vaughan, *Women's Work in the Civil War,* p. 168.

90. Ibid., pp. 338.

91. Culpepper, *Trials and Triumphs,* p. 349.

92. Historical Society of Pennsylvania, undated letter, John Mulhallan Hale Papers, 1837-1864, (Phi)1925.

93. *Med. Surg. Hist.,* part. 3, volume 1, *Med. Hist.* (Washington: GPO, 1888), p. 958.

94. Quoted in Culpepper, *Trials and Triumphs,* p. 326.

95. David L. Cowen and William H. Helfand, *Pharmacy: An Illustrated History* (New York: Harry N. Abrams, 1990), p. 236.

96. Brockett and Vaughan, *Women's Work in the Civil War,* p. 361.

97. Rable, *Civil Wars,* p. 128.

98. Metta Lou Henderson, *American Women Pharmacists: Contributions to the Profession* (Binghamton, NY: Pharmaceutical Products Press, 2002), p. 3.

99. Teresa Catherine Gallagher, "From Family Helpmeet to Independent Professional: Women in American Pharmacy, 1870-1940," *Pharm. Hist.* 31 (1989): 61-62.

Chapter 4

1. For details, see Henry N. Rittenhouse, "U.S. Army Medical Storekeepers," *Am. J. Pharm.* 37 (1865): 87-90.

2. *War Reb.,* serial 3, volume 2 (Washington: GPO, 1899): 67.

3. Ibid.

4. NA, "Records of the Adjutant General's Office, 1783-1920," RG 94, Box 137. Letter dated May 30, 1862, states: "The undersigned wholesale Druggists & dispensing Apothecaries of this City cordially unite in recommending to the Hon. Sec.^ty of War, Robert T. Creamer, also a Druggist of this City as an eminently fit & proper person for an appointment as one of the 'Medical Storekeepers.'" The document is signed by fourteen pharmacists and three physicians including the pioneer in vascular surgery Valentine Mott (1785-1865).

5. NA, RG 94, Box 137. Letter to the Surgeon General dated August 23, 1862.

6. NA, RG 94, Box 137. Letter dated August 25, 1862.

7. See *Directions Concerning the Duties of Medical Purveyors and Medical Storekeepers and the Manner of Obtaining and Accounting for Medical and Hospital Supplies for the Army* (Washington: GPO, 1863), p. 4. These were expanded and revised from Circular no. 12 issued from the Surgeon General's office on October 20, 1862.

8. NA, RG 94, Box 137. Letter to the surgeon general dated August 27, 1862. Creamer complained, "it seems impractical to draw up a proper bond without a knowledge of the duties of 'Medical Storekeeper,' as no instructions have been given in this matter, you will at once notice the force of this remark."

9. NA, RG 94, Box 137. Letter to the surgeon general dated October 8, 1862.

10. Rittenhouse, "Medical Storekeepers," 88.

11. Ibid., 89.

12. Ibid., 90.

13. Mary C. Gillett, *The Army Medical Department, 1818-1865* (Washington: GPO, 1987), p. 155.

14. The duties of medical purveyors are spelled out in Charles R. Greenleaf, *A Manual for the Medical Officers of the United States Army* (Philadelphia: J. B. Lippincott, 1864), pp. 112-134.

15. Gillett, *The Army Medical Department,* p. 160.

16. Hennell Stevens, "The Medical Purveying Department of the United States Army," *Am. J. Pharm.* 37 (1865): 93.

17. Ibid., p. 7.

18. Gillett, *The Army Medical Department,* p. 159.

19. Ibid., p. 5.

20. Ibid.

21. *Med. Surg. Hist.,* part 3, volume 1 *Med. Hist.* (Washington: GPO, 1888), p. 964. See also George Winston Smith, *Medicines for the Union Army* (1962; reprint, Binghamton, NY: Pharmaceutical Products Press, 2001), p. 8.

22. Joseph Janvier Woodward, *The Hospital Steward's Manual for the Instruction of Hospital Stewards, Ward-Masters, and Attendants, in Their Several Duties* (Philadelphia: J. B. Lippincott, 1862).

23. Ibid., pp. 43-44.

24. Ibid., p. 45.

25. Ibid., p. 82.

26. Ibid. pp. 42-43. It should be noted that as the war progressed, this number increased to three or four stewards per general hospital (see *Med. Surg. Hist.,* part 3, volume 1, *Med. Hist.,* 957).

27. Pennsylvania troops, for example, listed hospital stewards at regimental rather than company levels, revealing some regiments with no stewards, most with

one or two, and a few with three. See roster listings at <http://www.pacivilwar.com/>.

28. *Hospital Steward's Manual,* pp. 20-21.

29. Officinal comes from the Latin *officina,* a term meaning workplace. In pharmaceutical usage it was meant to signify those substances expected to be kept on hand by any well-stocked apothecary. The term was dropped from the seventh decennial edition of the *USP* (1890). For details see Lee Anderson and Gregory J. Higby, *The Spirit of Voluntarism: A Legacy of Commitment and Contribution: The United States Pharmacopeia, 1820-1995* (Rockville, MD: United States Pharmacopeial Convention, 1995), p. 23.

30. Woodward, *Hospital Steward's Manual,* p. 279.

31. Ibid., p. 271.

32. Ibid., p. 266.

33. Caswell A. Mayo, "The Military Pharmacist in the Civil War," *American Druggist and Pharmaceutical Record* 47 (1905): 343.

34. Charles Beneulyn Johnson, *Muskets and Medicine, or, Army Life in the Sixties* (Philadelphia: F. A. Davis, 1917), pp. 127-128.

35. *Official Roster of the Soldiers of the State of Ohio in the War of the Rebellion, 1861-1866,* volume 2 (Cincinnati: Wilstach, Baldwin, 1886), p. 420.

36. Transcription [by Michael G. Moon] of the Jonathon Wood Diary, July 1866. VFM 4730. Archival ms., Ohio Historical Society, Columbus, Ohio.

37. See letter by George E. Cooper, Medical Purveyor, dated September 2, 1861. NA, RG 94, Box 52.

38. An excellent survey of the problem of medical incompetence is available in Thomas P. Lowry and Jack D. Welch, *Tarnished Scalpels: The Court-Martials of Fifty Union Surgeons* (Mechanicsburg, PA: Stackpole Books, 2000). Surgeon John H. Brinton admitted that many of the contract physicians (literally acting assistant surgeons) were ignorant, had been long out of practice, or were outright charlatans. See John H. Brinton, *Personal Memoirs of John H. Brinton, Civil War Surgeon, 1861-1865* (1914; reprinted, Carbondale: Southern Illinois University Press, 1996), p. 66.

39. A. H. Hoge, *The Boys in Blue; or, Heroes of the "Rank and File"* (New York: E. B. Treat, 1867), p. 188.

40. Marilyn Mayer Culpepper, *Trials and Triumphs: Women of the American Civil War* (East Lansing: Michigan State University Press, 1991), pp. 347-348.

41. Diary entry for May 23, 1864, NLM, MS C 207, Winston, Thomas [transcripts of letters], "The Personal Papers of Dr. Thomas Winston, Union Army (1862-66)," Box 2.

42. Katharine Prescott Wormeley, *The Cruel Side of War with the Army of the Potomac* (Boston: Roberts Brothers, 1898), p. 109.

43. Edwin Witherby Brown, "Army Life in the War of the Great Rebellion: A True Record of His Service in the War for the Union," 2 volumes, Archival ms. Ohio Historical Society, Columbus, Ohio; 1: 6, 87-88, 119.

44. Ibid., 2: 50-51.

45. Ibid., 2: 51-52.

46. Thirty-two Letters of Spencer Bonsall to his wife Ellen, May 6 through June 22, 1862, and December 4 through March 26, 1863, Reynolds Historical Library, Lister Hill Library of the Health Sciences, University of Alabama at Birmingham.

47. Letter from Spencer Bonsall to Ellen Bonsall, February 6, 1862. For a more complete account of Bonsall and his letters, see Michael A. Flannery, "The Life of a Hospital Steward: The Civil War Journal of Spencer Bonsall," *Pharmacy in History* 42 (2000): 87-98.

48. For details, see Steven R. Moore and John Parascandola, "The Other Pharmacists in the American Civil War," *American Journal of Health-System Pharmacists* 57 (2000): 1276.

49. William Grace, *The Surgeon's Manual for the Use of Medical Officers, Cadets, Chaplains, and Hospital Stewards* (New York: Bailliere Brothers, 1864), p. 7.

50. Gillett, *The Army Medical Department*, p. 4.

51. Woodward, *Hospital Steward's Manual*, p. 13.

52. Civilian pay figures from Daniel E. Southerland, *The Expansion of Everyday Life, 1860-1876* (New York: Harper and Row, 1990), pp. 134-177 passim.

53. Gillett, *The Army Medical Department*, p. 182.

54. Mayo, "The Military Pharmacist in the Civil War," p. 343.

55. John N. Henry, *Turn Them Out to Die Like a Mule: The Civil War Letters of John N. Henry, 49th New York, 1861-1865*, edited by John Michael Priest (Leesburg, VA: Gauley Mount Press, 1995), p. 159.

56. Editorial Department, "Hospital Stewards," *Am. J. Pharm.* 37 (1865): 156-157.

57. Ibid., 157.

58. Philadelphia College of Pharmacy, Minute Book, pp. 50-51.

59. Quoted in Mayo, "The Military Pharmacist in the Civil War," p. 352.

60. Ibid.

61. "The Military Pharmacist," *American Druggist and Pharmaceutical Record* 48 (1906): 32.

62. *Kremers and Urdang's History of Pharmacy,* revised by Glenn Sonnedecker, Fourth Edition (1976; reprinted, Madison, WI: American Institute of the History of Pharmacy, 1986), pp. 346-347.

Chapter 5

1. Figures from James M. McPherson, *Battle Cry of Freedom: The Civil War Era* (New York: Oxford University Press, 1988) pp. 313, 336; and Allan Nevins, *The War for the Union,* volume 4, *The Organized War to Victory, 1864-1865* (1971; reprinted, New York: Konecky and Konecky, 2000), p. 254. Naval figures are from Ivan Musicant, *Divided Waters: The Naval History of the Civil War* (New York: HarperCollins, 1995), p. 57.

2. Mary C. Gillett, *The Army Medical Department, 1818-1865* (Washington, DC: GPO, 1987), p. 156.

3. For an excellent summary and discussion of Letterman's innovations, see Gordon W. Jones, "The Medical History of the Fredericksburg Campaign: Course and Significance," *The Journal of the History of Medicine and Allied Sciences* 18 (1963): 241-256.

4. Charles R. Greenleaf, *A Manual for the Medical Officers of the United States Army* (Philadelphia: J. B. Lippincott, 1864), p. 14.

5. Ibid.

6. Ibid., p. 13.

7. Ibid.

8. Charles Beneulyn Johnson, *Muskets and Medicine, or, Army Life in the Sixties* (Philadelphia: F. A. Davis, 1917), p. 129.

9. Ibid., pp. 129-130.

10. Ibid., p. 130.

11. Ibid.

12. Greenleaf, *Manual for Medical Officers,* pp. 139-140.

13. William Grace, *The Army Surgeon's Manual for the Use of Medical Officers, Cadets, Chaplains, and Hospital Stewards* (New York: Bailliere Brothers, 1864), p. 19.

14. See the letters of Spencer Bonsall to his wife Ellen, May 6 through June 22, 1862, and December 4 through March 26, 1863, Reynolds Historical Library, Lister Hill Library of the Health Sciences, University of Alabama at Birmingham.

15. NLM, MS F 45, HMD Manuscripts Oversized. U.S. Army Medical Purveyors Office, Baltimore, MD. Letters received, 1864-65. E. McClellan letters July 20, 1864 and July 22, 1864, volume 1.

16. NLM, Ibid., John C. Carter letter June 13, 1864, volume 1.

17. NLM, Ibid., J. H. Janway letter January 3, 1865, volume 1.

18. NLM, Ibid., "Assistant surgeon" letter October 3, 1864, volume 1.

19. NLM, Ibid., F. H. Patton letter August 31, 1864, volume 1.

20. NLM, Ibid., J. H. Shields letter November 11, 1864, volume 1.

21. NLM, Ibid., E. Buck letter January 20, 1865, volume 2.

22. John N. Henry, *Turn Them Out to Die Like a Mule: The Civil War Letters of John N. Henry, 49th New York, 1861-1865* (Leesburg, VA: Gauley Mount Press, 1995), p. 245.

23. Dennis B. Worthen, "The Pharmaceutical Industry, 1852-1902," *Journal of the American Pharmaceutical Association* 40 (2000): 589-591.

24. Williams Haynes, *American Chemical Industry,* 6 volumes (New York: Van Nostrand, 1947), *The Chemical Companies,* 6: 469.

25. Williams Haynes, *American Chemical Industry,* 6 volumes (New York: Van Nostrand, 1954), *Background and Beginnings,* 1: 239.

26. Ibid., 1: 215-216.

27. Details on prewar wholesale manufacturers are available in Ibid., 1: 215-218.

28. Dennis B. Worthen, "Frederick Stearns's Non-Secret Medicines," *Journal of the American Pharmaceutical Association* 41 (2001): 621.

29. Information on Rosengarten and Sons can be found in the Merck Archives, P & W files; and Williams Haynes, *Chemical Pioneers: The Founders of the American Chemical Industry* (1931; reprinted, Freeport, NY: Books for Libraries Press, 1970), pp. 26-41.

30. Merck Archives, interview with Adolph G. Rosengarten Jr. conducted by Leon Gortler, PWR files, p. 3.

31. Most material bearing upon the respective histories of these firms is located at the Merck Archives. In 1905, with the death of William Weightman, the company assets were merged with Rosengarten and became the Powers-Weightman-Rosengarten Company. In 1927 P-W-R was absorbed by Merck. For plant locations, mergers, and acquisitions details see Merck Archives, esp. the PWR files.

32. See Joseph W. England, "The American Manufacture of Quinine Sulphate," *American Journal of Pharmacy* 102 (1930): 702-713.

33. See "Articles of Copartnership," Merck Archives, PWR files, R6, 2.4.4, folder 8.

34. See "References to the Exhibits of Powers & Weightman and the Exhibitions of The Franklin Institute," Merck Archives, PWR files.   .

35. See the record for merchandise sales for the Upper Laboratory, 1853-1886, Merck Archives, PWR files. See also economic data in the "Valuation of grounds, building, and stationary apparatus of Upper Laboratory," Merck Archives, PWR ledger, R6, 2.6.2.

36. See, for example, Edward R. Squibb, "Spiritus Ætheris Nitrici," *Am. J. Pharm.* 4 (1856): 289-304.

37. Edward R. Squibb, "Apparatus for the Preparation of Ether by Steam," *Am. J. Pharm.* 4 (1856): 389-391.

38. These years are covered in detail in Lawrence G. Blochman, *Doctor Squibb: The Life and Times of a Rugged Individualist* (New York: Simon and Schuster, 1958), pp. 84-89.

39. Ibid., p. 86.

40. Ibid., p. 109.

41. Squibb's war years are well covered in Ibid., pp. 128-150.

42. George Winston Smith, *Medicines for the Union Army* (1962; reprinted, New York: Pharmaceutical Products Press, 2001), p. 39; see also Joseph Howland Bill's official report to Surgeon General Hammond reprinted in George Winston Smith, ed., "The Squibb Laboratory in 1863," *Journal of the History of Medicine & Allied Sciences* 13 (1958): 382-394.

43. Blochman, *Doctor Squibb,* p. 104.

44. Smith, "The Squibb Laboratory of 1863," pp. 383-384.

45. Quoted in Smith, *Medicines for the Union Army,* p. 40.

46. Smith, "The Squibb Laboratory," p. 383.

47. The entire preliminary report is reprinted in Smith, "The Squibb Laboratory," pp. 382-394.

48. Smith, *Medicines for the Union Army,* p. 29.

49. Blochman, *Doctor Squibb,* pp. 136-137.

50. George Winston Smith calls Maisch's work in the Squibb plant, "the most valuable preparation that Maisch could possibly have received for his position in the government laboratory"; see his *Medicines for the Union Army,* p. 73.

51. Editorial, "The United States Army Laboratory," *Am. J. Pharm.* 35 (1863): 283.

52. The Creamer affair is told in its entirety in Smith, *Medicines for the Union Army,* pp. 26-28.

53. Ibid., p. 31.

54. Ibid., pp. 31-32.

55. See biographical sketch in Joseph W. England, *The First Century of the Philadelphia College of Pharmacy, 1821-1921* (Philadelphia: The College, 1922), pp. 405-407.

56. Editorial, "The United States Army Laboratory," 283.

57. Editorial, "The U.S. Laboratory at Philadelphia," *Am. J. Pharm.* 35 (1863): 375.

58. Ibid.

59. For a biographical sketch, see Michael A. Flannery, "C. Lewis Diehl: Kentucky's Most Notable Pharmacist," *Pharm. Hist.* 39 (1997): 101-112.

60. C. Lewis Diehl, "United States Laboratory," *Am. J. Pharm.* 78 (1906): 560-561.

61. Ibid., pp. 573-574.

62. Smith, *Medicines for the Union Army,* p. 44.

63. Ibid., p. 45.

64. See an account of the fire and loss in Editorial, "The U.S. Army Laboratory at New York," *Am. J. Pharm.* 37 (1865): 234.

65. John M. Maisch, "Statistics of the U.S. Army Laboratory at Philadelphia," *Proc. APhA* 14 (1866): 272-278.

66. Ibid., p. 275.

67. Ibid., p. 278.

68. Smith, *Medicines for the Union Army,* pp. 112-113.

69. William A. Brewer, "Report of the Committee on the Drug Market," *Proc. APhA* 15 (1867): 267-307.

70. Ibid., p. 275.

71. Ibid.

72. Ibid.

Chapter 6

1. George Worthington Adams, *Doctors in Blue* (1952; reprinted, Baton Rouge: Louisiana State University Press, 1996), p. 240.

2. It had been noted that the so-called "miasmatic fevers" generally prevailed from mid-summer to the start of winter. See John T. Metcalfe, "Miasmatic Fevers" in *Military Medical and Surgical Essays Prepared for the United States Sanitary Commission,* edited by William A. Hammond (Philadelphia: J. B. Lippincott, 1864), pp. 207-234.

3. Quoted in Paul Steiner, *Disease in the Civil War: Natural Biological Warfare in 1861-1865* (Charles C Thomas, 1968), p. 54.

4. Ibid., pp. 67-81.

5. Ibid., p. 44.

6. Ibid., p. 128.

7. Ibid., p. 192.

8. Ibid., p. 218.

9. Contraction of malaria, today known to be a protozoan infection caused by the bite of the *Anopheles* mosquito, does not accord immediate and/or universal immunity. Whereas those in geographical regions frequently exposed to malarial infection often exhibit no or attenuated symptoms, those less exposed can become severely and *repeatedly* ill. Even today the molecular mechanisms underlying natural immunity to malaria are not clearly understood. For details, see the "Oxford Research on Childhood Disease: Malaria" at <http://www.well.ox.ac.uk/ich/malaria.htm>; and "WHO/TDR [World Health Organization/Tropical Disease Research] Database" at <http://www.wehi.edu.au/MalDB-www/who.html> (reviewed Feb. 6, 2001). Repeated attacks may even cause chronic malaria characterized by severe anemia, emaciation, enlargement of the spleen, weakness, edema of the ankles, and

a sallow complexion. See also *Stedman's Concise Medical Dictionary,* Second Edition (Baltimore: Williams and Wilkins, 1994), "Malaria" s.v.

10. On the Confederate defensive strategy, see James Ford Rhodes, *History of the United States from the Compromise of 1850 to the Final Restoration of Home Rule in 1877,* volume 3 (New York: Macmillan, 1907) see p. 398; and James M. McPherson, *Battle Cry of Freedom: The Civil War Era* (New York: Oxford University Press, 1988), pp. 336-337.

11. *Med. Surg. Hist.,* part 3, volume 1, *Med. Hist.* (Washington: GPO, 1888), p. 966. It would be wrong to conclude that ether was more commonly used than chloroform on the basis of the relative amounts distributed. In fact, about three-quarters of surgical cases where anesthesia was employed used chloroform. The reasons were the comparatively high volatility of ether and the need for less dosage with chloroform. According to anesthesiologist and Civil War historian, Dr. Maurice Albin, "In general, chloroform was the anesthetic agent of choice for the battlefield and sulfuric ether had its application in the general hospital stationed in the rear. While there is some local irritation from the inhalation of chloroform, there is considerably more with sulfuric ether and copious secretions result in the respiratory tract. This irritability is probably due to the fact that nearly three times as much sulfuric ether is used to achieve the same level of anesthesia where compared to chloroform, thus also indicating the potency of chloroform. . . . A special study in the *Med Surg. Hist.* of 597 cases anesthetized with chloroform, ether and the combination of chloroform and sulfuric ether illustrates the potency factor since about three times as much sulfuric ether was used to induce the anesthetic state." Letter from Maurice Albin, MD, to the author, May 29, 2003. For a complete discussion of anesthesia during the Civil War see Maurice S. Albin, "The Use of Anesthetics During the Civil War, 1861-1865," *Pharm. Hist.* 42 (2000): 99-114.

12. Wade Boyle, *Official Herbs: Botanical Substances in the United States Pharmacopoeias, 1820-1990* (East Palestine, OH: Buckeye Naturopathic Press, 1991), p. 57.

13. Sources of information include George B. Wood and Franklin Bache, *USD,* Eleventh Edition (Philadelphia: J. B. Lippincott, 1858); Alfred Stillé, *Therapeutics and Materia Medica,* 2 volumes (Philadelphia: Blanchard and Lea, 1864); and Henry Beasley, *The Book of Prescriptions,* Second Edition (Philadelphia: Lindsay and Blakiston, 1865).

14. Abstract [typescript] of Jack Dayton Key, "An Analysis of the U.S. Army Supply Tables Used During the Civil War Period," master's thesis, 1960, Kremers Reference Files, C46 (B)I, Madison, WI: American Institute of the History of Pharmacy.

15. *Med. Surg. Hist.,* part 3, volume 2, *Surg. Hist.* (Washington: GPO, 1883), p. 916. Items in the pannier included in the upper compartment 24 roller bandages, 1 yd. of isinglass plaster, 1 paper of pins, 2 yds. Bleached muslin, and 1 pair of scissors; the lower compartment contained 6½ oz. purified chloroform, 2 oz. fluidextract of ipecac, 2 oz. fluidextract of ginger, 2 oz. persulphate of iron, 12 doz. Compound cathartic pills, 12 doz. quinine pills (3 grs. ea.), 12 doz. opium pills, 12 doz. compound extract of colocynth (3 grs.) and ipecac ½ gr., 24 oz. whisky, 2 oz. tincture of opium, ¼ lb. patent lint, 1 medicine glass, 1 teaspoon, 1 small sponge, ¼ oz. silk for ligatures, 1 towel, and 6 corks.

16. These are pictured and described in Ibid., pp. 914-915.

17. See Erwin H. Ackerknecht, "A Plea for a 'Behaviorist' Approach in Writing the History of Medicine," *Journal of the History of Medicine and Allied Sciences* 22 (1967): 211-214.

18. Jeffrey S. Sartin, "Infectious Diseases During the Civil War: The Triumph of the 'Third Army,'" *Clinical Infectious Diseases* 16 (1993): 582; and Paul E. Steiner, *Diseases in the Civil War* (Springfield, IL: Charles C Thomas, 1968), p. 17.

19. *Med. Surg. Hist.*, part 2, volume 1, *Med. Hist.*, 42.

20. Ibid.

21. Alfred Stillé, Francis G. Smith, John Bell, John F. Meigs, and Samuel Lewis, *Report of a Committee of the Associate Members of the Sanitary Commission on Dysentery,* Sanitary Commission, M (Philadelphia: Collins, 1862), p. 6.

22. Ibid., p. 21.

23. Ibid., p. 26.

24. Ibid., p. 28.

25. Ibid., p. 38.

26. *Med. Surg Hist.,* part 2, volume 1, *Med. Hist.,* 68.

27. Ibid., pp. 41-100 passim.

28. Ibid., 100.

29. Stillé, *Therapeutics and Materia Medica,* 1: 166-167.

30. See, for example, *Gould's Medical Dictionary,* Fifth Revised Edition (Philadelphia: Blakiston, 1941), pp. 207-208. Bithmuth subnitrate is still listed as an antacid; see *The Merck Index,* Twelfth Edition (Whitehouse Station, NJ: Merck, 1996), p. 1327.

31. Charles Beneulyn Johnson, *Muskets and Medicine, or, Army Life in the Sixties* (Philadelphia: F. A. Davis, 1917), p. 162.

32. Ibid, p. 163.

33. NLM, MS B 347, HMD Ms., U.S. Army. New Hampshire Infantry Volunteers Regiment, 12th "Register and Prescription Book," 1865 1 Jan.-1865 Mar.

34. "Register and Prescription Book of the 110th Regiment, N.Y.S.V." on inside cover of U.S. Army Medical Department, "Register and Prescription Book," June-Aug., 1864, 152nd Ohio Volunteer Infantry. John C. Williamson Papers. BV 959, Box 2, Series 2331. Ohio Historical Society Archives, Columbus, Ohio.

35. Diary of Jonathon Wood, typescript transcription by Michael G. Moon, July 1866. VFM 4730. Ohio Historical Society Archives, Columbus, Ohio.

36. George M. Dixon, "Formulas, 1864-1868," volume 866, Ohio Historical Society Archives, Columbus, Ohio.

37. Steiner, *Disease in the Civil War,* pp. 17-18.

38. Ibid., pp. 219-221.

39. Andrew K. Black has indicated that incidents of malaria among black were considerably lower than among whites due to the fact that nearly all had previous exposure to malaria and had acquired either natural immunity or exhibited attenuated symptoms. See Andrew K. Black, "In the Service of the United States: Comparative Mortality Among African-American and White Troops in the Union Army," *Journal of Negro History* 79 (1994): 324-325.

40. See, for example, George Hayward, J. Mason Warten, S. Cabot Jr., S. D. Townsend, John Ware, and R. M. Hodges, *Report of a Committee of the Associated Medical Members of the Sanitary Commission on the Continued Fevers,* Sanitary Commission, K (Washington: GPO, 1862).

41. *Med. Surg. Hist.*, part 3, volume 1, *Med. Hist.*, 74-75.

42. Ibid., p. 76.

43. Ibid., p. 325.

44. Robley Dunglison, *A Dictionary of Medical Science*, new edition (Philadelphia: Henry C. Lea, 1874), pp. 416-420.

45. Lester S. King, *Transformations in American Medicine: From Benjamin Rush to William Osler* (Baltimore: Johns Hopkins University Press, 1991), p. 236.

46. Ibid.

47. Johnson, *Muskets and Medicine*, p. 159.

48. *Med. Surg. Hist.*, part 3, volume 1, *Med. Hist.*, 535, 541.

49. Stillé, *Therapeutics and Materia Medica*, 1: 618-619. Turpentine had a long and interesting history of use by the Civil War. For details, see John S. Haller Jr., "Sampson of the Terebinthinates: Medical History of Turpentine," *Southern Medical Journal* 77 (1984): 750-754.

50. *Med. Surg. Hist.*, part 3, volume 1, *Med. Hist.*, 541.

51. Hayward et al., *Report on Continued Fevers*, p. 7.

52. Ibid., p. 13.

53. Ibid., p. 22.

54. Ibid., p. 26.

55. John T. Metcalfe, *Report of a Committee of the Associate Members of the Sanitary Commission on the Nature and Treatment of Yellow Fever*, Sanitary Commission, Q (New York: Wm. C. Bryant and Co., 1862), p. 25.

56. John T. Metcalfe, *Report of a Committee of the Associate Members of the Sanitary Commission on the Nature and Treatment of Miasmatic Fevers*, Sanitary Commission, P (New York: Balliere Brothers, 1862), p. 15.

57. Ibid.

58. *Med. Surg. Hist.*, part 3, volume 1, *Med. Hist.*, 179.

59. Ibid., part 3, volume 1, 719-720.

60. For descriptions and treatments see Ibid., pp. 725-810.

61. Ibid., p. 807.

62. Ibid.

63. Ibid.

64. Austin Flint and three other members, *Report of a Committee of the Associated Medical Members of the Sanitary Commission on Pneumonia*, Sanitary Commission, J (Washington: McGill, Withrow, and Co., 1862), p. 22.

65. Ibid., p. 15.

66. Ibid., p. 17.

67. Alfred J. Tapson, "The Sutler and the Soldier," *Military Affairs* 21 (1957): 175-181.

68. Steiner, *Disease in the Civil War*, p. 28.

69. Ibid., pp. 58-59.

70. Letter to Carrie and Eddie, November 22, 1862, NLM, MC C 207, HMD, Winston Thomas [transcripts of letters], "The Personal Papers of Dr. Thomas Winston, Union Army (1862-66)," Box 2.

71. Letter December 6, 1862, Ibid.

72. *Med. Surg. Hist.*, part 3, volume 1, *Med. Hist.*, 657-661.

73. Ibid., p. 659.

74. *Med. Surg. Hist.*, part 3, volume 2, *Surg. Hist.*, 823.

75. Ibid.

76. Ibid., p. 830.

77. M. Goldsmith, *A Report on Hospital Gangrene, Erysipelas and Pyæmia, As Observed in the Departments of the Ohio and the Cumberlands,* Sanitary Commission, T (Louisville: Bradley and Gilbert, 1863), p. 5.

78. Ibid., pp. 78-84.

79. NLM, MS B 347, HMD Manuscripts. U.S. Army. New Hampshire Infantry Volunteers Regiment, 12th Register and prescription book, 1865 1 Jan.-1865 Mar.

80. NLM, MS F 51, HMD Manuscripts. U.S. Army, Hospital Dept., Fort Sumner, Maryland. "Prescriptions given to the sick and wounded, 1864."

81. *Official Roster of the Soldiers of the State of Ohio in the War of the Rebellion, 1861-1866,* 12 volumes (Cincinnati: Wilstach, Baldwin, 1886), 9: 170.

82. U.S. Army Medical Department, "Register and Prescription Book," June-Aug., 1864, 152nd Ohio Volunteers Infantry. John C. Williamson Papers. BV 959, Box 2, series 2331. Ohio Historical Society Archives, Columbus, Ohio.

83. *Official Roster,* 9: 182.

84. "Register and Prescription Book," John C. Williamson Papers.

85. Letter from Gideon Welles to L. M. Goldsborough, April 30, 1862, NA, RG 45, Box 210, Navy Subject Files.

86. Letter from William Keisworthy [?] to Rear Admiral John A. Dahlgren, October 20, 1863, Ibid.

87. Letter from J. L. Landner to Gideon Welles, Key West, September 12, 1862, Ibid.

88. Ibid.

89. All Gulf blockading squadrons reported outbreaks. See *Official Records of the Union and Confederate Navies in the War of the Rebellion,* series 1, volume 17, *East Gulf Blockading Squadron* (Washington: GPO, 1903), pp. 294-761 passim; series 1, volume 20, *West Blockading Squadron* (Washington: GPO, 1905), pp. 273-708 passim; series 1, volume 27, *Naval Forces on Western Waters* (Washington: GPO, 1917), 455-612 passim.

90. For details on yellow fever and its transmission, see World Health Organization, Fact Sheet 100 (reviewed August 1999), Web site <http://www.who.int/inf-fs/en/fact 100.html>.

91. Letter from Thomas Penrose to Lieutenant [Commander] Wainwright, June 8, 1862, National Archives, RG 45, Box 210, Navy Subject Files.

92. This information was explained to the author by Thomas J. Oertling, Marine Archeologist, at his podium presentation "The *Denbigh* Project: Investigations of a Civil War Blockade Runner at Galveston," October 18, 2002, Twenty-First Gulf South History and Humanities Conference, Galveston, Texas.

93. Letter from L. R. Boyce to H. K. Davenport, September 22, 1863; National Archives, RG45, Box 210, Navy Subject Files.

94. Ibid.

95. See letter from Gideon Welles to David D. Porter, November 14, 1862, *Official Records of the Union and Confederate Navies,* series 1, volume 25 (Washington: GPO, 1912), p. 561.

96. Samuel Pellman Boyer, *Naval Surgeon: Blockading the South, 1861-1866: The Diary of Samuel Pellman Boyer,* edited by Elinor Barnes and James A. Barnes (Bloomington: Indiana University Press, 1963), p. 219.

97. Ibid., p. 82.

98. Ibid., p. 317.

99. Ibid., p. 106.

100. Ibid., p. 165.

101. Records show high rates of illness, of which the following are examples: The steam sloop *Brooklyn* (commissioned for West Gulf Blockading Squadron) reported every one of its total complement of 386 men sick over the second quarter of 1862, and more than half its complement of 418 men during the second quarter of 1863. Similarly, a small vessel, the brig *Perry,* reported ninety admitted sick during the third quarter of 1862 out of a complement of eighty, meaning that at least statistically essentially everyone on board was sick once, some more. Statistics for illness aboard some selected ships are as follows: The U.S.S. *Philadelphia* admitted sick: 1861 = 154; 1862 = 251; 1863 = 313; 1864 = 429; 1865 = 738; the steamer *Lancaster* admitted sick: 1861 = 841; 1862 = 569; 1863 = 956; 1864 = 469; 1865 = 471; the steamer *Massachusetts* admitted sick: [records for 1861-1862 incomplete] 1863 = 150; 1864 = 186; 1865 = 253. See NA, RG52, Records of the Bureau of Medicine and Surgery, "Abstract of Sick Reports, No. 1 [U.S. Navy]," entry 29. The *Acacia* (commissioned December 8, 1863) reported 155 admissions to sick bay during its first full year of operation out of an average complement of seventy-six on board. Similarly, boats attached to the Mississippi squadron reported high sickness late in the war—e.g., the *Springfield* reported 101 admissions out of its average complement of fifty-two in 1863; 1864 reported 165 sick in an average complement of 105; and the *Silver Lake* sixty-five sick with an average complement of forty-six in 1863; 110 sick with an average complement of 127 in 1864; ninety-three sick with an average complement of 107 in 1865; the *Reindeer* reported ninety-five admitted sick out of its average complement of seventy-three in 1863; 1864 saw 144 sick out of an average complement of eighty-eight; in 1865 there were sixty-nine sick out of an average complement of eighty-six. See NA, RG52, Records of the Bureau of Medicine and Surgery, "Abstract of Sick Reports, No. 2 [U.S. Navy]," entry 29.

102. NLM, MS C 303, HMD Manuscripts, John Leavitt, "Letters to his wife concerning their son, a patient in Mansion House Hospital, Alexandria, Virginia, 1864.

103. William F. Norris, "Clinical notes on cases seen at the Douglas Hospital at Washington, DC during the Civil War," College of Physicians of Philadelphia. Unpublished document.

Chapter 7

1. On the background of calomel, see J. Worth Estes, *Dictionary of Protopharmacology: Therapeutic Practices, 1700-1850* (Canton, MA: Science History Publications, 1990), p. 34; and George Urdang, "Origin of the Term Calomel," *Journal of the American Pharmaceutical Association,* Practical Pharmacy Edition 9 (1948): 414-418.

2. For details on malaria, see World Health Organization, Fact Sheet 94 (revised October 1998), Web site <http://www.who.int/inf-fs/en/fact 94.html>.

3. Louis Goodman and Alfred Gilman, *The Pharmacological Basis of Therapeutics* (New York: Macmillan, 1941), pp. 923-927. See also James E. Robbers, Marilyn K. Speedie, and Varro E. Tyler, *Pharmacognosy and Pharmacobiotechnology* (Baltimore: Williams and Wilkins, 1996), pp. 155-158.

4. The early history of quinine, including the unraveling of the apocryphal tale of Francisca Henriquez Ribera, the Countess of Chinchon, whose purported cure from an attack of fever resulted from the administration of the bark to her in 1623, is given in Saul Jarcho, *Quinine's Predecessor: Francesco Torti and the Early History of Cinchona* (Baltimore: Johns Hopkins University Press, 1993). Apparently first dubbed *"pulvis Comitissæ"* (Countess powder), Linnæus, apparently accepting the legend, applied the genus name *Cinchona* in 1753 to the South American tree through an inadvertent misspelling of Chinchon. On these early accounts, see esp. pp. 12-26.

5. See Frederick L. Dorn, "On the Antiquity of Malaria in the Western Hemisphere," *Human Biology* 37 (December 1965): 385-393. Dorn persuasively argues that the genetic polymorphisms associated with malaria were absent in Native American populations.

6. Goodman and Gilman, *Pharmacological Basis of Therapeutics,* p. 903.

7. Unfortunately, quinine's antipyretic properties are relatively mild. The profound effects of quinine on malaria are due not to its febrifugal powers but to its specific action on the plasmodia responsible for the disease; see Ibid., 906.

8. Alexander Means, "Calomel—Its Chemical Characteristics and Mineral Origin Considered, in View of Its Curative Claims," *New Orleans Medical Journal* 1 (1845): 588-589.

9. For a detailed history of each of these movements, see the works of John S. Haller Jr.: *The People's Doctors: Samuel Thomson and the American Botanical Movement, 1790-1860* (Carbondale: Southern Illinois University Press, 2000); *Kindly Medicine: Physio-Medicalism in America, 1836-1911* (Kent, OH: Kent State University Press, 1997); and *Medical Protestants: The Eclectics in American Medicine, 1825-1939* (Cardondale: Southern Illinois University Press, 1994).

10. On the history of this sect see Harris L. Coulter, *Science and Ethics in American Medicine: 1800-1914,* Divided Legacy: A History of the Schism in Medical Thought, volume 3 (Washington, [DC]: McGrath Pub. Co., 1973); and the informative introduction in Francesco Cordasco, *Homeopathy in the United States: A Bibliography of Homeopathic Medical Imprints, 1825-1925* (Fairview, NJ: Junius-Vaughn, 1991).

11. Cordasco, *Homeopathy in the United States,* pp. xvii-xviii.

12. Alex Berman, "A Striving for Scientific Respectability: Some American Botanics and the Nineteenth-Century Plant Materia Medica," *Bulletin of the History of Medicine* 30 (1956): 7-31.

13. G. Price Smith, "A Few Chapters on Medical Reform," *Eclectic Medical Journal* 14 (1855): 446.

14. Ibid., 445.

15. Charles Wilkins Short, "An Introductory Address to a Course of Lectures on Materia Medica," *Transylvania Journal of Medicine and Associated Sciences* 6 (1833): 461.

16. William H. Cook, *The Physio-Medical Dispensatory* (Cincinnati: Wm. H. Cook, 1869), pp. 65-66.

17. Charles J. Hempel, *A New and Comprehensive System of Materia Medica and Therapeutics* (Philadelphia: W. Radde, 1859), pp. 398-399.

18. For details see Lois N. Magner, *A History of Medicine* (New York: Marcel Dekker, 1992), pp. 90-92, 201-202; and Sherwin B. Nuland, *The Mysteries Within:*

A Surgeon Reflects on Medical Myths (New York: Simon and Schuster, 2000), esp. pp. 109-134.

19. James Johnson, *A Treatise on Derangements of the Liver, Internal Organs and Nervous System,* Third Edition (London: Thomas and George Underwood, 1820), p. 55.

20. Among regulars, John Pechey had written about biliousness as a source of many ailments as early as the 1690s in his *Collection of Chronical Diseases* (London: Henry Bonwicke, 1692). Other noteworthy works discussing the primacy of the liver and "biliousness" in human disease with mercurous chloride as the remedy of choice include William Cullen, *Lectures on the Materia Medica* (London: T. Lowndes, 1773); Noah Webster, *A Collection of Papers on the Subject of Bilious Fevers* (New York: Hopkins, Webb and Co., 1796); John Faithhorn, *Facts and Observations on Liver Complaints and Bilious Disorders in General; and on Those Derangements of That Important Organ,* Second American Edition (Philadelphia: Hickman and Hazzard, 1822); and William Thomson, *A Practical Treatise on the Diseases of the Liver and Biliary Passages* (Philadelphia: Ed. Barrington and Geo. D. Haswell, 1842). Botanics also expressed their concern over liver function. Eclectics I. G. Jones and William Sherman, for example, sought to "relieve the spasmodic action of the duct" with hot hops or an "infusion of lobelia and boneset." Other suggested remedies comprised a hodgepodge assortment of botanicals including wild cherry, Culver's root, and dandelion. See their *American Eclectic Practice of Medicine,* 2 volumes (Cincinnati: Moore, Wilstach, Keys and Co., 1857-1858), 2, 269-337 passim.

21. Johnson, *A Treatise on Derangements,* p. 101.

22. For details see Edward J. Waring, *Bibliotheca Therapeutica, or Bibliography of Therapeutics,* 2 volumes (London: The New Sydenham Society, 1878-1879), 2, 485-486.

23. Goodman and Gilman, *Pharmacological Basis of Therapeutics,* p. 804.

24. A complete discussion of the persistence of calomel use in the nineteenth-century materia medica is available in John S. Haller Jr., "Medical Theory and the Use and Abuse of Calomel in Nineteenth Century America," *Pharmacy in History* 13 (1971): 27-33, 67-76.

25. Edward Parrish, *An Introduction to Practical Pharmacy,* Second Edition (Philadelphia: Blanchard and Lea, 1859), p. 604.

26. H. D. Schmidt, "On the Microscopic Anatomy, Physiology, and Pathology of the Human Liver," Confederate Medical and Surgical Journal 1 (1864): 49-54, 65-69.

27. Ibid., 69.

28. For example, see Jacob Bigelow, *A Discourse on Self-Limited Diseases Delivered Before the Massachusetts Medical Society at Their Annual Meeting, May 27, 1835* (Boston: N. Hale, 1835).

29. See, for example, James L. Brown, "On the Action of Mercury Upon the Liver," *Transactions of the Medical Society of New York* (1864): 267-279. These early doubters led others, such as Philadelphia physician Joseph Carson, to launch their own investigations. By 1870 Carson was convinced that Bennett's experiments were correct and that the characteristic green stools were *not* the product of calomel's action on bile production. See holographic letter by Joseph Carson, Historical Collections, Philadelphia College of Physicians.

30. For a complete discussion of the use of these substances see John S. Haller Jr., "Samson of the Materia Medica: Medical Theory and the Use and Abuse of Calomel in Nineteenth Century America. Part I," *Pharm. Hist.* 13 (1971): 27-34; Part II, *Pharmacy in History* 13 (1971): 67-76; and his "Use and Abuse of Tartar Emetic in the 19th-Century Materia Medica," *Bulletin of the History of Medicine* 49 (1975): 235-257.

31. Charles S. Tripler and George C. Blackman, *Hand-Book for the Military Surgeon* (Cincinnati: Robert Clark, 1861), p. 33.

32. Dyce Duckworth, "On the Modern Neglect of Calomel in Certain Diseases," *The Practitioner* 17 (1876): 1-6.

33. John King, "Calomel with the Regulars," *Eclectic Medical Journal* 22 (1863): 434.

34. John King, "A Home Thrust at Regular Medicine by the Surgeon General," *Eclectic Medical Journal* 22 (1863): 295.

35. E. P. Bennett, "Removal of Calomel and Tartar Emetic from the Supply List," *Ohio Medical and Surgical Journal* 6 (1863): 348.

36. *Transactions of the American Medical Association* 14 (1864): 32-33.

37. For specifications see "Charges and Specifications," *Medical and Surgical Reporter* 11 (1864): 378-379. The court-martial proceedings are covered in detail in Louis C. Duncan's two-part article "The Strange Case of Surgeon General Hammond," *The Military Surgeon* 64 (1929): 98-110, 252-262. See also Harvey C. Greisman, "William Hammond and His Enemies," *Medical Heritage* 2 (1986): 322-331.

38. *Defense of Brig. Gen'l Wm. A. Hammond, Surgeon General U.S. Army* (Washington, DC?: n.p., 1864), p. 3.

39. Joseph W. England, *The First Century of the Philadelphia College of Pharmacy, 1821-1921* (Philadelphia: The College, 1922), p. 467.

40. *Defense*, p. 4.

41. Ibid., p. 58.

42. For details see Mary C. Gillett, *The Army Medical Department, 1818-1865* (Washington, DC: GPO, 1986), p. 203.

43. "The Dismissal of Surgeon-General Hammond," *Medical Times & Gazette* 2 (1864): 706.

44. For an account see James Evelyn Pilcher, *The Surgeon Generals of the Army* (Carlisle, PA: The Association of Military Surgeons, 1905), pp. 55-57.

45. George Worthington Adams, *Doctors in Blue: The Medical History of the Union Army in the Civil War* (1952; reprint, Louisiana State University Press, 1996), p. 41.

46. Gert H. Brieger, "Therapeutic Conflicts and the American Medical Profession in the 1860's," *Bulletin of the History of Medicine* 47 (1967): 218.

47. See, for example, Gordon Dammann, *Pictorial Encyclopedia of Civil War Medical Instruments and Equipment* (Missoula, MT: Pictorial Histories Publishing, 1983), p. 46; William G. Rothstein, *American Physicians in the 19th Century: From Sects to Science* (Baltimore: Johns Hopkins University Press, 1972), p. 182; John Harley Warner, *The Therapeutic Perspective: Medical Practice, Knowledge, and Identity in America, 1820-1885* (1986; reprinted, Princeton University Press, 1997), p. 220; and James H. Cassedy, *Medicine in America: A Short History* (Baltimore: Johns Hopkins University Press, 1991), p. 29. Not everyone agrees with these

authors, admitting mercury's prominence in the armamentarium long after the Civil War. See, for example, Guenter B. Risse, "Calomel and the American Medical Sects During the Nineteenth Century," *Mayo Clinic Proceedings* 48 (1973): 63; and more recently, Roy Porter, ed., *The Cambridge Illustrated History of Medicine* (Cambridge: Cambridge University Press, 1996), p. 136.

48. *Med. Surg. Hist.*, part 2, volume 1, *Med. Hist.*, 718.

49. John M. Scudder, "The New Professor," *Eclectic Medical Journal* 34 (1874): 387. See also Harvey Wickes Felter, *History of the Eclectic Medical Institute, Cincinnati, Ohio* (Cincinnati: Alumni Association, 1902), pp. 129-130. The exact nature of this report cited by Scudder is unclear. Unfortunately, efforts to find Jeancon's original report have been unsuccessful. He is not mentioned among the sixty surgeons who responded to Hammond's questionnaire regarding his order (see "Treatment of Diarrhœa and Dysentery," *The Medical and Surgical History of the War*, volume 1, *Medical History*, part 2, p. 719) and the *Index-Catalogue of the Library of the Surgeon-General's Office. United States Army*, 16 volumes (Washington: GPO, 1880-1895), volume 7, 230, lists only his *Atlas of Human Anatomy* (Cincinnati, 1879).

50. Charles H. Hughes, "Surgeon General Hammond's Anti-Calomel Order," *St. Louis Medical and Surgical Journal* 1 (1864): 150.

51. Warner, *The Therapeutic Perspective*, p. 220.

52. David L. Cowen and Donald F. Kent, "Medical and Pharmaceutical Practice in 1854," *Pharm. Hist.* 39 (1997): 91-100. See esp. "Epilogue," p. 100.

53. E. N. Gathercoal, *The Prescription Ingredient Survey: Consisting of the Ebert Survey of 1885, The Hallberg Survey of 1895, the Hallberg-Snow Survey of 1907, The Charters Survey of 1926, the Cook Survey of 1930, the Gathercoal Survey of 1930, the U.S.P.-N.F. Survey of 1931-32* (Washington, DC: American Pharmaceutical Association, 1933). Occurrences are tabulated in an alphabetical listing. Calomel is listed on p. 94 under the heading "mercury chloride, mild."

54. Ibid. Total mercurial agents in all forms were prescribed in 1,016.8 instances per 10,000 occurrences in 1885. In 1907 they dropped to about half that of 1885 (516.8) and fall off markedly thereafter.

55. Warner, *The Therapeutic Perspective*, p. 67.

56. John D. Billings, *Hardtack and Coffee, or the Unwritten Story of Army Life* (Boston: George M. Smith, 1887), p. 176.

57. "Cinchonia vs. Quinia," *Proc. APhA* 7 (1858): 74-75.

58. Edward R. Squibb, "Extractum Cinchonæ (Containing Aromatics)," *Am. J. Pharm.* 35 (1863): 230-232.

59. John M. Maisch, "Statistics of the Army Laboratory at Philadelphia," *Proc. APhA* 14 (1866): 276.

60. *Med. Surg. Hist.*, part 3, volume 1, *Med. Hist.*, 184.

61. *A Report to the Secretary of War of the Operation of the Sanitary Commission*, Sanitary Commission, no. 40 (Washington, DC: McGill and Witherow, 1861), p. 50.

62. *Report of a Committee Appointed . . . to Prepare a Paper on the Use of Quinine As a Prophylactic Against Malarious Diseases*, Sanitary Commission, no. 31 (New York: Wm. C. Bryant, 1861). The commission happily reported the surgeon general's concurrence with the committee by the end of the year. See its December report in *A Report to the Secretary of War*, p. 50.

63. Edwin Witherby Brown, "Army Life. In the War of the Great Rebellion. A True Record of His service in the War for the Union." 81st O.V.I. Volumes 1230-1231. Ohio Historical Society Archives, Columbus, Ohio.

64. Quoted in Horace W. Davenport, "Such Is Military: Dr. George Martin Trowbridge's Letters from Sherman's Army, 1863-1865," *Bulletin of the New York Academy of Medicine* 63 (1987): 848.

65. Charles Beneulyn Johnson, *Musket and Medicine, or, Army Life in the Sixties* (Philadelphia: F. A. Davis, 1917), p. 97.

66. Billings, *Hardtack and Coffee,* pp. 175-176.

67. Paul Fatout, ed., *Letters of a Civil War Surgeon* (West Lafayette, IN: Purdue University Press, 1996), p. 59.

68. See William M. Straight, "Calomel, Quinine, and Laudanum: Army Medicine in the Seminole Wars," *Journal of the Florida Medical Association* 65 (August 1978): 627-643.

69. John W. Churchman, "The Use of Quinine During the Civil War," *Johns Hopkins Hospital Bulletin* 17 (June 1906): 175.

70. Ibid., p. 176.

71. Wade Boyle, *Official Herbs: Botanical Substances in the United States Pharmacopoeias, 1820-1990* (East Palestine, OH: Buckeye Naturopathic Press, 1991), p. 22.

72. George B. Wood and Franklin Bache, *USD,* Eleventh Edition (Philadelphia: J. B. Lippincott, 1858), pp. 226-273, 1233-1243.

73. Frederick William Headland, *The Action of Medicines in the System,* Third Edition (Philadelphia: Lindsay and Blakiston, 1859), pp. 382-383.

74. Editorial, *Am. J. Pharm.* 35 (1863): 93.

75. For an excellent review of this process, see Richard H. Shryock, "Empiricism versus Rationalism in American Medicine," *American Antiquarian Society* 79 (April 1969): 99-150.

76. Galen (129 A.D.-199 A.D.) was a physician from Pergamum whose humoural pathology dominated medical practice for centuries. Not until the Renaissance was Galen's authority in the healing art seriously challenged.

77. *Du Chaillu's Equatorial Africa* suggested three to four grains of quinine morning and evening, whereas the British Navy routinely gave sixty grains of Peruvian bark in one-half gill of wine. All quoted in the Sanitary Commission's *Report on Quinine,* pp. 11, 20.

78. Dale C. Smith, "Quinine and Fever: The Development of the Effective Dosage," *Journal of the History of Medicine & Allied Sciences* 31 (July 1976): 343-367.

79. *Med. Surg. Hist.* part 3, volume 1, *Med. Hist.,* 181.

80. William F. Norris, "Clinical Notes on Cases Seen at the Douglas Hospital at Washington, DC During the Civil War," College of Physicians of Philadelphia.

81. *Med. Surg. Hist.,* part 3, volume 1, *Med. Hist.,* 180.

82. Ibid.

83. Ibid., p. 539.

84. Ibid.

85. Goodman and Gilman, *The Pharmacological Basis of Therapeutics,* p. 910.

86. Ibid., p. 906.

87. Smith, "Quinine and Fever," 366.

88. Churchman, "Quinine During the Civil War," p. 180.

89. See the resolution passed in the *Proc. APhA* 10 (1862): 28-29.

90. E. R. Squibb, "Report on the Drug Market," *Proc. APhA* 11 (1863): 182.

91. The history of both firms is available at the Merck Archives, Whitehouse Station, New Jersey [finding aid locations given where possible]. In particular, see Adolph G. Rosengarten Jr., "An Interview for the Merck Archives Conducted by Leon Gortler . . . at Minder House, Wayne, Pennsylvania, November 22, 1988; "List of Articles Exhibited by Powers & Weightman at the U.S. Exposition, Philadelphia, 1876, Preceded by a Historical Sketch; "American Chemical Industries: The Powers-Weightman-Rosengarten Company," PWR R6 2.4.5; Articles of copartnership, John Farr and Co., PWR R6 2.4.4; typescript "Powers and Weightman, PWR R6 2.4.4 (folder 16). The best general account of quinine manufacture in the United States is Joseph W. England, "The American Manufacture of Quinine Sulphate," *American Journal of Pharmacy* 102 (1930): 702-713.

92. Churchman, "Quinine During the Civil War," p. 180.

93. Ibid.

94. Ibid., pp. 180-181.

95. Margaret C. Levenstein, "Vertical Restraints in the Bromine Cartel: The Role of Wholesalers in Facilitating Collusion," National Bureau of Economic Research Historical Working Paper Series, no. 49, July, 1993.

96. This is discussed at some length in George Winston Smith, *Medicines for the Union Army: The United States Army Laboratories During the Civil War* (1962; reprinted: Binghamton, NY: Pharmaceutical Products Press, 2001), pp. 93-97.

97. Ibid., p. 95.

98. Ibid., pp. 96-97.

99. Squibb, "Report on the Drug Market," p. 183.

100. Rene Leon de Milhau, "John Milhau," *Proc. APhA* 55 (1907): 581.

Chapter 8

1. Quoted in Norman Franke, "The Medico-Pharmaceutical Conditions and Drug Supply in the Confederate States of America 1861-1865" (Unpublished PhD dissertation, University of Wisconsin, 1956), p. 183.

2. Ibid., p. 184.

3. Ibid., p. 183.

4. Letter of appointment, Special Orders n. 300, December 23, 1862, Richmond, Virginia, Adjutant and Inspector General's Office, Alabama Department of Archives and History, SG17131, folder 18.

5. Letter from Besson to the Medical Purveyor's Office, Bristol, Tennessee, January 18, 1863 , Ibid.

6. Letter from "the undersigned citizens of Eufala" to the State of Alabama, January 16, 1864, Ibid.

7. H. H. Cunningham, *Doctors in Gray: The Confederate Medical Service,* Second Edition (1960; reprint, Louisiana State University Press, 1993), pp. 21-26.

8. Joseph Jones, "The Medical History of the Confederate States Army and Navy," *SHSP* 20 (Richmond: The Society, 1892), pp. 118-119.

9. Ibid., p. 120.

10. Cunningham, *Doctors in Gray,* p. 264.

11. *War Reb.,* series 4, volume 1 (Washington: GPO, 1900), p. 326.

12. Ibid.

13. Circular, April 12, 1862, National Archives, "War Department Collection of Confederate Records," RG 109, chapt. VI, volume 6.

14. Cunningham, *Doctors in Gray,* p. 146.

15. Ibid., p. 155.

16. Ibid.

17. Ibid., pp. 155-156.

18. T. N. Waul, "Report of the Committee Appointed to Examine into the Quartermaster's, Commissary, and Medical Departments," January 29, 1862, *War Reb.,* series 4, volume 1, pp. 883-891.

19. Ibid., p. 887.

20. Ibid., p. 888.

21. Ibid., p. 889.

22. Ibid., p. 890.

23. *War Reb.,* series 4, volume 1, pp. 421-424.

24. Ibid., p. 423.

25. Ibid., p. 423.

26. Franke, "Medico-Pharmaceutical Conditions," p. 68.

27. Letter from the surgeon general, Richmond, Virginia, March 18, 1862, NA, "War Department Collection of Confederate Records," RG 109, chapt. VI, volume 6. The order reads: "Medical Purveyors are instructed to confine their issues of medical supplies, for the future, except in unusual cases, in quantities sufficient for one month. This will obviate the necessity of so large a stock being kept on hand at the several depots, and it is hoped, diminish, if not altogether prevent, loss in the field from scarcity of transportation. Have such articles as cannot be procured in their vicinity, Purveyors will make, through this office, Requisition on the Purveyor at Richmond," S. Moore.

28. Letter from W. S. Lawton to William Prioleau, April 5, 1862, NA, "War Department Collection of Confederate Records," RG 109, chapt. VI, volume 6.

29. Quoted in Ibid., p. 70.

30. S. H. Stout, "Some Facts of the History of the Organization of the Medical Service of the Confederate Armies and Hospitals," *Southern Practitioner* 23 (1901): 197-199.

31. See, for example, Cunningham, *Doctors in Gray,* pp. 251-252, 260-266; George N. Malpass, "Medicine in the Confederate Army," *American Journal of Pharmacy* 115 (1943): 173-177; E. Robert Wiese, "Life and Times of Samuel Preston Moore, Surgeon-General of the Confederate States of America," *Southern Medical Journal* 23 (1930): 916-922; and Courtney Robert Hall, "The Influence of the Medical Department Upon Confederate Operations," *The Journal of the American Military History Foundation* 1 (1937): 46-54.

32. Chief surgeon for Pickett's division of the Army of Northern Virginia, despite praise for Moore's accomplishments in building from scratch a pavilion hospital system and boards of examination for physicians, noted that Moore could be inflexible and excessively stern. See Charles W. Chancellor, "A Memoir of the Late Samuel Preston Moore, M.D., Surgeon General of the Confederate States Army," *Southern Practitioner* 25 (1903): 634-643.

33. Letter from L. H. Lansar to J. P. Logan, April 4, 1862, NA, "War Department Collection of Confederate Records," RG 109, chapt. VI, volume 6.

34. Franke, "Medico-Pharmaceutical Conditions," p. 66.

35. Ibid., p. 68.

36. General Order no. 23 revoked all of the instructions emanating from Edward W. John's office, directing that "hereafter all reports will be made direct to the Surgeon-General, and all instructions will emanate from his office." Adjutant and Inspector General Cooper then rather tersely directed Johns to "send to the Surgeon-General's Office without delay all records, books, and papers connected with the duties assigned him under the above-named orders." See *War Reb.,* series 4, volume 2, 410-411.

37. Letter from John C. Stickney to George S. Blackie, Chattanooga, Tennessee, March 14, 1863, NA, "War Department Collection of Confederate Records," RG 109, chapt. VI, volume 750, Medical Purveyor. Army of the Tennessee, 1862-1863.

38. Letter by L. Guild, Medical Director's Office, Army of Northern Virginia, NLM, MS C 99. HMD. Latimer, Thomas Sargent. U.S. and Confederate Army medical papers.

39. William C. Davis, *Look Away!: A History of the Confederate States of America* (New York: The Free Press, 2002) p. 333.

40. Alfred Stillé, *Therapeutics and Materia Medica,* Second Edition, 2 volumes (Philadelphia: Blanchard and Lea, 1864), 1: 606.

41. For a complete history, see Harry W. Paul, *Bacchic Medicine: Wine and Alcohol Therapies from Napoleon to the French Paradox* (New York: Rodopi, 2001).

42. Letter from T. C. Howard to George S. Blackie, Atlanta, June 19, 1863, NA, "War Department Collection of Confederate Records," RG 109, chapt. VI, volume 750, Medical Purveyor. Army of the Tennessee, 1862-1863.

43. Ibid.

44. Letter from S. P. Moore to J. A. S. [James A. Seddon], January 5, 1864, *War Reb.,* series 4, volume 2, 1072-1073.

45. S. P. Moore, Surgeon General's Office, Richmond, Virginia, July 9, 1863, NA, "War Department Collection of Confederate Records," RG 109, chapt. VI, volume 750, Medical Purveyor. Army of the Tennessee, 1862-1863.

46. Letter from the *Richmond Sentinal* to the War Department, May 13, 1863, Ibid.

47. Letter from George S. Blackie to Samuel P. Moore, July 10, 1863, Ibid.

Chapter 9

1. Paul Steiner, *Disease in the Civil War: Natural Biological Warfare from 1861-1865* (Springfield, IL: Charles C Thomas, 1968), pp. 138, 192-194.

2. *Med. Surg. Hist,.* part 3, volume 1, *Med. Hist.* (Washington: GPO, 1888), p. 107.

3. See George Worthington Adams, *Doctors in Blue: The Medical History of the Union Army in the Civil War* (1952; reprinted, Baton Rouge: Louisiana State University Press, 1996), pp. 138, 214-215; and H. H. Cunningham, *Doctors in Gray: The Confederate Medical Service,* Second Edition (1960; reprinted: Baton Rouge: Louisiana State University, 1993), pp. 206-208.

4. S. H. Stout, "Some Facts of the History of the Organization of the Medical Service of the Confederate Armies and Hospitals," *Southern Practitioner* 24 (1902): 213.

5. Quoted in Cunningham, *Doctors in Gray,* p. 208.

6. *Stedman's Concise Medical Dictionary,* Second Edition (Baltimore: Williams and Wilkins, 1994), p. 1108.

7. For an interesting discussion of this phenomenon, see I. S. McGregor and Arnold Loewenstein, "Quinine Blindness," *The Lancet* (October 28, 1944): 566-572.

8. An excellent and succinct overview is available in Kumaravel Rajakumar, "Pellagra in the United States: A Historical Perspective," *Southern Medical Journal* 93 (2000): 272-277. The identification of niacin as the specific pellagra-preventing factor was first reported in Conrad Arnold Elvehjem, "The Isolation and Identification of the Anti-Black Tongue Factor," *Journal of Biological Chemistry* 123 (1938): 137-149.

9. Casimir Funk, *The Vitamines,* Second German Edition, trans. by Harry E. Dunn (Baltimore: Williams and Wilkins, 1922), p. 352.

10. S. H. Stout, "Some Facts of the History of the Organization of the Medical Service of the Confederate Armies and Hospitals," *Southern Practitioner* 23 (1901): 101-102.

11. More information on Chimborazo Hospital is available in J. R. Gildersleeve, "History of Chimorazo Hospital," *SHSP* 36 (Richmond, Virginia: The Society, 1908), pp. 86-94.

12. William H. Taylor, "Some Experiences of a Confederate Assistant Surgeon," *Transactions of the College of Physicians of Philadelphia,* third series, 28 (1906): 105.

13. John Samuel Apperson, *Repairing the "March of Mars": The Civil War Diaries of John Samuel Apperson,* edited by John Herbert Roper (Macon, GA: Mercer University Press, 2001), p. 119.

14. Ibid., p. 121.

15. Ibid., p. 225.

16. Ibid., p. 225.

17. Letter from George E. Weller to "Doctor," June 8, 1862, Southern Historical Collection, University of North Carolina at Chapel Hill, microfilm reel, 1512.

18. Ibid.

19. Letter from George E. Weller to his sister, March 4, 1864, camped near Smithfield, North Carolina, Ibid.

20. Ibid.

21. Quoted in Ivan Musicant, *Divided Waters: The Naval History of the Civil War* (New York: HarperCollins, 1995), p. 50.

22. Details of the blockade are given in Ibid, pp. 50-64.

23. "An Act Recognizing the Existence of War Between the United States and the Confederate States, and Concerning Letters of Marque, Prizes, and Prize Goods," in *The Messages and Papers of President Jefferson Davis and the Confederacy, Including Diplomatic Correspondence,* edited and compiled by James D. Richardson, 2 volumes (New York: Chelsea House, 1983), 1: 104-110.

24. Musicant, *Divided Waters,* p. 61.

25. Stephen R. Wise, *Lifeline of the Confederacy: Blockade Running During the Civil War* (Columbia: University of South Carolina Press, 1988), p. 24.

26. John W. Mallett, "How the South Got Chemicals During the War," *SHSP* 31 (Richmond, Virginia: The Society, 1903), pp. 100-102.

27. Maurice Albin, "The Use of Anesthetics During the Civil War," *Pharm. Hist.* 42 (2000): 102, 104.

28. Ibid., p. 102.

29. See Samuel Preston Moore's address to the Association of Medical Officers of the Army and Navy of the Confederacy, Richmond, Virginia, October 19-20, 1875, reprinted as "Address of the President of the Association," *Southern Practitioner* 31 (1909): 496.

30. Ibid.

31. C. C. Washburn, General Orders, no. 3, May 10, 1864, *War Reb.,* series 1, volume 39, part 2 (Washington: GPO, 1892), pp. 22-23.

32. For an interesting and thorough discussion of Confederate smuggling operations in Memphis, see Joseph H. Parks, "A Confederate Trade Center Under Federal Occupation: Memphis, 1862-1865," *Journal of Southern History* 7 (1941): 289-314.

33. Joseph Jacobs, "Some of the Drug Conditions During the War Between the States, 1861-5," *SHSP* 33 (Richmond, Virginia: The Society, 1905), pp. 171-173.

34. Holland Thompson, ed., *The Photographic History of the Civil War,* volume 4, part 2, *Prisons and Hospitals* (1911; reprinted, Secaucus, NJ: The Blue and Grey Press, 1987), pp. 241-242.

35. Letter from D. Camden deLeon to L. P. Walker, Montgomery, Alabama, April 8, 1861, *War Reb.,* series 4, volume 1, p. 212.

36. George S. Blackie in Atlanta happily reported that the cavalry of Nathan Bedford Forrest captured three four-mule army wagons of medicine worth $150,000; see *Photographic History,* p. 242.

37. Jacobs, "Some of the Drug Conditions," p. 165.

38. See, for example, Mary Elizabeth Massey, *Ersatz in the Confederacy* (Columbia: University of South Carolina Press, 1952), p. 116; and J. Hampton Hoch, "Through the Blockade," *Journal of the American Pharmaceutical Association,* new series, 1 (1961): 769-770.

39. Letter from J. P. Benjamin to Caleb Huse, Richmond, March 22, 1862, *War Reb.,* series 4, volume 1 (Washington: GPO, 1900), p. 1018.

40. Report of James A. Seddon, Secretary of War, October 1, 1863, *War Reb.,* series 4, volume 2, p. 845.

41. Report of James A. Seddon, Secretary of War, July 4, 1864, *War Reb.,* series 4, volume 3, p. 526.

42. Report of Lieutenant-Colonel Thomas L. Bayne, August 12, 1864, Ibid., p. 589.

43. Letter from R. W. Sanders, Quartermaster, to Lieutenant Colonel E. Surgent, Assistant Adjutant General, Selma, Alabama, November 6, 1864, Ibid., p. 790.

44. J. Hampton Hoch, "Tabulations of Selected Items," typescript from The Cowen Collection, American Institute of the History of Pharmacy, Madison, Wisconsin.

45. See Norman Franke, "Rx Prices in the Confederacy," *Journal of the American Pharmaceutical Association* new series 1, 12 (1961): 773-774.

46. Musicant, *Divided Waters,* p. 370.

47. Ibid.

48. Herbert M. Nash, "Some Reminiscences of a Confederate Surgeon," *Transactions of the College of Physicians of Philadelphia,* third series, 28 (1906): 133.

49. Norman Franke, "Medico-Pharmaceutical Drug Conditions and Drug Supply in the Confederate States of America, 1861-1865," (Unpublished PhD dissertation, University of Wisconsin, Madison, 1956), pp. 154-155.

50. Wise, *Lifeline of the Confederacy,* pp. 115.

51. Ibid., p. 139.

52. For the complete story of the capture of these three blockade runners, see Ibid., pp. 139-140.

53. Ibid., p. 140.

54. Musicant, *Divided Waters,* p. 370.

55. Report of Lieutenant-Colonel Thomas L. Bayne, August 12, 1864, *War Reb.,* series 4. volume 3, p. 590.

56. Musicant, *Divided Waters,* p. 370.

57. Norman Franke, "Medico-Pharmaceutical," p. 151.

58. This author's investigation turned up thirty-four out of fifty vessels carrying substantial medical stores. See NA, RG 45, Navy subject files, boxes 776, 781-784. Even higher figures are suggested by Sarita Bullard Oertling, "Emetics, Cathartics and Purgatives, Oh My!: The Cargo of the *Alice,*" unpublished manuscript, p. 1. Paper presented October 19, 2002, at the Twenty-First Gulf South History and Humanities Conference, Galveston, Texas.

59. Auction held September 30, 1863, at the Union Stores, Brooklyn, New York. See NA, RG 45, Navy subject files, box 783, folder 4.

60. Auction held April 8, 1863, at the Union Stores, Brooklyn, New York, Ibid., folder 3.

61. Auction held October 14, 1862, Ibid., box 776, folder 3.

62. This was *not* the famous C.S.S. *Alabama* sunk off the cost of France by the U.S.S. *Kearsarge* on June 19, 1864. See Wise, *Lifeline of the Confederacy,* pp. 286-287.

63. See "Catalogue Sale," November 28, 1863, National Archives, RG 45, Navy subject files, box 782, folder 1.

64. Ibid.

65. Letter from J. H. Graybill, Captain and Assistant Commissary of Subsistence, to Surgeon C. Terry, October 10, 1864, *War Reb.,* series 4, volume 3, p. 719.

66. Ibid.

67. Ibid., p. 720.

68. Surgeon W. A. W. Spottswood to S. R. Mallory, Secretary of the Navy, November 1, 1864, *War Reb.,* series 2, volume 2 (Washington: GPO, 1921), pp. 759-760.

69. Surgeon-General's Office, April 2, 1862, Richmond, Virginia, *War Reb.,* series 4, volume 1, p. 1041. This order was reiterated, it will be recalled, just a few days later in Circular no. 3; see p. 231.

70. Ibid.

71. Letter from W. A. Carrington to the Surgeon-General's Office, September 26, 1864, Richmond, Virginia, *War Reb.,* series 4, volume 3, p. 687.

72. Letter from R. Potts to the Surgeon-General's Office, October 3, 1864, Montgomery, Alabama, Ibid., p. 712.

73. Letter acknowledging receipt from Samuel Preston Moore to George S. Blackie, May 7, 1863, Richmond, Virginia, NA, RG 109, chapt. 6, volume 750.

74. M. B. Beck, "On Eupatorium and Serpentaria," *Confederate State Medical and Surgical Journal* 1 (1864): 137.

75. Massey, *Ersatz in the Confederacy,* pp. 121-122.

76. Samuel Preston Moore, "Address of the President of the Association of Medical Officers of Confederate States Army and Navy," *The Southern Practitioner* 31 (1909): 495.

77. Francis Peyre Porcher, *Resources of the Southern Fields and Forests* (Charleston, SC: Evans and Cogswell, 1863), p. 310.

78. Ibid., p. 486.

79. Ibid., p. 412.

80. *USP,* Fourth Decennial Edition (Philadelphia: J. B. Lippincott, 1863), pp. 4-63 passim.

81. Quoted in Patricia Spain Ward, *Simon Baruch: Rebel in the Ranks of Medicine* (Tuscaloosa: University of Alabama Press, 1994), p. 30.

82. Ibid.

83. Letter from Samuel Preston Moore to John C. Breckenridge, February 9, 1865, Richmond, Virginia, *War Reb.,* series 4, volume 3, p. 1074.

84. Ibid.

85. Franke, "Medico-Pharmaceutical Drug Conditions," p. 56.

86. Ibid.

87. John H. Felts and Robert W. Prichard, "Confederate Laboratory for Preparation of Medicines Near Lincolnton," *North Carolina Medical Journal* 39 (1978): 235-236.

88. Ibid., p. 235.

89. Ibid., p. 236.

90. Ibid.

91. Franke, "Medico-Pharmaceutical Drug Conditions," pp. 55-56.

92. Quoted in Ibid., pp. 57-58.

93. Ibid, p. 58.

94. Order of Samuel Preston Moore, July 9, 1863, Richmond, Virginia, NA, RG 109, chapt. VI, volume 750.

95. Letter from William H. Anderson to George S. Blackie, February 11, 1863, Montgomery, Alabama, Ibid.

96. Ibid.

97. Letter from J. J. Chisolm to George S. Blackie, January 27, 1863, Columbia, South Carolina, Ibid.

98. Letter from J. J. Chisolm to George S. Blackie, February 5, 1863, Columbia, South Carolina, Ibid.

99. Porcher, *Resources,* p. 26.

100. Letter from J. H. Zeilier to H. H. Prioleau, May 4, 1862. NA, RG 109, chapt. VI, volume 6.

101. Franke, "Medico-Pharmaceutical Drug Conditions," p. 62.

102. Quoted in Franke, "Medico-Pharmaceutical Drug Conditions," p. 64.

Chapter 10

1. See entry "Camp near Centreville, Va., Monday, Aug. 5, 1861," in John Samuel Apperson, *Repairing the 'March of Mars': The Civil War Diaries of John*

Samuel Apperson, Hospital Steward in the Stonewall Brigade, edited by John Herbert Roper (Macon, GA: Mercer University Press, 2001), p. 123.

2. Apperson, *Repairing the 'March of Mars'*, pp. 92-99. The reader is cautioned in consulting the published version of these prescriptions. Editor Roper's reading of these substances was sometimes incorrect, mistaking the cursive style of the double s for "ps" instead of the actual "ss," thus transcribing blue mass (i.e., mercury) into "blue maps." For details the actual documents should be consulted; see Apperson Family Papers, MS74-017, Special Collections Department, University Libraries, Virginia Tech.

3. Ibid., pp. 107-108.

4. Ibid., p. 119.

5. Ibid., p. 120.

6. Ibid., pp. 122-123.

7. Ibid., pp. 315-316.

8. Ibid., p. 325.

9. Ibid., p. 398.

10. Ibid., p. 464.

11. Robert E. Denney, *Civil War Medicine: Care & Comfort of the Wounded* (New York: Sterling Publishing, 1995), p. 208.

12. Ibid., p. 209.

13. Quoted in Ibid., p. 210.

14. Apperson, *Repairing the 'March of Mars'*, pp. 484-485.

15. Ibid., p. 488.

16. Surgeon B. W. Allen, Confederate Hospital Reports, 1862-1864 [two bound volumes in holograph], Reynolds Historical Library, University of Alabama at Birmingham (hereafter referred to as Casebook).

17. See letter explaining the casebook, signed B. W. Allen, Marietta, Ohio, August 4, 1880, Ibid.

18. Allen, Casebook, volume 1, pp. 68, 86, 124.

19. Ibid., volume 1, pp. 101-126 passim.

20. Ibid., volume 1, p. 205.

21. Ibid., volume 1, p. 217.

22. Ibid., volume 1, p. 219.

23. Ibid., volume 1, p. 222.

24. Ibid.

25. Ibid., volume 1, p. 234. Elixir of vitriol was an old and much favored remedy. Even as late as the 1880s the *USD* referred to Acidum Sulphuricum Aromaticum as a "valuable preparation, commonly called, *elixir of vitriol,* . . . a simplification of *Mynischt's acid elixir.* It is tonic and astringent, and affords an agreeable form of sulphuric acid for administration." See *USD,* Fifteenth Edition (Philadelphia: J. B. Lippincott, 1884), p. 110.

26. Allen, Casebook, volume 1, p. 236.

27. Ibid., p. 241.

28. Ibid., p. 242.

29. Ibid., volume 2, p. 246.

30. Ibid., volume 2, p. 252.

31. Ibid., volume 2, p. 254.

32. Ibid., volume 2, p. 256.

33. Ibid., volume 2, p. 257.

34. Ibid., volume 2, p. 258.

35. Ibid., volume 2, pp. 263-266.

36. Ibid., volume 2, p. 272.

37. Ibid., volume 2, pp. 300-301.

38. Ibid., volume 2, p. 332.

39. Joseph Jacobs, "Some of the Drug Conditions During the War Between the States," *SHSP* 33 (Richmond, Virginia: The Society, 1905), pp. 161-187.

40. Ibid., pp. 167-168.

41. William H. Taylor, "Some Experiences of a Confederate Assistant Surgeon," *Transactions of the College of Physicians of Philadelphia,* third series, 28 (1906): 105.

42. See, for example, in addition to Jacobs (note 39), John W. Mallett, "How the South Got Chemical During the War," *SHSP* 31 (Richmond, Virginia: The Society, 1903), pp. 100-102; C. J. Edwards, "Medical Expedients During the War Between the States," *The Southern Practitioner* 30 (1908): 533-535; and C. Kendrick, "Indigenous Plants Used by Southern People As Medicines During the War," *The Southern Practitioner* 31 (1909): 534-537.

43. Jacobs, "Drug Conditions," p. 175.

44. The diary, originally published in 1900, has since been reissued in Solon Hyde, *A Captive of War,* edited by Neil Thompson (Shippensburg, PA: Burd Street Press, 1996).

45. The status of hospital stewards as noncombatants was an unsettled question throughout the war. The Union apparently had a tendency to release stewards as noncombatants the same as they did surgeons, but the policy was carried out only on individual bases. When Colonel W. Hoffman, 3rd Infantry and Commissary General of Prisoners, suggested a general rule of noncombatant status for hospital stewards he quickly retracted, saying, "Please understand my letter of the 19th instant, in relation to hospital stewards, as applying only to the case of Hospital Steward Charles Whilan. The rule will not be adopted as general until it is ascertained that it will be observed by the authorities in Richmond." See letter from W. Hoffman to Major General George H. Thomas, March 4, 1864, *War Reb.,* series 2, volume 6 (Washington: GPO, 1899), p. 1091.

46. Hyde, *A Captive of War,* pp. 124-125.

47. Ibid., p. 139.

48. Ibid., p. 131.

49. Letter from J. Crews Pelot to E. D. Eiland, September 5, 1864, *War Reb.,* series 2, volume 7, pp. 773-774.

50. John M. Maisch, "Report on the Drug Market," *Proc. APhA* 12 (1864): 198.

51. Ibid.

52. Entry May 13, 1861, Thomas Potts James, Letterbooks, 1851-1863, (Phi) 885, Historical Society of Pennsylvania.

53. Letter from James to Burbower, September 9, 1861, Ibid.

54. Entry November 16, 1861, Ibid.

55. See, for example, Bern Anderson, *By Sea and by River: The Naval History of the Civil War* (1962; reprinted, [New York?]: Da Capo Press, 1989), pp. 225-232; and Ivan Musciant, *Divided Waters: The Naval History of the Civil War* (New York: HarperCollins, 1995), pp. 50-64.

56. See, for example, Frank L. Owsley, *King Cotton Diplomacy: Foreign Relations of the Confederate States of America* (Chicago: University of Chicago Press, 1959), pp. 229-240 passim; and Jochem H. Tans, "The Hapless Blockade, 1861-1865," *The Concord Review* 6 (1994): 13-30.

57. NA, RG 109, chapt. VI, volumes 621 and 630, Medical Purveyor's Office, 1862-1865. District no. 4, Macon, Georgia (formerly at Savannah, Georgia). Quinine sulfate is particularly absent from its later pages, and shortages are demonstrated even earlier: NA, RG 109, chapt. VI, volume 576, Medical Purveyor's Office, 1861-1863, Western Department, Memphis, Tennessee and Jackson, Mississippi. These, in particular, show drug receipts and disbursements becoming scantier and scantier.

58. Letter from L. Guild to S. P. Moore, August 8, 1864, NA, RG 109, chapt. VI, volume 642. RG 109, chapt. VI, volume 642, Medical Purveyor. Army of Northern Virginia, 1863-1865.

59. See Richmond, Virginia, May 9, 1865, "Inventory of *Captured* Medical and Hospital Supplies Remaining on Hand," Thomas S. Lattimer papers, MS C 99, NLM, History of Medicine Division.

60. See "Total supplies received at the Medical Purveyor's Office, 1862-65, Savannah, Ga.," NA, RG 109, chapt. VI, volume 580.

61. William Diamond, "Imports of the Confederate Government from Europe and Mexico," *Journal of Southern History* 6 (1940): 486.

62. Letter from B. P. Noland to I. M. St. John, April 16, 1874, in "Resources of the Confederacy in 1865—Report of General I. M. St. John Commissary General," *SHSP* 3 (Richmond: The Society, 1877), pp. 107-108.

63. Letter from J. T. Winnermore to G. S. Blackie, May 1, 1863, Augusta, Georgia, National Archives, RG 109, chapt. VI, volume 750.

64. Letter from J. J. Chisolm to G. S. Blackie, Charleston, SC, April 5, 1863, Ibid.

65. H. H. Cunningham, *Doctors in Gray: The Confederate Medical Service* (1958; reprinted, Baton Rouge: Louisiana State University Press, 1993), p. 161.

66. Jay Winik, *April 1865: The Month That Saved America* (New York: Harper-Collins, 2001), pp. 126-127. The report of Commissary-General I. M. St. John and testimony from several corroborating authorities associated with the Commissary office attest to the fact that no letter from General Lee requesting that rations be delivered to Amelia Courthouse was ever received. Lewis E. Harvie, president of the Richmond & Danville Railroad, the only supply line open for the Army of Northern Virginia, concluded that, "If the orders were sent to the Commissary Department, I presume they were intercepted or otherwise miscarried." For details, see "Resources of the Confederacy in 1865," *SHSP,* pp. 97-111.

67. Edwards, "Medical Expedients," p. 535.

68. See the sixteen-page pamphlet by Edwin S. Gaillard, *Medical and Surgical Lessons of the Late War* (Louisville: Louisville Journal Job Printers, 1868).

69. See, for example, Frank R. Freemon, *Microbes and Minnie Balls: An Annotated Bibliography of Civil War Medicine* (Rutherford, NJ: Fairleigh Dickinson University Press, 1993). Freeman claims that Porcher's *Resources of the Southern Fields and Forests* "contains nothing of modern medical importance" (p. 112). Similarly, see Norman Franke, "Medico-Pharmaceutical Conditions and Drug Supply in the Confederate States of America, 1861-1865," (Unpublished PhD dissertation,

University of Wisconsin, Madison, 1956), pp. 124; Franke's, "A Confederate Recipe Book," in *Three Essays on Formularies* (Madison, WI: AIHP, 1961), pp. 11-13; and David Madden, editor, *Beyond the Battlefield: The Ordinary Life and Extraordinary Times of the Civil War Soldier* (New York: Touchstone, 2000), p. 252.

70. Franke, "Medico-Pharmaceutical Conditions," p. 124.

71. Franke, "A Confederate Recipe Book," p. 13.

72. The sixty different plant genera in the "C.S.A Standard Supply Table of Indigenous Remedies" were checked against *Martindale: The Complete Drug Reference,* edited by Kathleen Parfitt, Thirty-Second Edition (London: The Pharmaceutical Press, 1999), a drug compendium of 4,336 monographs, 644 disease treatment reviews, and proprietary preparations from Australia, Austria, Belgium, Canada, France, Germany, Ireland, Italy, the Netherlands, Norway, South Africa, Spain, Sweden, Switzerland, the United Kingdom, and the United States. A total of twenty-two out of sixty were found listed, some with their own monographs.

73. Ibid., p. 1481.

74. Ibid., p. 1069.

75. Ibid., p. 1592.

76. Some modern studies on *Lobelia inflata,* for example, suggest that lobeline (its main alkaloid constituent) is a bronchial dilator. See Melvyn Werbach and Michael T. Murray, *Botanical Influences on Illness: A Sourcebook of Clinical Research,* Second Edition (Tarzana, CA: Third Line Press, 2000), pp. 137-138. *Polygala senega* does contain 5 to 10 percent triterpenoid saponines known to be active expectorants, see Varro E. Tyler, *Tyler's Herbs of Choice: The Therapeutic Use of Phytomedicinals* (Binghamton, NY: Pharmaceutical Products Press, 1994), pp. 97-98. Other items on the C.S.A. Indigenous Supply Table receiving favorable modern analysis are *Capsicum frutescans* as a topical preparation in skin irritations and post-amputation therapy, *Humulus lupulus* as a mild sedative, *Mentha piperita* as a nasal decongestant, *Uva ursi* in urinary tract infections, see Werbach and Murray, *Botanical Influences on Illness,* pp. 15-16, 70, 221-222, 569.

77. See David Madden, *Beyond the Battlefield,* p. 252.

78. Letter from Surgeon General S. P. Moore to R. Potts, Medical Purveyor, Macon, Georgia, Richmond, Virginia, December 5, 1863, *War Reb.,* series 4, volume 2, p. 1024.

79. See Samuel Logan, "Prophylactic Effects of Quinine," *Confederate States Medical and Surgical Journal* 1 (1864): 81-83.

80. George B. Wood and Franklin Bache, *USD,* First Edition (Philadelphia: Grigg and Elliot, 1833), p. 256.

81. George B. Wood and Franklin Bache, *USD,* Eleventh Edition (Philadelphia: J. B. Lippincott, 1858), p. 306.

82. W. T. Grant, "Indigenous Medicinal Plants," *Confederate States Medical and Surgical Journal* 1 (1864): 85.

83. Both plants contain salicin, which is converted by the body into salicylic acid, the basic substance from which acetylsalicylic acid (aspirin) is derived. See Andrew Pengelly, *The Constituents of Medicinal Plants: An Introduction to the Chemistry and Therapeutics of Herbal Medicines,* Second Edition (Muswellbrook, NSW: Sunflower Herbals, 1997), pp. 9-10.

84. Letter from the Surgeon General's Office to S. T. Latimer, October 26, 1864, Samuel Thomas Sargent Latimer papers, MS C99, U.S. and Confederate Army medical papers, folder 18, National Library of Medicine.

85. See, for example, John Redman Coxe, *The American Dispensatory,* Fourth Edition (Philadelphia: Thomas Dobson and Son, 1818), pp. 268-269; Benjamin Ellis, *The Medical Formulary,* Fourth Edition (Philadelphia: Carey, Lea and Blanchard, 1834), p. 188; and Robert Thomas, *Universal Formulary* (Philadelphia: Blanchard and Lea, 1856), pp. 259-260.

86. *Med. Surg. Hist.,* part 2, volume 1, *Med. Hist.* (Washington: GPO, 1879), pp. 105, 766.

87. J. C. Wharton, "A New Litmus Test Paper," *Confederate States Medical and Surgical Journal* 1 (1864): 54-55.

88. *USD,* Fifteenth Edition (Philadelphia: J. B. Lippincott, 1884), p. 495.

Epilogue

1. Robert E. Lee, General Order no. 9, April 10, 1865, *The Annals of America,* volume 9, *The Crisis of the Union, 1858-1865* (Chicago: Encyclopedia Britannica, 1976), p. 572.

2. George Winston Smith, *Drugs for the Union Army: The United States Army Laboratories During the Civil War* (1962; reprinted, Binghamton, NY: Pharmaceutical Products Press, 2001), p. 74.

3. See William A. Brewer, "Report of the Committee on the Drug Market," *Proc. APhA* 15 (1867): 267-307.

4. Ibid., 283.

5. Ibid., 284.

6. Dennis Worthen, "The Pharmaceutical Industry, 1852-1902," *Journal of the American Pharmaceutical Association* 40 (2000): 589-591.

7. Williams Haynes, *American Chemical Industry,* volume 1, *Background and Beginnings* (New York: Van Nostrand, 1954), p. 320.

8. The establishment of state pharmacy associations and pharmacy schools is listed chronologically in *Kremers and Urdang's History of Pharmacy,* Fourth Edition, revised by Glenn Sonnedecker (1976; reprinted, Madison: AIHP, 1986), pp. 379-380, 383-386.

9. Ibid., p. 325.

10. Chapter 10 of the "Handy Book for the United States Navy" dated 1917, being a textbook of instruction for the Hospital Corps Training Schools. This chapter gives a list of the common medicaments used in U.S. Navy Hospitals, including their synonyms, preparation, use, and dosage, in "World War I: The Medical Front." Available at <http://raven.cc.ukans.edu/~kansite/ww_one/medical/pharmacy/matmed.htm>.

11. Henry C. Fuller, *The Story of Drugs* (New York: The Century Co., 1922), pp. 148-149.

12. For further discussion, see Steward H. Holbook, *The Golden Age of Quackery* (New York: Macmillan, 1959), pp. 103-110; James Harvey Young, *The Toadstool Millionaires: A Social History of Patent Medicines Before Federal Regulation* (Princeton: Princeton University Press, 1961), pp. 96-100; and Michael A. Flan-

nery, " 'Good for Man or Beast': American Patent Medicines from 1865 to 1938 (with special reference to the South)," *Alabama Heritage* 59 (2001): 8-17.

13. See John P. Swann, "The History of Pharmacy and Estates of Pharmacy: Institutional Frameworks for Drug Research in America," *Pharmacy in History* 32 (1990): 3-11; and Harry M. Marks, *The Progress of Experiment: Science and Therapeutic Reform in the United States, 1900-1990* (Baltimore: Johns Hopkins University Press, 1997).

14. See David T. Courtwright, "The Hidden Epidemic: Opiate Addiction and Cocaine Use in the South, 1860-1920," *Journal of Southern History* 49 (1983): 57-72.

15. Mark A. Quinones, "Drug Abuse During the Civil War (1861-1865)," *The International Journal of the Addictions* 10 (1975): 1007-1020.

16. Ibid., p. 1018. The preponderance of women addicts is substantiated in Courtwright's study: see tables 3 and 4 in "The Hidden Epidemic," p. 61.

17. Quinones, "Drug Abuse," 1019.

18. For an excellent summary of the historiographical debate, see Philip Shaw Paludan, "What Did the Winners Win?: The Social and Economic History of the North During the Civil War," in *Writing the Civil War: The Quest to Understand,* eds. James M. McPherson and William J. Cooper Jr. (Columbia: University of South Carolina Press, 1998), pp. 174-200.

19,. John N. Henry, *Turn Them Out to Die Like a Mule: The Civil War Letters of John N. Henry, 49th New York, 1861-1865,* ed. John Michael Priest (Leesburg, Virginia: Gauley Mount Press, 1995), p. 436.

Bibliographical Essay

Preliminary Comments

Much of the research material for this book was obtained at the author's own institution, the Reynolds Historical Library of the Lister Hill Library of the Health Sciences, University of Alabama at Birmingham.* The author admits pride in the privilege of managing this collection, and it is no exaggeration to point out that the Reynolds Historical Library is one of the most extensive history of medicine collections in the southeastern United States and moreover possesses a Civil War collection equaled by few in this country. This is largely due to the generosity and indefatigable efforts of Arnold G. Diethelm, MD, Faye Fletcher Kerner Professor of Surgery at the University of Alabama School of Medicine and the source to whom this volume is dedicated.

That said, the researcher will find accessing material (both published and archival) in Civil War pharmacy a daunting task. As if the huge multi-volume compendia of published official records (see primary sources) are not enough, a seemingly unending sea of secondary sources roll off academic and trade presses annually on all aspects of this great American crucible. Fortunately, two titles can help chart these expansive bibliographic waters for those seeking health care information. First is Frank R. Freemon's *Microbes and Minie Balls: An Annotated Bibliography of Civil War Medicine* (Rutherford, NJ: Fairleigh Dickinson University Press, 1993). Freemon provides historians with 129 pages of published primary resources and ninety-four pages of secondary works in the field. Furthermore, his annotations provide the researcher with a handy guide of what to expect before consulting a title that only seems as if it might be of interest.

A second guide of importance relating to accessing primary sources is Kenneth W. Munden and Henry Putney Beers' *The Union: A Guide to Federal Archives to the Civil War* and Beers' companion *The Confederacy: A Guide to the Archives of the Government of the Confederate States of America* (Washington, DC: National Archives and Records Administration, 1998). The National Archives holds a massive amount of primary material relative

---

*This essay is not intended to be an exhaustive representation of every resource examined in the preparation of this book but rather is to serve as a general guide to those who may be interested in pursuing further studies in Civil War pharmacy.

to the war and a careful review of these two books will save the researcher considerable time in determining precisely what record groups to consult.

Published Primary Sources

Before examining Civil War pharmacy directly, it is essential to understand the therapeutic contexts in which that care was provided. This can be done by carefully reviewing the standard texts of the period. There are several authoritative guides: *The Pharmacopoeia of the United States of America,* Fourth Decennial Edition (Philadelphia: J. B. Lippincott, 1863); George B. Wood and Franklin Bache, *The Dispensatory of the United States of America,* Eleventh Edition (Philadelphia: J. B. Lippincott, 1858); George B. Wood, *A Treatise on the Practice of Medicine,* 2 volumes, Fifth Edition (Philadelphia: J. B. Lippincott, 1858); William Headland, *The Action of Medicines in the System,* Third Edition (Philadelphia: Lindsay and Blakiston, 1859); and Alfred Stillé, *Therapeutics and Materia Medica,* 2 volumes, Second Edition (Philadelphia: Blanchard and Lea, 1864). Once the theory and practice of medicine during the war are understood, pharmacy begins to take on some familiar forms as the material expression of nineteenth-century medical rationalism.

The number of published primary accounts bearing upon Civil War pharmacy is surprisingly large. They may be broken down into three basic categories: (1) narratives, published diaries, and casebooks of surgeons and assistant surgeons that give prescriptions, treatment regimens, and general pharmaceutical conditions during the war; (2) narratives and published diaries of hospital stewards; and (3) official correspondence and other documents related to the acquisition, distribution, or dispensing of medicines as well as those official materials bearing upon the administration of pharmaceutical functions for the Union and Confederacy.

Although there are many surgeons' accounts of the war, relatively few give any detailed information as to pharmaceutical conditions in camp and hospital and fewer still discuss their own therapeutic protocols. The historian searching for such gems is left to mine thousands of pages of narrative to uncover one or perhaps two precious jewels, an exercise that can be frustrating but rewarding in the end. Most are found in the official accounts and in various reminiscences and diaries of wartime experiences. Also of considerable assistance in determining the challenges of administering the Confederate medical corps was Samuel Preston Moore's posthumously published "Address of the President of the Association of Medical Officers of Confederate States Army and Navy," *The Southern Practitioner* 31 (1909): 491-498. Four articles focusing particularly upon drug conditions for the South and how shortages were dealt with are John W. Mallett, "How the South Got Chemicals During the War," *Southern Historical Society Pa-*

pers, volume 31 (Richmond, VA: The Society, 1903), pp. 100-102; Atlanta pharmacist Joseph Jacobs' "Some of the Drug Conditions During the War Between the States," *Southern Historical Society Papers,* volume 33 (Richmond, VA: The Society, 1905), pp. 161-187; C. J. Edwards, "Medical Expedients During the War Between the States," *The Southern Practitioner* 30 (1908): 533-535; and C. Kendrick, "Indigenous Plants Used by Southern People As Medicines During the War," *The Southern Practitioner* 31 (1909): 534-537. For accounts by Confederate surgeons, see William H. Taylor, "Some Experiences of a Confederate Assistant Surgeon," *Transactions of the College of Physicians of Philadelphia,* third series, 28 (1906): 93-121; and the next article in that issue, Herbert M. Nash, "Some Reminiscences of a Confederate Surgeon," pp. 122-144.

In the second category—published reminiscences of hospital stewards— four book-length diaries stand out. First is Solon Hyde, *A Captive of War* (Shippensburg, PA: Burd Street Press, 1996). Hyde, a hospital steward of the 17th Ohio Volunteer Infantry captured at the Battle of Chickamauga, offers a unique perspective by providing a considerable amount of information on his pharmaceutical duties and drug conditions at Libby, Pemberton, Danville, and Andersonville prisons. Two diaries of Union stewards are Charles Beneulyn Johnson, *Muskets and Medicine* (Philadelphia: F. A. Davis, 1917); and John N. Henry, *Turn Them Out to Die Like a Mule: The Civil War Letters of John N. Henry, 49th New York, 1861-1865,* edited by John Michael Priest (Leesburg, VA: Gauley Mount Press, 1995). For a hospital steward's view from a Confederate perspective see John Samuel Apperson, *Repairing the 'March of Mars': The Civil War Diaries of John Samuel Apperson, Hospital Steward in the Stonewall Brigade,* edited by John Herbert Roper (Macon, GA: Mercer University Press, 2001).

The official records and correspondence are in many respects the most important group to consider. For the Union the massive *Medical and Surgical History of the War of the Rebellion (1861-1865),* 2 volumes in 6 (Washington: Government Printing Office, 1870-1888) is essential, especially the three-part *Medical History* volumes. These contain virtually all of the U.S. Army Medical Department reports and statistical analyses of the various diseases that plagued the armies of both eastern and western theaters of the conflict. In addition, hundreds of case studies with medicinal regimens are listed in this work. This is arguably the single most important title in Civil War medicine. *The War of the Rebellion: A Compilation of the Official Records of the Union and Confederate Armies,* 70 vols. in 128 (Washington: Government Printing Office, 1880-1901) is also very useful, but especially so for Confederate records. This compendious work is subdivided into four series, and has been variously titled *Official Records of the Union and Confederate Armies.* Despite the general nature of the material found therein, a careful perusal of the comprehensive index will yield considerable documents related to medical and pharmaceutical topics, especially the three volumes in series 4. For information on the blockade, naval operations, and the naval medical corps, see the *Official Records of the Union and Confederate Navies of the War of the Rebellion,* 30 volumes (Washington: Government Printing Office, 1894-1922).

Another important source relating to the Confederate Medical Department is the brief but not insignificant run of the *Confederate States Medical and Surgical Journal.* Published under the editorial direction of Dr. James B. McCaw, this serial began in January of 1864 and continued up through February of 1865. It gives many valuable accounts of medical conditions in the South, including much discussion on the indigenous materia medica.

One final resource specific to the Confederacy should be mentioned; it is the enormously valuable "Documenting the American South" Web site of the University of North Carolina at Chapel Hill <http://docsouth.unc.edu/> where many extremely helpful primary sources are available full-text, online. Circulars, reports, and handbooks from the Surgeon General's Office are available, including Francis Peyre Porcher's *Resources of the Southern Fields and Forests* (Charleston, SC: Evans and Cogswell, 1863).

The regulations and duties of hospital stewards are available in Joseph Janvier Woodward, *The Hospital Steward's Manual* (Philadelphia: J. B. Lippincott, 1862). Although this is a U.S. Army publication, the responsibilities of stewards in the Confederacy were largely a mirror image of those found in this book and therefore are useful in seeing how pharmacy care was delivered in the military in general.

Lastly, the context of pharmacy in America is provided in the *Proceedings of the American Pharmaceutical Association* (hereafter *Proceedings*) and the *American Journal of Pharmacy* (hereafter *Journal*). Especially useful were the following: Edward R. Squibb, "Report on the Drug Market," *Proceedings* 11 (1863): 175-195; John M. Maisch, "Report on the Drug Market," *Proceedings* 12 (1864): 187-205; William A. Brewer, "Report of the Committee on the Drug Market," *Proceedings* 15 (1867): 267-307; John M. Maisch, "Statistics of the U.S. Army Laboratory at Philadelphia," *Proceedings* 14 (1866): 272-278; Henry N. Rittenhouse, "U.S. Army Storekeepers," *Journal* 12, third series (1865): 87-90; and two other articles in that issue by Hennell Stevens, "The Medical Purveying Department of the United States Army" (91-98) and Edward R. Fell, "The Pharmaceutical Department of a U.S.A. Hospital" (107-112).

Unpublished Primary Resources

The archival materials from Virginia Tech (home of the Virginia Center for Civil War Studies), University of North Carolina at Chapel Hill, Ohio Historical Society Archives, the National Library of Medicine, the National

Archives, Merck Archives, the Alabama Department of Archives and History, and the University of Alabama at Birmingham were utilized in preparing this book. Each of these repositories brought important information and perspectives to this study. Virginia Tech holds several diaries of surgeons as well as the Apperson diary; the UNC Chapel Hill has a number of records of hospital stewards on microfilm; the Ohio Historical Society is fortunate to have several regimental prescription books along with diary accounts by hospital stewards; the Medical History Division of the National Library of Medicine in Bethesda, MD, holds a number of important files related to Civil War pharmacy, especially those of Medical Purveyor Thomas Sargent Latimer. The National Archives (Archives I in Washington, DC) also hold a rich store of pharmacy-related materials. Particularly useful are the Navy subject files (Record Group [hereafter RG] 45) that contain shipboard medical reports as well as the prize sales records of captured blockade-runners. These contain lists of items along with their sale prices and offers particularly detailed records of medicinal substances attempting to be smuggled through the Union squadrons and their relative values. Also helpful were files from RG 52, RG 94, and RG 109. Merck Archives located in Whitehouse Station, New Jersey, holds the extant records of Rosengarten and Sons and Powers and Weightman, the two largest pharmaceutical manufacturers during the war. Two manuscripts in addition to those already mentioned are the letters of Spencer Bonsall, hospital steward of the 81st Pennsylvania Volunteers, and the hospital reports and diary of B. W. Allen, who served as surgeon at the Confederate hospital in Charlottesville, Virginia. Both belong to the Reynolds Historical Library mentioned earlier.

General Secondary Sources on the Civil War

The number of general accounts of the Civil War is legion and, it would seem, growing daily. Of those, a few stand out. For years the classic treatment was James Ford Rhodes' *History of the United States from the Compromise of 1850 to the Final Restoration of Home Rule at the South in 1877*, 7 volumes (New York: Macmillan, 1906-1907). For the present study, however, two titles have been especially helpful in giving much-needed context to the military and political events of the Civil War. They were Allan Nevins' *War for the Union*, 4 volumes (1971; reprinted, New York: Konecky and Konecky, 2000); and James M. McPherson's *Battle Cry of Freedom: The Civil War Era* (New York: Oxford University Press, 1988). Other helpful books have been Richard E. Beringer et al., *Why the South Lost the Civil War* (Athens: The University of Georgia Press, 1986); Jay Winik, *April 1865: The Month That Saved America* (New York: Perennial, 2001); and William C. Davis, *Look Away!: A History of the Confederate States of America* (New York: The Free Press, 2002).

In order to understand the medicinal situation in the Civil War, the critical nature of naval operations must be appreciated. Bern Anderson's *By Sea and by River: The Naval History of the Civil War* (1962; reprinted, New York: Da Capo Press, 1989) is a good general naval history of the war that has stood the test of time. Especially helpful for understanding the extent and character of the Union blockade and the privateers who sought to elude it are two books: Stephen R. Wise, *Lifeline of the Confederacy: Blockade Running During the Civil War* (Columbia: University of South Carolina Press, 1988); and Ivan Musicant, *Divided Waters: The Naval History of the Civil War* (New York: HarperCollins, 1995).

On women's role during the war see George C. Rable, *Civil Wars: Women and the Crisis of Southern Nationalism* (Urbana: University of Illinois, 1989); and on the United States Sanitary Commission, in which women played such an important role, see William Quentin Maxwell, *Lincoln's Fifth Wheel: The Political History of the United States Sanitary Commission* (New York: Longmans, Green, 1956).

Secondary Sources in Pharmacy and Medicine

The two best general texts on the history of pharmacy are *Kremers and Urdang's History of Pharmacy,* fourth edition, revised by Glenn Sonnedecker (1976; reprinted, Madison, American Institute of the History of Pharmacy, 1986) and David L. Cowen and William H. Helfand's *Pharmacy: An Illustrated History* (New York: Harry N. Abrams, 1990). In medicine, several titles have been particularly helpful in preparing the present study. For a general overview of the period, see Richard Harrison Shryock, *The Development of Modern Medicine: An Interpretation of the Social and Scientific Factors Involved* (1947; reprinted, Madison: University of Wisconsin Press, 1979); William G. Rothstein, *American Physicians in the 19th Century: From Sects to Science* (Baltimore: Johns Hopkins University Press, 1974); and John S. Haller Jr., *American Medicine in Transition, 1840-1910* (Urbana: University of Illinois Press, 1981). Extremely useful in tracing out the changing concepts of disease entities and their etiologies—especially with regard to fever—and the complex nuances between the rational and empirical perspectives of the period is Lester S. King's *Transformations in American Medicine: From Benjamin Rush to William Osler* (Baltimore: Johns Hopkins University Press, 1991).

Only a few titles directly covering Civil War pharmacy are available. Most important of these are Norman Franke, "The Medico-Pharmaceutical Conditions and Drug Supply in the Confederate States of America 1861-1865" (Unpublished PhD dissertation, University of Wisconsin, 1956) and George Winston Smith, *Medicines for the Union Army: The United States Army Laboratories During the Civil War* (1962; reprinted, Binghamton,

Printed and bound by CPI Group (UK) Ltd, Croydon, CR0 4YY

17/10/2024

01775661-0002

NY: Pharmaceutical Products Press, 2001). As part of the centennial anniversary of the Civil War, the American Institute of the History of Pharmacy featured a symposium titled "Pharmacy Looks Back at the Civil War Years." Participants included George Winston Smith, Ernst Steib, J. Hampton Hoch, and Norman Franke, and three of the four papers were published in the *Journal of the American Pharmaceutical Association* 1(12) (1961): 763-774. More recently see a brief but informative and well-referenced article by Guy Hasegawa, "Pharmacy in the American Civil War," *American Journal of Health-System Pharmacy* 57 (2001): 475-489. This has since been reprinted as part of a special Civil War issue of *Pharmacy in History* 42 (2000) that also contains Michael A. Flannery, "The Life of a Hospital Steward: The Civil War Journal of Spencer Bonsall" (87-97) and Maurice Albin, "The Use of Anesthetics During the Civil War, 1861-1865" (99-114).

An important part of Civil War pharmacy—perhaps *the* important part—relates to the impact the war had on the industry. The single most useful guide is Williams Haynes, *American Chemical Industry,* 6 volumes (New York: Van Nostrand, 1945-1954), especially volume one, *Background and Beginnings: 1609-1911* and volume six, *The Chemical Companies.* A less detailed analysis is available in Jonathon Liebenau's *Medical Science and Medical Industry: The Formation of the American Pharmaceutical Industry* (Baltimore: Johns Hopkins University Press, 1987).

The dearth of published secondary literature will send the researcher to medical histories of the war in order to fill in gaps and lend important detail to much of the pharmacy story. In this regard the two classic sources are George Worthington Adams' *Doctors in Blue: The Medical History of the Union Army in the Civil War* (1952; reprinted, Baton Rouge: Louisiana State University Press, 1996) and its companion, H. H. Cunningham's *Doctors in Gray: The Confederate Medical Service* (1958; reprinted, Baton Rouge: Louisiana State University, 1993). Another valuable book that adds substantial detail to the Adams work is Mary C. Gillett's *Army Medical Department, 1818-1865* (Washington, DC: Government Printing Office, 1987).

Because the materia medica was tied directly to the diseases most prevalent in the Civil War, an understanding of the scourges of that conflict is essential. Here the best source in print is Paul Steiner, *Disease in the Civil War: Natural Biological Warfare in 1861-1865* (Springfield, IL: Charles C Thomas, 1968). Also helpful in giving a modern clinical perspective to Civil War illnesses is Jeffrey Sartin, "Infectious Diseases During the Civil War: The Triumph of the 'Third Army,'" *Clinical Infectious Diseases* 16 (1993): 580-584. For details on diseases among African-American troops, see Andrew K. Black, "In the Service of the United States: Comparative Mortality Among African-American and White Troops in the Union Army," *Journal of Negro History* 79 (1994): 317-333.

Conclusion

Research into Civil War pharmacy is an exercise not so much in finding the source materials as it is an effort in ferreting out from a mass of material that which seems to tell the story best and explain the conditions most honestly, directly, and fully. For the North, official accounts, diaries, and other personal reminiscences in books old and new amply supplement the official sources. For the Confederacy a slightly different situation exists. Although the unpublished papers of the Surgeon General's Office were destroyed on the night of Richmond's evacuation, April 2, 1865, the South—even in matters of medicine—seems to have gone out of its way to record its memories of the war. Confederate surgeon-veterans collectively sought to write their own account. Under the direction of Joseph Jones, they published it as "The Medical History of the Confederate States Army and Navy," *Southern Historical Society Papers,* volume 20 (Richmond, VA: The Society, 1892), pp. 109-166. Despite their best efforts, the final product lacks a coherent narrative and flow and seems to have suffered from the curse that besets most projects initiated by well-intentioned societies: Data is gathered and roughly cobbled together with little analysis or context to the events described.

Numerous reminiscences over and above those already mentioned have been added to the corpus of available material on Civil War pharmacy. Every former Confederate surgeon, it seems, wanted to hold forth on his view of the war. There was Samuel H. Stout, Medical Director of the Army of the Tennessee, who published his memoirs as "Some Facts of the History of the Organization of the Medical Service of the Confederate Armies and Hospitals," in *The Southern Practitioner* (volumes 22-25) running some twenty-three parts from 1900 to his death in 1903; Claudius H. Mastin, "The Medical Profession in the War," *Southern Historical Society Papers,* volume 13 (Richmond, VA: The Society, 1885), pp. 476-480; Hunter Holmes McGuire, "Progress of Medicine in the South," *Southern Historical Society Papers,* volume 17 (Richmond, VA: The Society, 1889): 1-21; even a preacher's version in James H. NcNeilly "Recollections from One, Who Though Not a Surgeon, Was with Them All the Time," *The Southern Practitioner* 22 (1900): 415-420.

Most of these articles need to be read with a certain degree of caution. The passage of time alone clouded many memories, and there is a distinct leitmotif of the Lost Cause in the painful but passionate assertions of their sacrifices and noble efforts to heal. No doubt their privations and struggles were many, but the realities and nature of those sacrifices often seem clouded in the mists of nostalgic reverence. These accounts can be clarified by carefully comparing the recollections (often published forty or even fifty years after the war) with the actual correspondence, casebooks, reports, and prescription books of the period. In looking over the vast body of wartime reminiscences of medical staff, one is reminded of a comment made by the Southern agrarian poet Allen Tate who said, "One must entertain the paradox that the South has enjoyed a longer period of identity in defeat than it might have been able to preserve in victory." Having spent the past two-and-a-half years plowing through these records, Tate's assertion seems compelling.

Index

Page numbers followed by the letter "f" indicate figures; those followed by the letter "t" indicates tables.